The Life and
Times of
GEOFFREY
BARROW
DOWLING

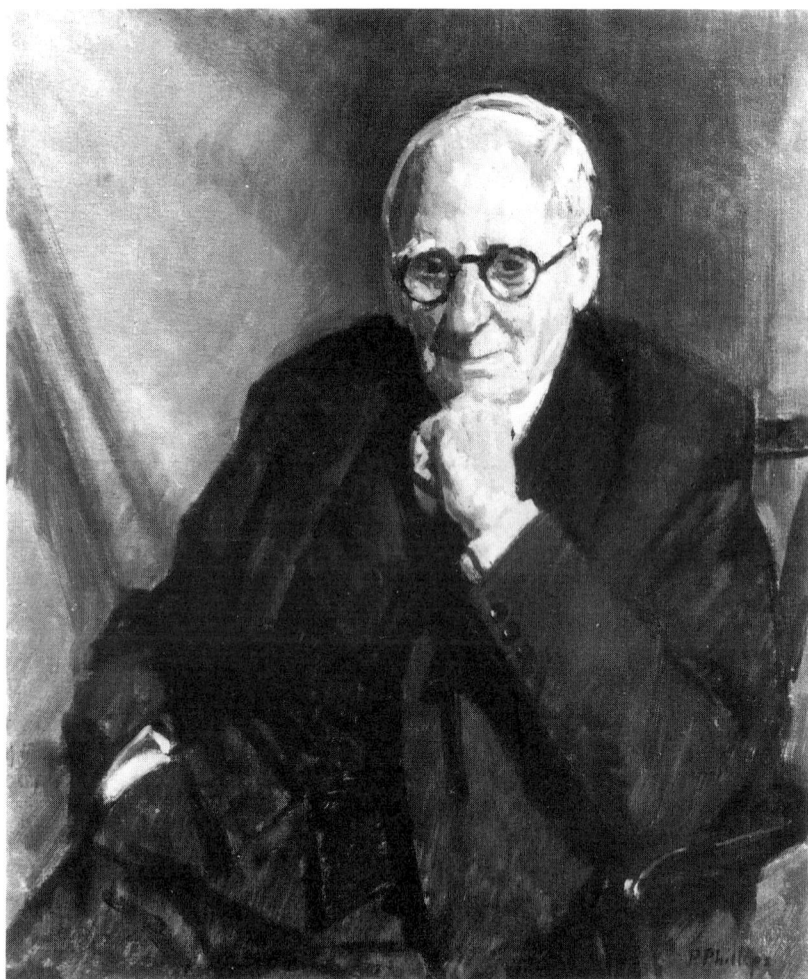

FRONTISPIECE Geoffrey Barrow Dowling
by the late Patrick Phillips

The Life and
Times of
GEOFFREY
BARROW
DOWLING

Charles Calnan

OXFORD
Blackwell
Scientific
Publications

© 1993 Charles Calnan
Published by
Blackwell Scientific Publications
Editorial Offices:
Osney Mead, Oxford OX2 OEL
25 John Street, London WC1N 2BL
23 Ainslie Place, Edinburgh EH3 6AJ
238 Main Street, Cambridge
  Massachusetts 02142, USA
54 University Street, Carlton
  Victoria 3053, Australia

Other Editorial Offices:
Librairie Arnette SA
2, rue Casimir-Delavigne
75006 Paris
France

Blackwell Wissenschafts-Verlag
Meinekestrasse 4
D-1000 Berlin 15
Germany

Blackwell MZV
Feldgasse 13
A-1238 Wien
Austria

First published 1993

Set by Excel Typesetters Company,
Hong Kong; printed in Great Britain
at the Alden Press, Oxford,
and bound at the
Green Street Bindery, Oxford

DISTRIBUTORS

Marston Book Services Ltd
PO Box 87
Oxford OX2 ODT
(*Orders*: Tel: 0865 791155
      Fax: 0865 791927
      Telex: 837515)

USA
Blackwell Scientific Publications, Inc.
238 Main Street
Cambridge, MA 02142
(*Orders*: Tel: 800 759-6102
           617 876-7000)

Canada
Times Mirror
Professional Publishing, Ltd
5240 Finch Avenue East
Scarborough, Ontario M1S 5A2
(*Orders*: Tel: 800 268-4178
           416 298-1588)

Australia
Blackwell Scientific Publications
(Australia) Pty Ltd
54 University Street
Carlton, Victoria 3053
(*Orders*: Tel: 03 347-0300)

A catalogue record for this title
is available from the British Library

ISBN 0-632-03505-6

Contents

List of Plates
(facing page 152)

Preface

SOON AFTER Dr G.B. Dowling died in 1976, many of the dermatologists who had been most closely associated with him in the last 25 years of his life felt strongly that he had been inadequately rewarded. A few years previously an approach had been made to the Prime Minister's Office, recommending him for a knighthood. But it failed. He was too old. It should have been made 20 years earlier.

There were numerous obituaries but they seemed inadequate. Dr George Findlay of Pretoria, South Africa, and I discussed the idea of writing about the man who had played such a major part in our lives for 25 years. And so we started on a task which has taken 10 years to finish.

There was little printed matter on which to work, although George Findlay was remarkably successful in searching out numerous family members in South Africa and much documentation. He contributed a chapter on 'The Dowlings in Cape Town'. In addition he kept more than 100 personal letters from Dr Dowling. It is unfortunate that he died in 1990 from a lymphoma, but his wife has made all his collected material available to me.

In 1964, Mr Robert Moody, a solicitor in Bristol wrote 'An Account of the Knapp Family of Gloucestershire and Their Descendants'. It was published privately and circulated to the living descendants, of whom he is one. He has kindly allowed me to summarize it in the present volume, and it provided the genealogy of the Dowling family back to the sixteenth century.

The rest of this book is what is now known as oral history. Most of the content has been obtained by interview with Dr Dowling's many medical colleagues, friends, family members and relations. They are too numerous to mention by name individually. I am especially grateful to them all for their generous help, understanding and co-operation in the task over the past 10 years. I particularly wish to thank Dr Dowling's four children and members of the Fawcett and Paterson families.

I acknowledge the permission of various editors and publishers of books and journals in allowing me to quote from their publications.

They include the *British Journal of Dermatology*, the *Transactions of the Saint John's Hospital Dermatological Society*, the *British Medical Journal* and the *Lancet*, as well as the histories of the George Inn, Huntercombe Golf Club, and the Lord Mayor Treloar Hospital and College.

There can be no doubt that Geoffrey Dowling was the greatest dermatologist in Britain in the twentieth century. He lived through most of the century, and was responsible for the renaissance of British dermatology in the second half of the century, which continues to the present day.

C.D. Calnan

Chapter 1
The Knapp Family

SILVESTER Knapp of Winterbourne in Gloucestershire was born about 1590. Winterbourne was then a small village situated to the north of Bristol but is now virtually annexed to the expanding city. When Silvester was born Queen Elizabeth I was on the throne of England and the village was set in the depth of pleasant Gloucestershire countryside.

Whether or not he was actually born in Winterbourne is uncertain but on 15 January 1615 he was married in the parish church there to Martha Middleton. They had three children — James, Matthew and John. Matthew died when he was not much over 30 years of age and John also died as a young man in July 1641 — shortly before the Civil War broke out.

James Knapp (the first) survived both his younger brothers. He was a yeoman* and lived in Southmead(e), which is now a suburb of Bristol but at that time was a small village not far from Winterbourne. His wife Sarah bore him 10 children, five boys and five girls.

James Knapp (the first) died in 1680. He made his will on 18 August in 'the twentieth yeare of the Rayne of our Soveraigne Lord King Charles the Second Anno Dom 1668' (loyally calculating the period of King Charles's reign from the execution of his father in 1649 and not from the restoration of the monarchy in 1660). His will was proved in the Prerogative Court at Canterbury on 12 September 1680.

His eldest son John, yet another yeoman, married a woman called Mary and they had at least six children. Towards the end of the seventeenth century he built a new house at Harry Stoke and acquired much other property in his lifetime.

The house at Harry Stoke was handsome, as is known from the description of it and its list of contents by his brothers William and Matthew, with the help of a certain William Gingell. It was then (and still is by English law) necessary to make an inventory of his/her goods

---

* A yeoman was a person qualified by possessing free land of an annual value of forty shillings to serve on juries and to vote for the knight of the shire, etc., essentially a landowner, farmer or person of middle class engaged in agriculture.

I

on the death of any person. His 'new dwelling house' at Harry Stoke consisted of a hall (which would have been a fairly large room where guests would have been entertained and where meals would probably have been eaten), the parlour, the kitchen, the parlour chamber (which was the bedroom over the parlour), the hall chamber and the best chamber.

In the cheese loft there were 1600 cheeses and some table linen! His most valuable possessions, however, were 18 cows, three yearlings, a bull and two tons of hay, all of which were valued at £60. One of the cows, called Beauty, which was specifically mentioned in his will, was in the keeping of his son James.

John and Mary Knapp had six children, two boys and four girls. His elder son, John, apparently died without having any children, since his house, Windmill Tutt, eventually belonged to the son of his younger brother, James. This brother, James Knapp (the second), was probably the only surviving son of John Knapp. He was a yeoman at Westerleigh, a village near Winterbourne. He married a woman, also called Mary, like his mother, and they had at least five children. He died in 1749 but his wife lived for a further 15 years.

James and Mary had five children, three boys and two girls. The eldest was William, who was the founder of the family at Oldbury-upon-Severn; the youngest was James, who was the founder of the family at Thornbury. Their brother Thomas was a cooper at Westerleigh. The two girls were Anne, who died young in 1734, and Sarah, who married Charles Godwin, a sawyer of the city of London.

The two brothers, William and James, both decided to leave the Winterbourne area, where their family had farmed for more than a century. James became a blacksmith and moved some six miles north to settle in Thornbury. He married and had at least seven children, but lost his wife from smallpox, an all too common disease at that time. She was the eldest child of a Thornbury cordwainer and not a farmer's daughter, so had almost certainly never had cowpox.

The elder brother, William, lived for a short time at Almondsbury, just a few miles from Winterbourne, and it was there that he married 22-year-old Charity Andrews. Soon after his marriage, William moved from Almondsbury to Oldbury. Their son was baptized in the ancient church there on 3 May 1730. Oldbury is a low-lying village, reached by narrow roads winding across the flat marshy land divided into willow-bounded fields. The notoriously damp atmosphere of Oldbury did not suit Charity Knapp and she died in August 1732, being buried in the churchyard at Iron Acton near her parents' home.

Within a year or two, William remarried. His second wife was Elizabeth Linke, who had grown up in Oldbury and was presumably used to the damp climate of the Vale of Berkeley. William and Elizabeth returned to live and run the farm at Oldbury. They had two children, Elizabeth and William. Their daughter married William Virgo, a local yeoman, in 1759, had several children and died in 1801. Their son was born in 1745, and inherited his mother's family (Linke) house at Oldbury. He married Elizabeth Russell at Tytherington and from this union were descended the Knapp family of Oldbury to the present century.

William Knapp (the elder) suffered increasing ill health and made his will when only 45 years of age, in 1751. He died in 1753 and his body was taken back to the ancestral burial ground at Winterbourne. His widow Elizabeth was only 38 years old at the time and spent the next few years bring up her two children. Her stepson Thomas had recently married and was no longer her responsibility. Six years later, in 1759, her father Thomas Linke died and she inherited his land at Oldbury. In the following year she was married again, to Richard Russell, who was more than 20 years younger than herself. Nevertheless, this marriage lasted for 35 years, until she died at the age of 80 and was buried at Oldbury on 24 August 1795.

Thomas Knapp, the only child of William and Charity, was baptized at Oldbury church on 3 May 1730. When he was 21 he married Elizabeth Nelmes at Rockhampton, a village just north of Thornbury. Her father, Thomas Nelmes, was a wealthy yeoman and she inherited his property. Her husband acquired additional land by purchase, including six acres known as Gilder Meadow from Mr John Gaynor, an apothecary in Thornbury. In 1764 he bought land at Oldbury for £383, which was a considerable sum at that time.

Thomas and Elizabeth had only two children. The first was a boy, christened Robert at Thornbury church in 1752. The second was a boy named Thomas, but he died at the age of five and was buried at Oldbury church.

Robert Knapp was a farmer, like most of his ancestors. He owned a good deal of land and so he probably had little or no manual work to do himself but was the manager and supervisor of the several holdings. At the age of 21 he married Jane Cox in the great church at Thornbury.

She was the only daughter of a wealthy landowner, Thomas Cox, who lived at Kingston, which was a hamlet close to Thornbury. The fathers of the bride and bridegroom were first cousins, so the couple had probably known each other since childhood. Thomas Knapp's mother, Charity, was a sister of Thomas Fox's mother, Anne. The father of these two sisters was Robert Andrews of Iron Acton. Both Robert and Jane Knapp had inherited some land at Iron Acton, via their respective parents, from Robert Andrews and all of the land eventually passed to their only child and heiress, Elizabeth.

When Robert died at the age of 49 in 1801, his widow Jane was a wealthy woman, at least by county standards. In Fosbrooke's *History of Gloucestershire*, which was published in 1808, she is described as one of the principal landowners in the Thornbury area. By this time, her only brother William and her father had died and she had inherited all their property. One can see a marble monument to the memory of her parents and brother in Thornbury church.

Robert had made his will just three years before his death. Since his daughter Elizabeth was not married in 1798, he made provision for her specifically in case she should die without leaving any children. It was said that he had but this one child and so it was she and her children who inherited all the wealth and land accumulated by this branch of the Knapp and Cox families over 100 years.

After Robert Knapp died in 1801, the house at Shipperdine must have been a lonely place for Jane and her daughter Elizabeth. They moved to Kingston, possibly to her father's old house. Elizabeth was married in 1806 to John Barrow, who was eight years older than herself, and they had four children, two boys called Thomas and Robert and two girls called Sarah Frances and Jane. The boys were named after their two great grandfathers — Thomas Cox Barrow and Robert Knapp Barrow.

Elizabeth's mother Jane Knapp lived another 12 years of widowhood and made a very lengthy will before she died in 1818, for there was a lot of property to be disposed to the grandchildren. She left Robert a silver tankard marked 'R.K.' and Thomas one marked 'J.C.' and a watch. All the rest of her plate was divided between the four grandchildren. Thomas was to receive all the casks at her house at Shipperdine and Robert all those at her Kingston house. Her servant Warren Hopkins must have been a faithful retainer. To him she gave the bedclothes and bed on which he usually slept in her house, as well as her smallest oak table, a deal table, three ash chairs and the best of her brass pots and tea kettles. After various pecuniary legacies to friends and servants, she gave £500 to Thomas Cox Barrow, to be placed as a clerk to an attorney, and £500 to Robert Knapp Barrow, to be placed as an apprentice to a surgeon and apothecary. It is interesting that as early as 1815 wealthy farmers and landowners had a wish to put their sons into the professions of law and medicine. This was not mentioned in Robert Knapp's will and so it may have been entirely Jane's idea. In fact, neither of the legacies were used for the purpose intended, although in later life Thomas might have benefited from some legal training.

So the name of this branch of the family changed on 7 January 1806, when Robert and Jane's only child, Elizabeth, married John Barrow. He was a member of a long-established Oldbury family. The name Barrow is one that appears frequently in the parish registers over the previous three centuries.

Three of their four children, Thomas, Jane and Robert, all married and had descendants continuing up to the present time. Thomas Cox Barrow was born in 1806. He married Mary Ann Perry. Her father Richard Perry was a grandson of Henry Creswicke of Hanham Court near Bristol, who was a mayor of Bristol in the seventeenth century. A portrait of Sir Henry Creswicke (and portraits of Sir Francis Creswicke and Lady Elizabeth Creswicke) were donated to the city of Bristol by M. Carlos Brossel, the son of a Belgian judge, who had married Florence Louise Barrow, one of Elizabeth and William Barrow's children.

Thomas Cox Barrow of Shipperdine kept a series of personal notebooks, which he had first used as school-books. Two of these and a bundle of letters were discovered in a solicitor's office in Thornbury. They provide a lot of information about him and his way of life in the years from 1823 to 1850. Into these notebooks he copied out essays on such subjects as filial piety and benevolence. On 5 August 1826 he was staying with a Mr Tilbrook at Horningham in Wiltshire, where he wrote out a long poem of a passionate nature extolling the virtues of a girl called Matilda. On one occasion in 1829 he was living in Chepstow and while there he copied out the first three scenes of Act I of Roach's edition of *Hamlet*. On another occasion, together with his wife, Mary Ann, he composed an epitaph for the tomb of Doctor Edward Jenner, who had made the observation that milkmaids who had had cowpox were never afflicted by smallpox. From this he proceeded to inoculate people deliberately with cowpox material from cows and proved that it was effective prophylaxis against smallpox. This discovery must have been widely recognized in Gloucestershire long before it was appreciated by doctors in the rest of the country and the world.

After 1830 he recorded a lot of his farming activities in his notebooks. For example, in a field known as Eight Leaze, he planted no less than 197 apple trees and each rank of this new orchard is carefully mentioned, with the names of all the apples. There are other details of the tasks carried out by the men working for him and their meagre wages. In May 1840 he made a note that a particular half-day was very wet when John Jones and Stephen Hopkins were planting potatoes!

It was now that Thomas Cox Barrow began to fall on bad times. He had inherited much from his parents, was brought up in comfortable surroundings and married into a well-established and distinguished family. His income was derived partly from the rents of the landed holdings which he had inherited and partly from cider production and the sale of withy. Withe or withy is a tough flexible branch, usually from willow or osier and used for binding up bundles of various materials in the country, or basket-making. In 1840 in his notebook he made a 'calculation of what withy came to'. In that year Mr Cox hauled 447 bundles to Bristol and John Cornock, Mrs Adams and Mr Cox brought a further 47 bundles. At 1/6d (one shilling and six pence) a bundle, £37 was produced. In 1844, when the men carted 170 bundles into Bristol, they left Shipperdine at midnight and took with them food and drink and four shillings to pay expenses.

In one year, from Lady Day (25 March) in 1845 to Lady Day in 1846, he reckoned to receive £403.10s.0½d from rents. But it seems doubtful if all of the rents were paid in full. One must remember that the 1840s were bad years for farmers, with acute agricultural depression. They were known as the Hungry Forties, with the well-described potato famine and all its devastating hardship and resultant emigration.

It is not surprising, then, that Thomas was in constant financial difficulties. As the dreadful decade progressed, he got deeper and deeper into debt and his notebooks and letters provide ample evidence of this. He decided that the only way to satisfy his creditors was to assign the money from his future rents to his solicitor. This was John Thurston, one of his kinsmen and one of the Thornbury family who had traditionally provided the lawyers in the district. Thomas's dire position is perfectly illustrated in the following letter, which he wrote on 17 July 1849 to Messrs Wyld's of Bristol:

> Gentlemen,
>
> I have seen my Solicitor today respecting Mr Hippisley's letter in regard to your demand of me. Having signed over to my Solicitor part of rents due next September which will enable him to pay you £20 Mr Hippisley does not seem satisfied with this arrangement but demands the whole in October, or security for the same — Now Gentlemen I regret to say I have no security to offer except personal — the whole of my property is in my wife's marriage settlement and I see it useless to engage to do what is out of my power to fulfil by promising to pay you the whole in October. I have above said you will have £20 in September. I will also assign another £20 to my Solicitor to pay you in March. Mr Hippisley's expense shall be paid in September with your £20. If I can possibly manage to pay the remainder between then and March I will endeavour to do so. Trusting to your reply.
>
> I am Gentlemen
Your obliged and obedient servant
Thos. Cox Barrow

Thomas sought help from his solicitor but without success. In one letter Thurston wrote to him apologizing for not being able to let him have £5 at present, assuring him that he would most willingly do so if it had been in his power and informing him that he was doing all he could to provide him with a loan.

It is likely that Thurston found Thomas a difficult client to deal with and in December 1849 wrote him the following letter:

> Dear Sir,
>
> Mr Baker surprised me this morning by delivery of an a/c against you for £21.8s.2d with account of Weeks, the Coalman for £7.13s.11d. You will recollect that when I undertook with Mr Hippisley to pay Messrs Wyld's debt that you gave me authority on Baker to receive the whole of the rent from him. I have received £35.0s.0d. only to pay Messrs Wyld's some £24 with £10 to pay Ellis exceeding this by £6. You also said I was to receive £15 myself. Of this I say nothing. Pray let me see you at your earliest convenience.

Jones's matter remains in *statu quo*.

I have not heard from Mr Buchan.

Yours truly

O. Edward Thurston

But apparently Thomas was unwilling or unable to take the advice and did not go to see his solicitor. For, about a month later, he received the following letter, dated 14 January 1850, from Thurston:

> My Dear Sir,
>
> Do allow me to call your attention to the copy of Mr Lloyd's letter on the other side. It will be much better to settle the matter at once without again putting it off and it will according to your statement be necessary for me to go through these accounts with Mrs Barrow. I can, if convenient and on hearing from you, see you at Shipperdine any day this week excepting on Thursday for this purpose.
>
> At the same time, perhaps you will allow me to call your attention to the Annuity now due to Mr Barrow, Senior.
>
> My dear Sir
Yours truly
O. Edward Thurston

In his beleaguered circumstances, Thomas also sought help from his father, John Barrow, who was living with daughter Sarah Frances at Span Cottage. He wrote to him as follows:

26 February 1850

> My Dear Sir,
>
> Finding the liberty considering recent events which have taken place in your worldly prosperity and that has now placed me in the present position, being in a measure compelled to rely upon parental affection, I crave your humble pardon by politely requesting you will assist me in my emergency having paid your money and left myself in want as my creditor to whom your money was due having now pressed me. By complying, my Dear Sir, with my request, you will confer an obligation not easily erased from my mind. Reflect for a moment as to my simple petition — I have assisted you when in my power and have no other person to call upon on this earth but yourself. May Almighty God give you a feeling heart towards myself and

children and cause you to act the part of a Father and a Christian before you go into that bourne from which no traveller returns. I repeat again that 'tis no more than your duty to act as a man towards me your eldest son.

I write to you with proper and consistent feeling and I trust that my humble petition will meet with your generosity.

I remain with every duty of respect and proper feeling as a son.

Yours affectionately,
T.C. Barrow

He probably spent a long time composing this letter and it clearly caused him a great deal of pain and heart-searching. One cannot be certain that he actually sent it. In one of his notebooks he had made a copy of another letter dated 18 March 1850, which he presumably felt was an improvement on the previous effort. The wording was almost the same but there were some significant differences. It began with 'My Dear Father' instead of 'My Dear Sir', which seemed too formal. He also changed the last paragraph to 'I write to you with proper and consistent feelings and I trust that my humble position will coaless with your noble generous heart which you always possessed.'

One wonders what his father's response was to whichever of the two letters was sent. It is doubtful if it was favourable, because Thomas already appeared to have defaulted on his annuity payments to his father, to which his attention had been drawn in Thurston's letter. Presumably some of the land which he had inherited was charged with an annuity payable to his father. There is evidence in his notebook that Thomas expected to have a further £40 a year when his father — his 'old man' — died, as shown by the following note in his accounts one year:

Baker's rent £120 per annum	120.00.00
Prewett's Goodings	59.15.00
Withy	25.00.00
Cottage	4. 4.00
	208.19.00
Cider	80.00.00
	10.00.00
When old man goes	40.00.00
	338.19.00

Whether it was because of his financial difficulties or for other reasons, his marriage was apparently not going well at the time. His wife, May Ann, had moved out of his house in 1849 and was living elsewhere, while the children stayed at Shipperdine. One of Thomas's creditors indicated to him that he might be able to pay when Mrs Barrow returned. In one of his notebooks there is the draft of a pleading letter to his wife, dated 6 December:

> My Dear Mary Ann,
>
>   It appears an age since we last had the happiness of seeing each other. I should think ere this I must be almost forgotten. Time frequently weans the affection from the desired object of its admiration thereby producing a chilly coldness which in the end dwindles into perfect dislike and inanimate feelings.
>
>   However, we will not dwell upon this mournful subject but say come home and be happy with your Husband and children . . .

One can only guess at the causes of Thomas's marital and money problems. He may have been inefficient, just not practical, or a weak character. But he was appreciative of the kindness and generosity of others. For instance, when Long, Kelling and Nowell of Yate wrote to him, asking for payment of 'our small account', he wrote in pencil on the letter, 'This must be attended to as soon as possible having been treated with the greatest kindness.' On another occasion, he wrote 'Rob not a poor man of his right but give him his due. Do thy duty to every man and with proper judgement decide with regard to work so as not to injure.'

He may also have been an alcoholic, since he seems to have had a number of disputes over wine. He was only 27 years of age in 1832 when he carried on an acrimonious correspondence with a Henry Perry of Henbury, who was presumably one of his wife's relations. In a letter dated 27 September 1832, Henry Perry wrote to Thomas:

> Sir,
>
>   I will presume myself to be in error in regard to the bottle of port wine — rather than submit to receive the intended insulting unmannerly ungentlemanly epithet expressed in your communication of yesterday — although it would emanate from the individual I so utterly dispise.
>
>   Yours etc.
>   Henry Perry

Strong words indeed, and one might imagine they were final, but on the very same day he wrote again to Thomas as follows:

> Sir,
>
> I have sent you the wine and Brandy, the latter I had not forgotten but intended forwarding it with the etceteras you will now receive from me — the earliest opportunity which offered. In regard to a 'Bottle of Port Wine from Frenchay' I beg to protest against never having such there from but perfectly bear in mind a bottle of port I had from you during your residence at Wyck for which I gave you one of sherry in return.
>
> I am perfectly aware of your deficiency of memory and therefore, excuse the defalcation in this respect and lest imagination of your having lent me such and received *equivalent therefore* should over hang you I have sent you a bottle of excellent flavour to quaff away *reminiscences* of old and tried friends — You will receive a *Halster Barke* etc. by my servant having no desire to retain one *gift* more than another such as Scythe Chain or be charged therewith in your *acct consent* — I am quite aware there is something more even now in the Shape of a *Gift* which your memory may serve you with namely a *quadrupedal* one yet should I ever be tainted with this I happily can bestow on you a Roland for an Oliver.
>
> Yours etc.

How would this abrasive dispute end? Did it continue? There is no record and we shall never know.

There seems little doubt that Thomas did enjoy drinking. Two of the poems which he copied into his notebooks are entitled 'The Glasses Sparkle' and 'A Bacchanalian Tribute by a Gouty Old Commodore'. The lines from one include the following:

> *The day is gone the night's our own*
> *Then let us feast the soul;*
> *If any paid or care remain*
> *Why, drown it in the bowl!*

Some of his drink bills were quite considerable. He was evidently a good customer at the Windbound, a public house on the banks of the River Severn. One of his accounts there amounted to £4.8s.7½d. for the purchase of brandy, rum, gin, whisky and beer, at a time when brandy cost 3/9d a pint and gin cost 3s a bottle.

He had to borrow money from a Mrs Morgan, who was one of his tenants (her rent was four guineas a year). In the six months from October 1849 to April 1850 he had borrowed from her £29.3s.11d. for coal, spirits and beer. She delivered an account to him for this and he conscientiously made a note on the back that it must be paid immediately. He immediately set off a year's rent against the account and paid £1.8s.0d. in part payment for coal, but one wonders when she received the balance.

His tailor, as one might expect, was also owed money. At Christmas 1849, an account for £4 had not been paid to Mr Hutstein of 28 College Green, Bristol. The 1840s were hard times and there must have been many other gentlemen like himself in a similar position. About the same time, his brother Robert Knapp Barrow was selling parts of his estates, presumably as a result of financial pressures.

Thomas must have devoted quite a lot of time to making the entries in his notebooks. They were not only concerned with business matters. For instance, one page contains a 'recipe to make a salade worthy of a Man of Taste'. Another page shows a long account of the 'sepia or cuttlefish'. Yet other pages contain a copy of a lengthy letter from a friend in Upper Canada in 1833.

One of his valuable possessions, which has survived to this day, was his Book of Common Prayer, which he had presumably inherited, because it was purchased by his ancestor Thomas Cox of Kingston in 1757. It is now is the possession of one of Thomas Cox Barrow's great-grandsons, namely M. Carlos Brossel of Brussels. The following rather curious lines were apparently written by Thomas Cox on the first page of the book:

> When Jesus was crucified
> The Jews asked him if he shook.
> Jesus answered and said: Whosoever hath
> These Lines shall never be troubled with Ague or fever.

On the following page there is a statement that Thomas Cox died in 1808 and Elizabeth Barrow in 1815, with the comment 'She was granddaughter of the above Thos. Cox of Kingston and only Child of Robert and Jane Knapp of Shipperdine in the Parish of Rockhampton, Gloucestershire.'

Thomas himself died in 1868 at the age of 62 and was buried at Oldbury. He and Mary Ann had three daughters but no sons. The girls were called Elizabeth, Mary Ann Jane and Emily Charlotte. The eldest, Elizabeth, was born on 1 December 1832 at Frenchay and baptized at Thornbury. She was seven years older than Mary Ann and 12 years older than Emily Charlotte.

In 1855, Elizabeth married William Dowling from Over Wallop in Hampshire. Her sister married Alfred Dowling, who may well have been his brother. William Dowling came from a family long established in that part of Hampshire. In the churchyard of St Peter's, Over Wallop, there is a large table tomb, surrounded by railings, commemorating William Dowling, who died in 1849, and his wife Harriet, who died in Kensington nine years later. An earlier William Dowling was the minister of St Andrew's Church at Nether Wallop and was buried under the chancel there in 1680.

Elizabeth and William Dowling spent their early married life at Over Wallop. He died at Basingstoke in 1900. They had nine children, several of whom left the area when they grew up, and the family became quite widely dispersed. One of the daughters, Florence Louise (1863–1946) married a Belgian judge (M. Brossel) and they had two sons, Andrew and Carlos. The youngest of Elizabeth's children, Sydney, became a parson in Leicestershire and died in 1962.

Another of their children was Thomas Barrow-Dowling, who was born at Over Wallop on 31 May 1861 — the father of Dr Geoffrey Barrow Dowling.* He was a musician and a Fellow of the Royal Academy of Music. Trained in Salisbury, he was first organist at St Philip's, Regent Street, and then organist and choirmaster at St George's Cathedral in Cape Town.

Before sailing for South Africa, he married Caroline Marion (Minna) Grant, in 1888. She was born on 22 December 1870 at Sibdon in Shropshire. Her father died in America before she was born. Her early education was at Saint Boniface School in the Isle of Wight, where she received her first training in pianoforte. On one occasion she obtained poor marks in a music examination and was severely punished at home. She made up her mind never to tell her mother about anything again. She did not get on well with her grandmother in Sibdon, so the opportunity of marriage at 18 and emigration to Cape Town was an attractive prospect.

---

* The Cape Town family always used a hyphen in their name, but when Geoffrey came to England he dropped it.

Chapter 2
The Dowlings in Cape Town. I

by GEORGE FINDLAY

GEOFFREY Barrow Dowling's parents were both professional musicians. His father, Thomas Barrow-Dowling, arrived in Cape Town from England in the year 1888. He was then 27 years old, and brought with him his 18-year-old bride, born Minna (Marion) Grant. He had accepted the post of organist at St George's Cathedral, Cape Town. Their family of seven children were all born there, including Geoffrey in 1891.

Visiting South Africa in 1959, Geoffrey Dowling set out to rediscover his birthplace in a lodging off Queen Victoria Street. 'House gone — no plaque,' he announced with a twinkle. Probably it was Poplar Lodge in Perth Street, where a tall block of flats now stands. They also lived at Thornhayes, at 5 Belvedere Avenue, Oranjezicht, and perhaps also at 10 Hof Street Gardens. Both these lovely buildings have survived. The latter, called Newport House today, has been restored with wonderful taste by its present owner.

For a full 38 years, until he died in 1926, Geoffrey Dowling's father was a prominent figure in the musical world of Cape Town. Minna Barrow-Dowling outlived her husband, and wielded her influence in that city for half a century.

There may be no obvious relationship between the parents' activities in music and their son's in dermatology, but I think I can show that each was doing in his way a comparable job. Their personal gifts were shared, and they often dealt with analogous problems. Musical life in the Cape was in transition, and the Dowlings struggled to maintain high standards, to prevent disintegration, and to adapt, in a critical period, to expansion and reorganization.

DR THOMAS BARROW-DOWLING

Thomas Barrow-Dowling (1861–1926) was mostly spoken of as 'the Doctor'. This title dated from December 1903, when the Archbishop of Canterbury, Dr Randall Davidson, had awarded him the degree of Doctor of Music. In the register of degrees held at Lambeth Palace, the grounds for conferring it are cited: 'In consideration of his knowledge, ability and success in the practical Department of Music and of his having occupied with distinction the position of organist of the Cathedral Church of St George...' His musical sponsors recommending the Lambeth doctorate were Sir George Martin, organist of St Paul's Cathedral, Sir Hubert Parry of the Royal College of Music, and Sir Walter Parratt, Master of the King's Musick. Dowling could not afford the doctoral robes, but 40 of his pupils and friends clubbed together to present them to him as a mark of their esteem.

Geoffrey Dowling was rightly proud of his father's musical achievements. He may well have been present when the Archbishop of Canterbury conferred the degree of Doctor of Music. Geoffrey retained in his possession his father's certificate and the royal seal which accompanied it. He once told me what a privilege it was to have grown up in the midst of musical church services, despite the dismal fact that 'musicians generally are rather poor'. Life for such people required an unremitting effort merely to keep going, though at the time, in Europe and Britain, the prospects of a musical career were often bleaker.

Compositions and services

One wanted to know something about 'the Doctor's' tastes, performances and creativity. Dowling's known compositions are few — two school songs, a choral 'Amen' for use after the blessing at the end of the service, and an incomplete manuscript of a masque, entitled 'The Progress of Prosperity'. This was written in celebration of the opening of the first Parliament of the Union of South Africa in 1910. His only published composition was a piano solo, which appeared in the late 1880s, called *Chastelar*, and was described as a Gavotte de Concert in E minor, dedicated to his fiancée.

Going through the musical services, anthems and organ recital programmes from Dowling's cathedral career, the present incumbent of the post, Mr Barry Smith, admires the effort but disparages the taste by the standards of today. He finds that they represent Victorian church music 'at its lowest ebb'. Dowling's organ recital programmes show how the organ often had to serve as the sole regular, and inexpensive, source of every kind of music. Programmes were laden with bizarre, popular and maudlin transcriptions, which had little to do with the musical literature of the organ as an instrument in its own right. Barry

Smith writes: 'Barrow-Dowling was not without the spirit of a musical pioneer. Perhaps one of the most amazing achievements of his whole career was a performance of Bach's St Mathew Passion in St George's Cathedral on 20 March 1894 — the first in Cape Town, and possibly the first in the whole of the African Continent...no mean achievement...in those early days...With this performance Barrow-Dowling established a tradition of an annual Passiontide performance which was maintained.'

Before Dowling arrived in Cape Town, the musical activity outside the churches consisted of somewhat desultory glee clubs, choral groups, amateur instrumentalists and a regimental band. An oratorio was sometimes performed, and concerts were made up of overtures, solos, glees and pieces accompanied on the harmonium, etc.

Barrow-Dowling's first loyalty went to the cathedral, but his musical activities spread far beyond. Beatrice Marx wrote: 'The "old Doctor" had his finger in every musical pie.' He transplanted, maintained and developed the British musical traditions of his time in a small community. 'No choral conductor has had his success,' she claimed. Margaret van der Post said that 'until the formation of the Cape Town Orchestra (in 1914), Dr Barrow-Dowling and his wife had done more to keep music alive in Cape Town than any one else'. Such words are obviously not merited without great personal sacrifice, and much of his hard-earned cash must have been ploughed back into the purchase of music. Professor Percival Kirby, himself a pupil of Charles Villiers Stanford, once told me that he had bought a large valuable collection of full scores, notably of the Handel oratorios, from the Dowling estate.

Dowling was also known to have engaged and imported soloists from elsewhere at his own financial risk, so as to ensure the worth of his performances. They often stayed as house guests with the Dowlings. Geoffrey Dowling recalled the names of John Harrison, Lloyd Chandos, Signor Foli and Sir Charles Santley. I took Geoffrey Dowling and his mother somewhat by surprise by letting them hear the voices of Harrison, Davies and Santley once more from my own library of historic gramophone records.

Choral practices

Barrow-Dowling triumphed as a conductor and organizer. He believed most in an active, unremitting and systematic cultivation of musical interest. Kindred activities in the hands of others were, he found, associated with 'a life of not very long duration'. The fitful existence of a certain choral group he chose to ascribe to a 'temperamental aberration ... with an odd little manner of effacing itself every now and then'. Thus he benefited from the fusion of several separate choir groups of adult amateurs.

Where should constructive efforts be directed? Dowling would answer: 'What an invaluable asset to the musical culture of the country the systematic training of children in singing can be.' He sought the sympathetic support of the Ministers and Directors of Education, and arranged choir practices in schools throughout the Cape Peninsula. It seems that schoolteachers were much relieved at not having to train school choirs. In many places they had neither the time nor the experience to do this successfully. These classes entered in many public competitions for the challenge shields. As Barrow-Dowling once said, 'May I unobtrusively remark that one of the shields remained 10 or more years with our high school singing classes, which I was privileged to direct at the time.' It seems that these school choirs were always occupied with pageants, charity matinées and other functions. Their combined efforts were seen in a massed choral work for 600 children's voices, which Dowling produced in 1909 — Gabriel Pierne's *Children's Crusade*. Behind a strict manner, a genuine fondness for the young shone through his efforts to get the best out of musical instruction for them.

From the pupils' point of view, I have heard more reference to Dowling's gruff and fierce ways than anything about the music itself. They dared not try tricks on him. I have met a number of old ladies, today in their eighties, who are still awe-inspired by their memories of him — 'Dr Barrow-Dowling was a holy terror', 'He was a bad-tempered old devil', 'Dictatorial'. A 90-year-old aunt of mine, herself a professional musician and a product of the Royal College of Music in Hubert Parry's day, put down Dowling's lack of a kind and easy manner to a limp, which he was obliged to correct with a walking-stick and a built-up boot. 'It seemed that he could strike you with his stick.' 'Take six order marks,' he once said to a refractory class of girl singers.

Organist

Dowling supervised the design and installation of the Cape Town City Hall organ in 1905, and held the post of city organist until its future seemed secure in other hands. He was also the last to perform on the old cathedral organ in 1890, and the first to inaugurate its successor and to supervise the coming of the present organ in the new cathedral in 1909.

These landmarks were commemorated in some precious pieces of contemporary journalism. In 1890, 'After the evening service Mr Barrow-Dowling's recital was more than usually emotional. The "Harmonious Blacksmith" was the closing number, and never did that fascinating creation of Haydn [*sic*] express itself in a stronger and sweeter flood of melody. It seemed to sob itself out at the last; and the accomplished organist is said to have shed a silent tear as he turned the gas down on the keyboard to be seen no more.' Strange, with Dowling's legendary lack of sentiment!

With the next organ, 'Mr Barrow-Dowling was waiting by the unopened keyboard. The Dean addressed the organist as "Dear Brother in Christ" and formally entrusted to him the minstrelsy of the Church by handing him the key of the organ, having full confidence in his skill and judgment.' Mendelssohn, Guilmant and Bach followed. 'Like all fugues,' the reporter said of the Bach, it was 'attractive to those who delight in classical music'.

The Hill organ which followed, in 1909, was also first used by Dowling, and it is employed in a practically unaltered condition today.

One of his last organ pupils and a singer in the choir, the late Geoffrey Mark Hussey, told me that Dowling had a fine feeling for the organ, which he inculcated in his pupils. He was a first-rate organist, and overcame his leg lameness by various tricks and pre-settings. He was a demanding person, insisting on what was musically 'right'. Everything had to be ready promptly, with no 'messing about'. On the boys and girls in the choir, he was uniformly tough and unforgiving, though just. It was because of his essential rightness and justice that one could not have hard feelings towards him. One day Hussey took the liberty of playing some light jazzy item on the cathedral organ. An unexpected and terrible bellow came from somewhere beneath. Dowling had heard this transgression. The desecration cost Hussey his bursary, but by then he had learned enough to get a church organ post, which helped pay his way through college.

Orchestral conductor

Another body which Barrow-Dowling conducted from 1894 until 1911 was the Cape Town Musical Society — a body of instrumentalists rather than an orchestra. 'With my appointment,' he wrote, 'the status of the concerts was entirely changed, and an orchestral programme was established upon modern lines.' He praised the leader, who 'bore with my peculiarities with patience, fortitude and singular ability'. The programmes included a number of violin concertos (Mendelssohn, Max Bruch, Vieuxtemps), and various solos accompanied by Mrs Dowling. Looking through the Society's minutes, one detects an elasticity and yet a great firmness in Dowling's attitudes.

As he had command of the choral and orchestral resources, the programmes over the years were full and rich. The sacred works of Mendelssohn and Handel were in the lead, but performances of the works of Mozart, Haydn, Berlioz, Gounod, Rossini, Elgar, Hubert Parry, Coleridge-Taylor, Arthur Sullivan and Villiers Stanford were prominent as well.

By today's standards of taste and interest, all of these works should still be attractive. Other compositions were given the chance to do well. These included the works of John Francis Barnett, Sterndale Bennett, Alexander Mackenzie, Gaul, Spohr, Gade, Smart and Gadsby. At least they were given a hearing and not ignored. For the important choral concerts, the published programmes contained the entire book of words of the vocal parts.

Problems arose with the orchestra. It faltered, and Dowling thought that it was 'not fitting to enter into the reasons'. One would have to guess what these were, but the finances of the Cape Town Municipality were probably among them.

By 1912 and after, two great changes came about in Cape Town. The Municipal Orchestra was founded under Theo Wendt, and the South African College of Music was started, to be run presently by W.H. Bell. Both were from London, where Bell had also been a pupil of Stanford. Wendt's daughter tells how Dowling saved her father from being interned in the First World War, when a burst of spy-fever led to some wild accusation of his being an Austrian.

Portraiture

Philip Tennyson Cole, the British portrait artist, painted Dowling in his doctoral robes. From this picture one can imagine the truth of Beatrice Marx's comments about him — a striking appearance, with dark eyes, beetling brows, white hair and a stentorian voice which quelled conversation.

There is also a splendid cartoon of Barrow-Dowling by D.C. Boonzaaier, which I have been assured is amazingly true to life. Having known the eldest Dowling daughter, Mrs Anderson, the colouring and facial mould of father and daughter coincide accurately to my mind. The original cartoon is in the keeping of the Owl Club, Cape Town's replica of the Savage Club, of which he was a proud member.

Filling in the character sketch, Theo Wendt's daughter says that Dowling was not a man to be lightly offended; he was a rather intimidating personality, often gruff and sarcastic, but also generous and hospitable. In spite of his lameness in one leg, which in no way interfered with his organ-playing, he had physical stamina which made him 'better off than others with two healthy legs'. Those who joined him on rambles or mountain climbs would find themselves hard put to keep up with him. On these walks, he was usually surrounded by his dogs, which were as disciplined as the choir singers.

Reading some of his essays and reports, we seem to be listening to the characteristic Dowling voice, recognizable by a brand of modest self-assurance, as met with in some of his children. He spoke his mind, as long as it did not prejudice his local ideals. He found that, 'the South African War rather knocked things about', but it did not interrupt the flow of activities — lessons on harmony and counterpoint, lectures and lessons in singing, the organ and the pianoforte. Of a visiting Italian opera company, he remarked: 'some fine voices, and a *very inefficient* management'. He spoke of the famous singer Sims Reeves as having given 'two rather pathetic concerts'.

Denouement

Slowly Dowling handed over his many-sided activities to others as they came along — the orchestra, the academic teaching, the post of city organist. Closest to his heart and last to be abandoned were the Cape Town choral societies. When his health was breaking down in 1925, he could continue as their conductor no longer. As the turmoil of his busy life settled, people came more clearly to realize what he had meant to them.

In an illuminated address, signed amongst others by the British conductor Leslie Heward, the choral societies expressed their esteem and regard for Dr Barrow-Dowling: 'We wish to thank you for the time given and the energy and patience exercised in your work with us as well as the knowledge you have imparted to us during the practice of the various oratorios etc. produced by you in the past 36 years... Many old members have happy recollections of past triumphs under your guidance and can testify to the added interest which your work has given to their lives.'

Death in 1926

Barry Smith has collected some obituary notices which single out Dowling's enduring characteristics — freshness, unwearying enthusiasm, long sacrifice, devotion, disapproval of slackness, praise for merit and endeavour, a love of his art, and a person remembered with deep affection. One writer said: 'It would indeed be difficult to find any other single person whose influence has had such effect in building up a refined taste throughout the country.'

Dowling's last professional stronghold was the cathedral. When he died after 38 years as organist and choir-master, a memorial plaque was inscribed with the words:

> By the vigour of his personality, his power of leadership and his unflagging zeal, he made music a noble accompaniment to worship and did worthy service to the City of Cape Town. Lest a devoted musician, faithful friend and loyal citizen be forgotten, this tablet is placed by those to whom he was well beloved.

'GRANNY' — MINNA BARROW-DOWLING (M.B.D.)
1870–1962

There are not many alive today who have much to tell about 'the Doctor'. If he was a 'character', then it is hard to know what word might apply to his spouse, Dr Geoffrey Barrow Dowling's mother. I think I can claim to be perhaps the only dermatologist who actually knew her.

As a young bride, 'Granny' probably formed the plan of copying the Doctor in as many ways as she could. Before her birth, her father, whom she always said was a Scottish Grant although he was English, had been killed in America by an electric eel. Her Shropshire grand-mother is reputed to have been so fierce that marriage and emigration to South Africa provided a welcome escape for the young girl.

People found it hard to understand how two personalities such as the Doctor and Granny remained together for a lifetime. In between the birth of her children she slipped off to take her piano licentiate in London. She mastered the art of playing the cathedral organ, and accompanied the choirs at oratorio rehearsal. She acted as accompanist and hostess to visiting artists (often playing all the accompaniments from memory), and stood staunchly by Dr Barrow-Dowling's interests at all times.

The best part of Minna Barrow-Dowling's life was thought to belong to her time as a journalist. For 14 years she held the post of music and theatre critic of the *Cape Times*. She wrote notices almost daily, covering activities in the theatre, giving advance notices of pro-grammes, reporting on concerts, attending shows at the Railway or the Seaman's Institute, vaudevilles, fancy dress balls, wireless recitals, performances by bands on the pier, shows in pavilions and in parks, and the comings and goings of performers of every kind, besides any other newsy items. In the specimens of her writing which I have seen, she was uniformly pleasant, but essentially non-committal in most of what appeared in the paper.

For the last 34 years of her long life, she stayed with her son Edward ('Bunny') and his wife, born Prisca Hutton, who was the most agreeable daughter of a Dorsetshire parsonage, and a St Thomas's-trained nursing sister. To give an impression of the aftertaste left in that household by Granny, I am able to draw on a devastating store of recollections supplied with the utmost finesse by the late Prisca Barrow-Dowling.

There is no doubt that Granny enjoyed her time in East Africa. In 1935 she wrote an account of her experiences for a magazine:

> My life in East Africa began nine years ago in Tanganyika with a safari from Tanga to Arusha, which to me was of immense interest after the older civilisation of the Cape, where travelling is easy, roads good and hotels frequent. Everything was different,

primitive and tropical. Our route lay first through beautiful forest country. Monkeys chattered in the trees, bright hued birds made unfamiliar sounds, and the road rendered sticky by recent rains was impossible. The car skidded, turned right round and exemplified perfectly the old comedy slogan of the three speeds of a Ford car — slow, damn slow, stop! The car was actually a Chrysler, but the motor vehicle has yet to be built which will negotiate black cotton soil without misbehaving itself. It was all very amusing and later in the day very exciting, for we travelled through country stiff with rhino and buffalo. We were unfortunate for we saw none.

In the evening Mount Kilimanjaro, magnificent, massive and snow covered, stood out quite clearly in brilliant moonlight, a never-to-be-forgotten sight. Later several lion relieved the monotony of a shocking road. They gazed at our headlights and we gazed at them. Then they pursued their leisurely way into the bush and we went on. Lion are usually the least aggressive of East African big game as far as humans are concerned, but I can quite truly say that on no safari of which I was ever a member has a gun been used or even thought of; and as time went on I saw elephant, rhino, buffalo, leopard, giraffe and all the smaller varieties at close quarters.

In due time, muddy, wet through, but none the less thrilled, we came to Arusha. Nestling on the foothills of Mount Maru, and only 30 miles away from Kilimanjaro, Arusha is very lovely; a little green oasis, well watered and well wooded.

But Arusha was not for me and as soon as possible I turned my face towards Nairobi, 200 miles away. The opportunity came delightfully with another safari, as far as Uganda via Nairobi. That was a marvellous trip, made sometimes in good weather, sometimes in bad. The great north road by which we travelled is I might say a courtesy title. The road was narrow with frequent deep drifts, sandy and rock bottomed. We inevitably stuck, not once but many times; but we unloaded, pushed and laughed, and in the end got through.

On safari one takes what comes and gets some enjoyment out of the mishaps. During that journey I had to correct many times my previous impressions of British East Africa as a hot, steamy country, invariably green and with enormous yearly rainfall. In the first 200 miles we passed over arid land, stony, uncultivated and inhospitable, but the track (still the great north road), which lies at the base of the Ngong Hills, was scenically beautiful though dangerously narrow. Today all that is altered. A new and safer road has been constructed, and the drifts are concrete and easily negotiable.

I shall say little about the safari to Uganda. The scenery was varied and some of it very dull. No-one I think could ever fail to be impressed with the first view of Victoria at Jinja and the Ripon Falls, the actual source of the Nile. I was deeply impressed and, in thinking of the travel part of my East African life, I never forget that Lake Victoria is as large as Ireland, and that its shores are bounded by the three territories, Tanganyika, Kenya and Uganda. At Jinja I saw many crocodiles and hippos. In fact we used to wander among the bamboos at night in full view of the huge beasts. They never worried us.

From the first moment I entered Nairobi and enjoyed my first sundowner at the New Stanley Hotel I felt that I had come to a friendly place — a place where I could make a home and find congenial work. I was right in both cases. The first person to meet me in Kenya had been associated with me on the staff of the *Cape Times* and had even shared my home in Cape Town. So we gladly renewed the association and made a home together in a new country.

I acquired a thoroughbred Cairn terrier, my faithful companion for nearly eight years, and later was given a grey parrot which came from the Belgian Congo and could speak French and a few words of Swahili. He soon learnt to speak English and, oddly enough, was devoted to the Cairn.

During my first week in Nairobi I became organist of All Saints Cathedral, an appointment which I kept for five years, and was also attached for bi-weekly talks on music, the latest issues of gramophone records and various other subjects, to the Nairobi Broadcasting Company. I learnt to know 'This is 7LO Nairobi, Kenya calling' almost as well as my own name. It was always a keen pleasure to talk to an unseen audience with the hope that someone in the outlying districts would enjoy both the music and the talks. Later the talks broadened into lectures on things theatrical as well as musical. These were given at the

MacMillan Library, an up to date literary institution which may be counted as one of Nairobi's cultural assets.

Nairobi is a town of surprises. Shortly after I arrived, the Editor of the *East African Standard* rang up and asked me if I would write the criticism of *Hamlet*. I gasped a little because somehow *Hamlet* seemed out of place in Equatorial Africa, but naturally I accepted my first offer of journalistic work in Nairobi, and accepted it with gratitude. I suppose I went to the full rehearsal prepared to scoff but I certainly remained to admire. The play was presented by The Railway Players, and most excellently produced by James Master, also of the Kenya and Uganda Railways. Some of the players are in Nairobi today and are still continuing the good work for Red Cross funds. Mr Master has raised by his productions since the beginning of the War £3000 for the Red Cross.

To return to *Hamlet*, this was the beginning of a very happy association with the amateur and professional players in Nairobi, and equally of my association with the *East African Standard*.

It seems extraordinary that in the very heart of Africa Shakespearean Festivals should be held yearly, and held with success. During the eight years of my work in connection with these Festivals *Hamlet*, *Julius Caesar*, *Twelfth Night*, *King Lear*, *A Midsummer Night's Dream*, *The Taming of the Shrew* and *As You Like It* were all produced in turn and always in conjunction with the Shakespearean play chosen for the Matriculation examination. Some of the productions were better than others but on the whole the standard was very high.

Side by side with the more serious drama, modern plays were presented by different producers and now, in Military Nairobi, revues and pantomimes and plays of an altogether higher type are the order of the day.

I enjoyed everything wholeheartedly, but I enjoyed most things in Kenya and for the first time I lived in an almost perfect climate, never too hot and never too cold. Cultural life is growing apace in Kenya and I am dwelling at some length on this because I want to correct the impression that Kenya is the gay, giddy and irresponsible country it is generally thought to be. It would be absurd to compare the musical life in Nairobi to that of Cape Town but there is an excellent Musical Society with quite a good little orchestra, a string quartet and some good soloists. Oratorios are given from time to time and there is a general urge among those who are interested towards a more comprehensive artistic life.

Five years ago I was given the priceless opportunity of flying to England. I will not go into the details of that journey because it has been written up time and again, but to me it was a glorious adventure; I am just as well in the air as on terra firma and I suffered none of the inconveniences common to many air travellers.

Uganda from the air looked like an emerald country, which with its huge annual rainfall it really is; Lake Victoria in respect of its size was a revelation, and even the Sudan had its charm, lovely sunsets, huge herds of elephant and other game. We were fortunate in having 24 hours in Alexandria, the interesting city of many tongues, and incidentally it was good to be at sea level again. The Mediterranean on that sunny October day was at its finest.

In four months I was back in Nairobi and I soon settled down to work again on the *East African Standard*. I only left it with sincere regret to come to South Africa again.

I have been asked to compare life in Central Africa with life in the larger centres of the Union. It is a little difficult because Cape Town, in which I spent so many years, is so much older and so very much larger. One lived there very much the same formal life that is offered in large centres in England, and as the population grew so did the formality. Nairobi in comparison is tiny, and a small community is always more friendly than a large one. Life is much freer and in some ways safer. I was able to drive long distances by car alone at night without the slightest fear and, as far as the domestic problem is concerned, servant troubles are a rare occurrence. My boys were with me for the greater part of my stay in Kenya, and there is a very just and efficient system of registration. In fact all the amenities of life are in Kenya, including all-electric houses and well built flats with refrigerators, electric water systems, stoves and heaters. Also there are many beauty spots such as Nyeri on the foothills of Mount Kenya where Lord Baden Powell spent the remaining years of his life.

I say very little about the Military conditions of present day Nairobi. Everyone is doing war work and incidentally making things as pleasant as possible for South African and other troops which pass through on their way north.

Altogether I found life very good in Kenya, and when I came away I left a large circle of true friends. My great hope is that some day I may go back again to renew many pleasant associations and perhaps put in some more work for the *East African Standard*.

This account shows that, although Granny Barrow-Dowling expected her sons to look after her when her husband died, she was more than capable of being independent, and was well equipped to do so.

'Bunny' Barrow-Dowling, according to his widow and his daughter, showed many of the Dowling characteristics. Bunny hated the word charm. 'Be natural — that's enough,' he would say. He was helpful to many more people than they knew of, and was described as one of nature's gentlemen. He was indeed a gentle person, who could be fierce at times without losing his temper. He was also tremendously liked by children, who would flock when they saw him coming.

Bunny met his future wife in East Africa. When they considered marriage, Bunny's brother warned her, 'If you want to get married, you had better do so before mother comes.' To this Prisca answered, 'If Bunny is the sort of man who listens to his mother first, I'd rather not have him.' Quite right, they told her, 'but you haven't met our mother.'

Granny expected her sons not to marry, so that they could look after her. In due time she arrived from the Cape, complete with Steinway piano, to settle on her sons in Tanganyika. Her first words on meeting the engaged couple were: 'All right, I've forgiven you.'

If this is what she expected of her sons, her daughters came in for criticism and dislike continually. Prisca said that Granny hated women and femininity in any shape. A dog lover and keen supporter of the SPCA, Granny would proclaim, 'The more I see of women, the more I like dogs.'

Prisca claimed that the Dowlings in general were not marrying types. Granny never nursed her babies and had no time for children unless they showed some talent or promise. On producing a baby, she would hand it over to a wet-nurse and get on with her professional work. Prisca said, 'The real trouble with Granny was that she was too clever for a woman.' In the house she was hopelessly incompetent. Once, on making a steak and kidney pie, the kitchen looked as if she had done a full day's cooking.

Granny acted as if she had droves of servants at her bidding. She would be inclined to command attention at a doorway, making queenly entrances, and hold court with visitors. A strict chaperoning system was also applied to parties. If a party in the house went on too long, she'd come in and play 'God Save the King' and expect it to break up. Once she had to play the anthem three times before the guests took the hint.

I asked Prisca how Granny came to develop such airs. 'I have no idea, except that she was an awful snob. When everybody kissed her on her eightieth birthday, she said she never dreamed she would ever be kissed by the butcher.'

Only their tolerance and good nature saved them from fights, though clashes were not unknown. Once when Prisca was out, Granny changed round the furniture.

'What on earth has happened?' asked Prisca.

'I was tired of the things as they were'.

'Well,' said Prisca, 'I'll go back to town, and when I come back I expect to see the furniture where I like it.'

This was the only way with her — she had to be outmanoeuvred.

Other members of the family told me that Granny was found to be a bad loser and had little sense of humour. She was never seen to laugh or cry. Unswerving resolve was her watchword; it was her aim to see that what must go through went through regardless. Her principles and sense of Victorian proprieties were to be maintained at the expense of all else.

She died at the home of her son, Edward, in Borrowdale near Salisbury, Rhodesia (now Zimbabwe), on 5 May 1962 at the age of 92. He had kept his promise to look after her since his father died 36 years earlier.

When she died, the obituaries were as numerous and as laudatory as for her husband. She had become as well known and as famous as him in the Cape, entirely on her own merit, using all the talents as a pianist, organist and journalist with which she was endowed. A colleague wrote in the *Cape Argus* (9 June 1962):

> It saddened me to read of the death of Mrs Minna Barrow-
> Dowling. Cape Town had much to be grateful for to Dr Barrow-

Dowling, forceful choirmaster and organist at St George's Cathedral, and the pretty young wife he married at 18 and brought to Cape Town from England.

They had seven children — five of them still living — but Mrs Barrow-Dowling's hands were not too full to keep her from augmenting the family income by teaching the piano. She would pedal about the town on her bicycle to give lessons and she played for rehearsals when her husband was training the Choral Society for some work in the City Hall.

To sing oratorios with the Choral Society the Barrow-Dowlings would bring principals from Europe. They were truly the pioneers of the rich musical life Cape Town has today.

The happiest years for Mrs Barrow-Dowling, I think, were the 16 she spent as musical and dramatic critic of the *Cape Times*. In her little office overlooking St George's Street at tea time one might have met Marie Tempest or Irene Vanbrugh with a member of parliament who was hoping to see the editor next door or senior journalist. Hers was an excellent brew of tea and she knew how to make conversation sparkle.

Mrs Barrow-Dowling was 92 when she died and not many of her contemporaries are left.

But through her children she kept abreast of Cape news and was warmly welcomed when she came back on visits. In the middle thirties she went to live in Tanganyika with her son 'Bunny' and was on the staff of the *East African Standard* in Nairobi, until she retired from active journalism.

Another colleague included some of her strongly held opinions: 'Ninety two year old Mrs Minna Barrow-Dowling hates rock 'n roll. "I'm a musician," she said. "If there's one thing threatening the continuance of good music it is this jazz and swing and the fact that children are brought up to it. They listen to such tripe." '

A great lady indeed.

Chapter 3
The Dowlings in Cape Town. II

GEOFFREY Dowling's eldest sister (Minna, 'Bino') was a schoolteacher who went to work in Windhoek, South West Africa, when there was a call to the Union for teachers. She met and married John Anderson, one of seven children of George Beattie Anderson, who was born in Kennethmont, Aberdeenshire, and went out to South Africa to work for the London Missionary Society shortly after being ordained in Scotland.

During three years of courtship they both worked in the medical field during the devastating influenza epidemic of 1919. They were married from the Barrow-Dowling home in Cape Town and the service was in St George's Cathedral, where her father played the organ. They returned to Windhoek and lived in the north-west corner and adjacent wings of the Alte Feste Fort behind the Horse Statue; today it is a museum and national monument. They had three children — Barbara, born in 1921, John, born in 1923, and David, born in 1927.

Bino's future husband was a teacher at the Graaf Reinet High School in 1914 when he decided to do his stint and join the South African forces under General Botha. After an eventful campaign in the south, the South African forces eventually reached Windhoek in 1915. He pleaded with the military authorities to be allowed to remain in that town in order to inaugurate the first South African school in the territory. He then continued to dedicate his life, in the only way he knew, to his teaching which he loved. Oubaas Andy, Ou Skot, became an educational legend in his time, and nobody was more proud of him than John, his eldest son.

John, Geoffrey's nephew, was musically inclined from early child-hood onwards and indeed as time passed the interest in music became intense. The reason for this perhaps strange, almost fanatical interest in music is not difficult to understand as both his parents hailed from musical families. Indeed, on his mother's side, music was the life-work of both parents. There are undoubtedly few people of the Cape Town of yesteryear still alive today who would not have known, and in all probability have been taught by, either Grandpa or Grandma Barrow-

Dowling, and many were subject to his strict baton in the Cape Town Orchestra in whose inauguration he played the major role.

John Anderson, the nephew, writes:

Dr Barrow-Dowling's activities were, musically, all-embracing, for, in addition to his training of the cathedral choir, he had many private pupils for singing, pianoforte and organ, as well as being responsible for the choral training of many of the schools in the Cape Peninsula.

Prior to the 1914 war, he was instrumental in presenting the biennial Festive Concerts, which were a great feature in Cape Town's musical life. He introduced such artists as Agnes Nicholls, Perceval Allen, Edna Thornton, Lloyd Chandos, John Harrison, William Green, Charles Knowles and Albert Archdeacon. Amongst the choral works performed were *The Messiah, Elijah, The Dream of Gerontius, The Golden Legend, Caractacus* and Gabriel Pierne's *Children's Crusade*; this last was a monumental work involving a chorus of 600 voices, when the combined choral societies were augmented by all the Doctor's school choirs. For this performance, the composer wrote him a personal letter of thanks from Paris.

Dr Barrow-Dowling owed a great deal of his success to his wife, who, as official accompanist to the combined choral societies and a fine musician in her own right, had proved a tower of strength in these crowded years.

In addition to her private pupils, to whom she taught pianoforte and singing, and the bringing up of a family of four sons and three daughters, she found time to study and master the organ, an accomplishment which was put to excellent use later in her career.

Minna Barrow-Dowling was a gifted musician and born accompanist. From 1896 to 1911, she recurs constantly in this role in the records of the Cape Town Musical Society under her husband's conductorship. During these years, she became also the official accompanist to the combined choral societies and a tremendous help to her husband in the production of the Festival oratorios.

Throughout the years, her intellectual qualities had not passed unnoticed. In 1918 she was appointed Musical and Dramatic

Critic to the *Cape Times*, by Sir Maitland Park, the Editor. With a natural flair for journalism, her wide musical knowledge and her love of the theatre, the next 14 years were perhaps the fulfilment of her career. An exacting critic, she was scrupulously fair in her remarks. Of all the great composers, Brahms was to her the Master.

In 1932 family affairs compelled her departure for East Africa where, in Nairobi, she joined the newspaper, the *East African Standard*. For some years she was also organist and choirmaster of the Cathedral of the Highlands. She returned to South Africa in 1939.

In the last 20 years of her life, rheumatism in her hands gradually took its toll and brought to an end her piano playing and accompanying, a source of great sorrow to her.

A great lover of animals, she organised many concerts in aid of the SPCA, a cause to which she was devoted.

Among John Anderson's earliest memories of their lovely old home in Cape Town, 10 Hof Street, virtually in the grounds of the Mount Nelson Hotel and below the Helmsley Hotel, was the magnificent old oak door, probably one of the finest in the city, which can still be seen to this day. This opens on to the garden path leading to the house, which stands back from the street. Another very vivid recollection is that of a veritable 'pound' of dogs of all sorts and sizes. They were all very well trained and extremely obedient. A masterly 'beddy-byes' or 'walkies' would see an avalanche of canines either disappearing to their kennels in the back yard, or making excitedly for the front door, whichever was the command. There were, conservatively, nine at any one time; but the numbers used to change, varying proportionately with the stray element finding their way into the Dowling home from all corners of the city. Entrée seemed to be automatic. They had never had it so good!

An incident at the wedding luncheon of John's parents is perhaps worth recording. The table was graced with two trifles: one for the abstemious Anderson end of the table, the other for the Dowling contingent. Grandfather Dowling liked his trifle adequately laced with sherry. The two trifles, unfortunately, landed up at the wrong ends of the table and, while Grandfather Anderson was demanding the recipe, Grandpa Dowling nearly had a cadenza. He somehow managed to keep calm (under the circumstances, a feat in its own right), while transfer was made and he was dished up with the alcohol edition, much to John's parents' relief.

Dr Barrow-Dowling was an irascible old gentleman who, as a perfectionist, used to become short-tempered when things did not run according to plan, especially when he was conducting. There was one memorable occasion in the City Hall when an embarrassed flautist in the Cape Town Orchestra committed the ultimate sin by blowing a 'lost note' in a moment of total orchestral silence. 'You fool!' echoed around the vast auditorium, much to the amusement of all, after which the orchestra continued unabated!

John Anderson still remembers how his grandparents entertained many well-known international artists, for most of whom they had been the intermediary in persuading them to visit his country. These artists constituted a unique celebrity line-up for a country which, in those days, was far removed from the hub of musical activity in the northern hemisphere, and where travel was still slow, tedious and difficult. Many of them stayed at the Hof Street family home. The grandchildren, of course, as impressionable youngsters, found them to be extremely interesting and exciting, although it was only later that John really recalled them. Most were still enjoying acclaim in Europe and North America at the time. This fact helped immeasurably to propagate enthusiasm and a love of music in the offspring of a family steeped in it. Some of the more notable artists in the list are:

> Paderewski and his wife, Helena, in March 1912
> Henry Irving, May 1913
> The Quinlan Opera Company, July 1913
> Oscar Berringer, Freda Godfrey and H. Warrington-Smith
>   (during the First World War)
> The Edward Donnally American Dramatic Company, 1918
> Marie Tempest, 1919
> Anna Pavlova, 1920
> Irene Vanbrugh, 1923
> Moiseivitch and his wife, Annie, June 1930
> Jascha Heifetz, 1923

John Anderson joined the South African Air Force soon after the outbreak of the Second World War. With initial training completed, he moved up to Cairo and then to Tunis and Naples in Italy, where he was posted to the Royal Air Force 145 Spitfire Squadron.

He took part in the Allied campaign progressing northwards in Italy but was finally shot down about 30 miles from Bologna. He landed by parachute and was soon snatched by an 18-year-old boy, Giuseppe Bernardi, from the searching German troops. He was befriended and looked after by an Italian peasant family before moving on and reaching the Allied lines after some two months. Sadly, two days after his departure, unknown to John, Giuseppe was caught by the Germans, interrogated and handed over to a brutal gang of Italians, who murdered him. A short time later John returned to a Spitfire squadron, but was again shot down and parachuted from 400 feet. This time he was rescued by troops from the Fourth Polish Division, only a few weeks before the end of the War in Italy.

In 1950, with a fellow pilot who had been shot down, John Anderson returned to Italy on a motor bike to look for and thank the Italian families who had looked after them. They found them and, having been tearfully reunited, heard the sad news about Giuseppe Bernardi. When back in England John Anderson broadcast to Italy on the Italian service of the BBC, together with Giuseppe's younger brother, Quinto, who was aged 10. About this time there was a move to make his story into a film. A draft film script was submitted by the Alexander Korda Studio to John Anderson. To his surprise the sex of some of the leading characters had been changed 'for box office appeal'. John rejected it, much to the chagrin of the film people, and they refused to alter their script. So the film was never made.

After the war John went to Dublin to qualify as a doctor, and then worked as a general practitioner in Lusaka (in partnership with Dr Raymond Oliver, now a dermatologist in Johannesburg). He married Elizabeth Herbert and they have three children, Gail, Susan and Christopher, who is a doctor and was recently in England doing some postgraduate work with his wife Elizabeth.

John Anderson's sister Barbara (Geoffrey's niece, Mrs Havelock Cross) has two children, James and Sandra. John's brother David is a lawyer in Bulawayo, Zimbabwe: he is married to Salvia Clews and they also have two children, Colin and Gillian.

Geoffrey Dowling's younger brother Edward (like so many South Africans he had a nickname, and his was Bunny) was born in 1902. He was married to Prisca Hutton. Her father, Arthur Bertram Hutton, was the Vicar of Loders, a small town two miles from Bridport in Dorset, as well as the village of Dottery about four miles away. He took evensong every Sunday afternoon. He had a grave dug by the church at both places, but was buried close to the church door at Loders, as was his wish.

Prisca had trained as a nurse at St Thomas's Hospital, where she had met Geoffrey, then a senior dermatologist. From there she joined the Overseas Nursing Association and went out to Dar es Salaam, where she met Geoffrey's youngest brother, Duncan, who was in the Tanganyika Police. After six months she was sent to Arusha on the coast, where she met Thomas, who was then manager of a coffee plantation.

Edward had promised to make a home for his mother after her husband died in Cape Town in 1926. He married Prisca Hutton and, three days after they returned from their honeymoon, his mother arrived in Arusha (with her piano). They had two children — Margaret, who married Roy Harris and had two children, Helen and Richard, and Elizabeth, married to Leigh Lautenbach.

Edward was trained as an accountant in Scotland and had worked in Tanganyika before returning to Vereeniging on the Cape in 1939. From there he moved to Salisbury, Rhodesia, where he was company secretary at Stewart and Lloyds Ltd for several years. He died in 1966, just three years before he was due to retire.

He was a prominent Rotarian and public-spirited to a degree. Many were the calls upon his services to various 'good causes', and never did he fail to give them unstintingly. He was an outstanding organizer of carol services. He was a member of St Luke's Anglican church in Que Que, where he was organist during the years he lived there.

Bunny was a noble character with qualities of humility, sincerity, loyalty and unselfishness above the average. Possibly his most out-standing quality was his avid desire to give service to his fellow men. He gave his help quietly, without fuss or ostentation. He was modest in the extreme, kind, courteous and generous. Bunny was widely loved and respected by all. Wherever he went he made friends; he seemed to have that special gift. He never lost his affection for the Mother City of Cape Town, with its old tradition, the mountains and the beauty and grandeur of the coastline and hinterland. The gift of music was inherent in him, from his parents. He became a pianist and organist of con-siderable ability. His early death left a memory among his friends of a sterling character, a staunch friend and a most charming personality. He loved young people and was never happier than when in their company.

His wife, Prisca, returned to South Africa and often stayed with her sister-in-law Bino, before she died in 1975. Prisca died in 1984.

Geoffrey also had a younger sister, Marjorie, born in 1902, but she fell from a balcony at home and died in 1905.

Geoffrey's brother Thomas was born in Cape Town on 25 September 1895. Soon after the outbreak of the First World War he joined up and took part in the South West Africa Campaign. Immediately that was over, he accepted a commission and went to England. He became a lieutenant in the Royal Navy Volunteer Reserve, and served as a machine-gun officer in the 63rd Royal Navy Division. He was posted to France and was in action at the second battle of Arras in April 1917. It was at the battle of Grauvelle on 4 April 1916 that he won the Military Cross for gallantry in action. He subsequently transferred to the Machine Gun Crops and was promoted to captain in 1918. After the Armistice in November 1919 he served with the Army of Occupation in the Rhineland. He was finally demobilized in July 1919.

During his time in England he often stayed with the Fawcetts at 66 Wimpole Street, and would have seen a lot of Geoffrey, who was then a young doctor at Guy's Hospital.

After the war he went to East Africa. For a short time he ran a gold-mine, which was unfortunately not profitable, and later a sisal estate. At one time he was manager of a coffee plantation at Arusha in Tanganyika. While there he invited his younger brother Edward to come and stay with him. Edward had trained as an accountant in Scotland. At that time, there was only one accountant in Arusha, and he had recently been invalided home after a severe heart attack.

In Nairobi Thomas met his future wife Sylvia Barnard; her brother was a mining engineer there and she went out to spend a holiday with him. Sylvia and Thomas were married in Marseilles on 4 March 1939.

When the Second World War started in September 1939, Thomas joined the Royal Air Force, and Sylvia became a private secretary at the Air Ministry. They had earlier managed the Elford Leigh Hotel, outside Plumpton in Devon. It was taken over during the war by an orphanage, Nazareth House. Thomas served with the RAF Regiment at Tavyn in South Wales. After the war it was not easy to keep the hotel going and in 1949 they sold it, to return to South Africa, but he always regretted leaving England. Back in the Cape Thomas bought the Links Hotel at Kowie West near Port Alfred, where he died on 10 February 1975.

Thomas and Sylvia had three children. Jacqueline was born in 1942 at Shipston on Stour, Diana at Stratford-upon-Avon in 1947 and Marjorie in Grahamstown, South Africa, in 1949. Jacqueline studied speech and drama at Cape Town University, and then spent a few years as a teacher in Scotland. When she returned to Cape Town she worked for Reader's Digest. She married Richard Hamilton Wege in Johannesburg in 1972. He is a photographer, specializing in food photography, on which he has published two books. They have one son, Timothy.

Jacqueline was very fond of her Uncle Geoffrey. When in England she often spent evenings with him at Festival Hall concerts and Royal Academy exhibitions. She sometimes stayed with him at 52 Ravenscourt Gardens, listening to music and enjoying his famous cottage pies!

When Thomas died in 1975 Sylvia returned to England and lived with her brother, Ralph, at Stratford-upon-Avon. She died in August 1989.

Chapter 4
The Fawcetts

MINNA BARROW-Dowling spent her childhood in Shropshire with her bereaved mother at the house of her grandmother, who was quite a strict disciplinarian. She developed Minna's musical knowledge and talent, but may have been too strict. When she performed badly in an examination she was punished quite severely. So it was not surprising that she welcomed the offer of marriage at 18 and a future life in far away Cape Town.

Understandably, she was homesick and had great difficulty in accepting life in South Africa. Although her husband never returned to England, being totally absorbed in his musical career, Minna made more than a dozen return visits and once spent six months in London to take her LRAM at the Royal Academy. On these visits she mostly stayed with the Fawcetts. Mrs May Fawcett (née Baxter) was her first cousin and they had always been firm friends.

When Minna's husband was awarded his Doctorate of Music in November 1903, the decision was made to send Geoffrey to school in England. It is very likely that his mother accompanied him to make all the arrangements. They would have sailed together from Cape Town to Southampton on one of the Union Castle Liners, and then been met off the boat-train at Waterloo Station by Mrs Fawcett.

It is possible that Geoffrey and Mrs Fawcett attended the ceremony at Lambeth Palace and received his father's certificate and seal of the D.Mus. degree, before starting school in England and the rest of his childhood in the Fawcett household. The Fawcett and Dowling families were to be closely associated all their lives.

John Fawcett was born in 1866, the son of John Bisdee Fawcett, who was an underwriter at Lloyds of London. One of his grandfathers was a merchant navy captain, who retired to farming in Cumberland. And his great-grandfather was one of Admiral Lord Nelson's lieutenants at the Battle of Trafalgar on 21 October 1805.

John was the second eldest of seven children, and the eldest son. Very shortly after her last child was born, his mother died, presumably of puerperal septicaemia. He was 11 years old at the time, and was regarded as the leader of the orphaned family. Bereaved, with seven children under the age of 12 years to bring up and educate, his father became increasingly depressed. Within a year, he took his own life. But, as was usual in those days, family support was available and assumed the burden. The children were 'adopted' by Robert Grant and his wife, John Bisdee Fawcett's sister, who had no children of their own. They sent John and probably his brothers to be educated at Dulwich College. John retained a lifelong devotion to his school and many years later became a Governor of the College.

He decided to become a doctor, and entered Guy's Hospital Medical School in 1885, graduating with the London MB.BS degree in 1890. He must have been an exceptional student; he passed the MD examination a year later and soon after the MRCP and the FRCS. When he was elected FRCP in 1902, he joined the still select band of doctors who had qualified by examination to be Fellows of both the Royal College of Surgeons of England and the Royal College of Physicians of London.

He was elected to the staff of Guy's Hospital as physician in 1899, and was Dean of the Medical and Dental Schools there from 1900 to 1903. He had a broad background of training in pathology, particularly morbid anatomy and biochemistry, having held a research scholarship to work with Dr (later Sir) Edward Gowland Hopkins, who won the Nobel Prize for his discovery of vitamin C. John Fawcett was known at Guy's Hospital for his thoroughness and meticulous attention to detail. He was strongly conservative, and had a reputation for absolute reliabilty and integrity. His nickname was 'Honest John'. His outpatient sessions and ward rounds were often prolonged, and he never allowed any other duties or responsibilities to prevent him from attending them; he was a stickler for punctuality.

His peers, as well as his students, nurses and junior staff, rated him highly. When the chairmanship of the Medical Committee at Guy's Hospital became a decision by voting rather than seniority, he was elected unanimously and remained Chairman until he retired. The post was important because the Chairman was the intermediary between the medical staff and the Governors of the Hospital.

For nine years (1920–1929) he was the representative of the Royal College of Physicians on the Senate of the University of London. He had been elected to the Council of the College in 1920, and became a College Censor in 1921, being appointed Senior Censor in 1923. The President of the College is elected annually by secret ballot at a meeting of Fellows in the College on the first Monday after Palm Sunday. When Sir Humphrey Rolleston was elected President in 1922, it is widely believed that John Fawcett was the runner-up.

This was the man who was to have such an influence on the formative years and career of Geoffrey Dowling.

He married May Fleming Baxter in 1899 when he was 33 years of age, in the same year that he was appointed a physician to Guy's Hospital. His first child, Robert, was not born until 1907, when he was 40, and his daughter Alice was born in the following year. So, when Mrs May Fawcett received Geoffrey in 1903, she regarded him as a son and he grew up as a kind of elder brother to Robert and Alice, who were some 15 years younger.

The Fawcetts certainly cherished Geoffrey and were responsible for his education at Exeter Cathedral Choir School and Dulwich College. They lived at 66 Wimpole Street, where Dr Fawcett saw his private patients. It was said that each consultation there took one to one and a half hours, and he never saw a patient unless they had been referred from their own family doctor. He kept meticulous handwritten notes, and always wrote letters to the referring doctor in his own neat script. To his children he always appeared as a very serious man.

The Fawcetts as foster-parents could not have been more kind and generous, and Geoffrey was forever grateful. He often said that he owed them a great deal, and he was to be able to reciprocate their kindness in later years. But it is doubtful if Geoffrey would have shared the view of the Victorian and Edwardian eras that 'your schooldays are the happiest days of your life'.

When they were grown up Robert and Alice went on holiday to South Africa and stayed with the Barrow Dowlings in Cape Town, just before Geoffrey's father died. His mother was working as a theatre and music critic on the *Cape Times* newspaper. She struck the young Fawcett children as reactionary and very right-wing, in present-day language. At the end of their holiday they returned to England on one of the Union Castle ships together with Minna Barrow-Dowling. The journey lasted about three weeks. Being young they gradually became disenchanted with their 'aunt'. On the ship was Miriam Ryle, the wife of Professor John Ryle, who was in contrast very left-wing in her views of society.

Robert Fawcett became an articled clerk in the prestigious firm of accountants, Price Waterhouse and Company. He stayed there for some 15 years, before being appointed as Company Secretary to Aero Research Limited in 1944. The firm was taken over by Ciba of Basle, Switzerland, in 1947. This was a new company set up in Duxford, Cambridgeshire, to manufacture epoxy resin and other synthetic resin products. Epoxy resin had been developed by a Swiss dentist, but he sold it to the Ciba Company before the Second World War. Robert Fawcett remained with the Company until he retired 25 years later, and lived in Ickleton, a delightful village just a few miles from Duxford. He married Anne Fairlie-Clarke in 1933, and had three children.

Although Dr John Fawcett retired at the compulsory age of 60 from the staff of Guy's Hospital in 1926, he continued in private practice at 66 Wimpole Street. In 1934 he sold the house in Wimpole Street and moved to 10 Chester Terrace; soon after he gave up private practice. Because of the heavy air bombardment in 1940 the Fawcetts left London and lived in various country homes until 1943. Their house was damaged in an air raid; so their daughter Alice gave up her job and took the lease of a flat in St John's Wood Road with the intention of making a home for her parents for the rest of their lives. While the flat was being prepared the Dowlings had them to stay at Porchester Terrace.

John Fawcett had suffered from a duodenal ulcer for decades, and underwent a lot of medical and surgical treatment. His general condition deteriorated, and he was admitted to a nursing home. He died there on 18 February 1944 at the age of 77. A splendid obituary was published in *Guy's Hospital Reports*.

May Fawcett continued her stay with the Dowlings for a short time, where she had a minor stroke, after which she moved into a nursing home. Later in the same year she had a massive stroke and died on 21 August 1944.

Their stay, some months before Simon was due, was a great strain on Geoffrey's wife, May, but she made sure that they were as comfortable as possible. Every meal was carefully prepared, particularly tea, which was always prettily laid out in the drawing-room. There is no doubt that both she and Geoffrey were pleased that they were able to provide care and comfort to the Fawcetts in their final illnesses. Geoffrey always felt a great indebtedness to them. In her will May Fawcett bequeathed him a legacy of £2000, which was set aside to pay for Simon's education, and a handsome antique desk. Alice later gave them the Beckstein piano that Geoffrey's mother had enjoyed playing when she was in London and Simon continues to enjoy it until this day.

Robert and Anne Fawcett's eldest son Thomas is a timber technologist and lives at Newbegin, Beverley, Yorkshire. He has three children. Their second son, John Patrick, is a self-employed architect (ARIBA) and lives in Cambridge. He designed his parents' house at Ickleton, near Saffron Walden.

Their daughter, Teresa Sloden, lives in London with her husband and three children. She is Secretary to the Victorian Society. At one time she was an art student and later became an art historian.

Robert Fawcett's sister, Alice, lived for much of her life with her parents, and was unmarried. She did various jobs, including some time as a psychiatric social worker. She was a gay, cheerful, loving and impulsive person with many friends, including Geoffrey Dowling's children. In later years she owned and ran a hotel in Devon; May often went to stay there with Simon. Tom was her godson. In later years she became gravely crippled with arthritis, and died in 1977.

Chapter 5
The School

GEOFFREY Barrow Dowling began his schooling in Cape Town at Diocesan College (Bishops), one of the oldest and still most distinguished schools in South Africa.

In 1903 he was taken away and sent for his further education to England. The reasons for this move are quite obscure, since none of his younger brothers went to school in England. Several have been put forward. First, he may have expressed a wish to enter the Royal Navy, and his father agreed to let him go to London and apply for entry to Dartmouth. Dr George Findlay in researching the family origins in South Africa suggested that Geoffrey did not do well at school, and his mother believed that the teachers were more responsible for this than her son. One cannot believe that he was a 'difficult' boy at school or at home. And he could not have been backward because he won a Form Prize at Bishops between 1901 and 1903. A third suggestion is that he was not a physically strong child, and that he was sent to school in England for health reasons. It seems unlikely that the climate in England would have been healthier than in Cape Town at the beginning of the century. But photographs do show that Geoffrey had a lighter and smaller physique than his brothers, although there is no record of his having had any major illness in childhood. If it was for health reasons, it was scarcely a success. When he returned at the age of 19, his (favourite) sister May was astonished at the change in her brother. He left as a fine exuberant boy, and returned as a thin, quiet and introspective young man.

Marriage and emigration to South Africa may have been an escape for Minna Barrow-Dowling, but she did not enjoy her early years in Cape Town. She never entirely settled there and maintained strong contacts with her relations in England. She asked May Fawcett (a cousin) and her husband Dr John Fawcett in London to take Geoffrey into their home (they had no children of their own at the time), and to arrange his schooling in England.

So Geoffrey was packed up with his trunk and personal possessions, and sailed from Cape Town, possibly with his mother, who took the

chance to go to London. With Dr Fawcett's help he applied for a place
at the Royal Naval College at Dartmouth. He went up for an interview
at the Admiralty in Whitehall. It was not a success. His parents in
discussion with the Fawcetts then arranged for him to go to Exeter
Cathedral Choir School. A letter of recommendation from his father
would have been enough to ensure his acceptance, and Dr Barrow-
Dowling almost certainly knew some of the members of staff there.

His departure from London by train from Paddington Station to
Exeter for his first term as a boarder was accompanied by all the
anxieties and apprehension of so many English boys leaving home for
the first time. But for Geoffrey it was worse. His mother was not there
to see him off, only a substitute in the form of Mrs Fawcett; no doubt
she did her best, but it could not be the same. From Exeter railway
station it was a short distance to the school. The memory of that
journey up the hill by slow horse-drawn cab was indelibly engraved on
Geoffrey's memory. Years later on a visit to Exeter he told one of his
daughters of the misery and loneliness amounting almost to despair.
Nothing else would ever be as deeply depressing.

We know little of his time at the school there as a boarder, but he
probably grew to enjoy it because of the musical environment. Having
grown up in a musical household with his parents in Cape Town, he
must have started with some advantage over the other boys. In later
years he would listen to the BBC broadcast of Handel's *Messiah* every
Christmas and sing every word with the performers, because he had
done it so many times before as a child.

On 2 May 1906 he began four years of public school as a boarder in
Orchard House at Dulwich College in south-east London. Dr Fawcett
had no doubt decided where he should go, and presumably his parents
in Cape Town were readily persuaded by such an enthusiastic and loyal
former pupil. Dulwich was the best in John Fawcett's eyes, and at this
time he was himself childless.

Like many boys from South Africa, Geoffrey enjoyed most sporting
activities, and represented Orchard House at rugby, football and cricket.
In gymnastics he represented the Science team when they beat the
Classical Engineering and Modern sides, and was a member of the
Orchard House team when they won the House Cup against Blew
House and Ivyholme. At cricket he was recognized as a bowler more
than a batsman and took wickets in a match for the Science team

against the Classical team. Sports reporters for the college magazine
(*The Alleynian*) did not mince their words when criticizing standards of
play, as can be seen from the following account of a rugby Final House
Match when Blew House trounced Orchard, for whom G.B. Dowling
was playing at right wing three-quarter.

> Played on Monday, February 28th. A very surprising game, the
> Orchard offering no sort of resistance to their somewhat heavier
> opponents. The Orchard kicked off uphill, and play soon settled
> down in their half, where, with the exception of one burst by
> Lowe, it remained for the rest of the game. Two minutes from
> the start Green, feinting smartly, ran in near the posts. Bathgate
> added the necessary points, 5–0. Doulton kept up the pressure,
> but Dowling saved well, and Shand relieved with a kick. Then
> weak tackling by Lowe let Broad in for an unconverted try, 8–0.
> Immediately afterwards King was penalised for 'picking out' and
> Bathgate landed a goal, 11–0. Orchard now rushed to half-way,
> but Blew House brought it back and Broad scored again, 14–0.
> Blew House continued to press strongly, Curry keeping up the
> pressure with some excellent kicks. Hereabouts G.D. Baxter was
> laid out and half time arrived.
>
> After the resumption, the game became a procession. Blew
> House scored an unconverted try from a forward rush, and
> then Broad added three unconverted tries, 26–0. With 20
> minutes still to play, Reincke scored far out, and Bathgate kicked
> a fine goal, 31–0. Even considering the state of the ground,
> the Orchard were feeble in the extreme. King and Lowe were
> practically useless while Shand, although continually making his
> presence felt, was little real good to the side. G.D. Baxter and
> Curry both played good games at back.
>
> The following were the teams:
> BLEW HOUSE: H.D. Curry (back); E.G. Gabain, A.C. Green,
> D. Davis, P.C. Braddon (three-quarters); F.H. Broad and A.J.
> Reincke (halves); V. Bose, H.W. Benson, J.M. Bathgate, E.H.
> Scott, J.A. Paterson, J.E. Warner, E.C. Cartwright, A.N. Bocock
> (forwards).
> THE ORCHARD: G.D. Baxter (back); G. Dowling, C.N. Lowe,
> E.G. Shand, E.E. Baxter (three-quarters); J.F. King and W.E.

Evans (halves); G.W. Bentley, J.M. Marlowe, J.S. Roberts, G.L.
Eyre, A.L. Harman, H. Chai, J. Criswick, E.W. Waite (forwards).
H.F. Hose, Esq., kindly acted as referee.

Having come from Cape Town as a member of a large family of
children, Geoffrey was now an only child in the Fawcett household.
Although he had had three years as a boarder in Exeter, the change to
Dulwich must have been somewhat intimidating. But he formed a
friendship in those years at Dulwich which was to have a profound
effect on him for years to come.

There were three Paterson brothers — James, Agar and Richard — at
the school, and one of them was in the same class with Geoffrey. He
spent many weekends and part of the school holidays with the boys
and their sister, Anna, at the Paterson home. When all three boys
died in the Great War, Geoffrey continued to be part of their family
and developed a lifelong friendship with Anna and her husband and
their children. Although he continued to live at 66 Wimpole Street with
the Fawcetts, the Paterson's house must have seemed more like a family
home, with the four children much closer to him in age. By the time he
was leaving school at the age of 18, Robert and Alice Fawcett were still
young children.

Geoffrey left Dulwich at the end of the summer term in July 1910,
with what feelings one can only imagine. In February of that year one
of the college's distinguished old boys, Sir Ernest Shackleton, returned
to deliver a lecture on his *Nimrod* Expedition to Antarctica in 1909.
There is little doubt that Geoffrey would have been present.

In some of the school holidays Dr and Mrs Fawcett arranged for
him to stay with various relations of his parents. One was his father's
brother, Uncle Sidney, who was a clergyman and lived in the Old
Rectory at Ravenstone in Leicestershire. He married Caroline Lancaster,
and they had one daughter, Emily Caroline, known to all as Maimie.
She devoted most of her life to her father, acting as housekeeper in the
Old Rectory. Her father, Sidney, died in 1962 at a great age. Finally,
Maimie herself married Lancelot Bennett, who was an elderly widower.
After a few years he had a stroke and was nursed by Maimie in her own
bungalow for the last few years of his life. One of her few friends and
relatives was Mrs Woods, her cousin's eldest daughter and the mother
of Doctor Paul J. Woods of Boston, Lincolnshire. Maimie lived in a
small semi-detached bungalow; when she died, Mrs Woods was named

as her 'next of kin' by her general practitioner. Consequently Mrs Woods had the responsibility for organizing the disposal of her estate, since she had not made a will. The solicitors made strenuous efforts to contact all the known family. After several years, the estate was divided into equal shares and allocated to the descendants of her uncles and aunts as indicated in the family tree. The total estate was not large, as Maimie lived in greatly reduced circumstances. It amounted to £33,441.04. Four of the beneficiaries were Geoffrey Dowling's children, who each received £418.01 in 1989.

Another of Geoffrey's relations was a cousin, Fred Crump, who lived in Hampshire and was especially kind to Geoffrey. Yet another lived at Field Dolling Hall, near Blakeney in Norfolk; years later Geoffrey took Jane to see the house. And sometimes he stayed with Mrs Nelson, who was one of his mother's sisters. He liked her and years later she gave him a handsome antique desk, which he passed on to his daughter Jane after her marriage.

Chapter 6
Guy's Hospital

DR JOHN Fawcett was entirely responsible for Geoffrey's early career. After he left school, like many boys of his age, Geoffrey was undecided about what he should do in life. He went home to Cape Town for a long holiday, and must have discussed the possibility of doing medicine with his parents. On his return Dr Fawcett may have said to him, 'If you cannot get into the Navy, come to Guy's Hospital and be a doctor.' Geoffrey was only too delighted to accept, and he entered Guy's Hospital Medical School in 1911. He had apparently not had very good school reports from Dulwich College and must have been pleased at the suggestion. There were no special entrance requirements at the time, apart from an ability to pay the fees.

He had some difficulties with passing the preliminary examinations but persisted. At that time there was virtually no limit to the number of times that one could attempt the examinations. In fact right up till 1939 a small number of 'chronic' students were a feature of most medical schools. They were never 'difficult' or querulous people; in fact they often had the very personal qualities which would help them to be successful general practitioners. They played a big part in the social and extracurricular activities such as hospital rags, the students union, rugby for the Hospitals Cup, the Medical School Club and its bar. But in 1916 the war situation for the Allied armies in France was desperate. Medical students were encouraged to join the Armed Forces. Geoffrey volunteered with several of his colleagues, including John Conybeare. He joined up as a trooper in the King Edward's Horse Regiment. The Regiment was raised in 1901 as the 4th County of London Yeomanry (the King's Colonials). It originally comprised expatriates from the dominions and colonies, with squadrons affiliated to the dominions by name. The title was changed to 'King Edward's Horse (the King's Overseas Dominions Regiment)' in 1910. In 1913 it was judged that the Territorial Force terms of service were not entirely suitable for the regiment; accordingly it was transferred to the Special Reserve, thereby losing its yeomanry status.

On mobilization two regiments were formed almost immediately.

From April 1915 to June 1916 individual squadrons of the 1st King Edward's Horse served in France as divisional cavalry. They were regrouped as a corps cavalry regiment. The regiment served in Italy from December 1917 to March 1918. On return to France it was once more split up and squadrons served separately until the end of the war. The 2nd King Edward's Horse served in France from May 1915 to May 1916, not always as a complete unit. In June 1916 it was reinforced by a section of the 21st Lancers and regrouped as a corps cavalry regiment, and as such served until August 1917. The regiment was then broken up and the personnel largely absorbed into the Tank Corps. King Edward's Horse remained in the Army List until disbandment in 1924.

After initial training, Trooper Dowling was sent with the Expeditionary Force to France. He served there for two years, until the Armistice in 1918. There is little doubt that he liked Army life as a trooper. He learnt to ride and enjoyed looking after the horses. But mishaps do happen. On one occasion his horse broke loose in the night and found its way to a large store of oats. Next morning the horse looked like a barrage-balloon! In France each trooper had to serve as cook for his group of men, taking it in turns for a week at a time. Trooper Dowling used to cook them pancakes, which were very popular!

His brother Thomas, who had come over from South Africa to join up, had a distinguished war record, being awarded the Military Cross. But Geoffrey remained a trooper without even attaining non-commissioned rank. This may seem surprising, but his humility was such that apparently it did not occur to him to apply for a commission as an officer. Perhaps he had a sense of inferiority as a colonial. Maybe he did not feel that he was in the officer mould. He was not involved in much 'action', the cavalry being mainly held in reserve. But he survived.

Scarcely any of the younger (Dowling Club) generation can recall Dowling ever talking about the war ('his war'), although he was always ready to talk about 'their war' of 1939–1945. One of the few is Wolf Tillman. During the 1950 Dowling Club visit to Belgium, he took Dr and Mrs Dowling in his car from London, but she stayed in Brussels, while Dowling and Tillman made the return journey by themselves. They had been to a reception given by the British Council and, although they had to leave it early in order to catch the boat at Dunkirk, they were both very cheerful. Suddenly Dowling saw a signpost 'Ypres' and this really moved him. He told Tillman that he interrupted his medical studies in 1916 and volunteered for service as a trooper. Would Tillman mind making a short diversion? The experiences of over 30 years back became very vivid. Having lived through a war himself it was easy for Tillman to understand how much this short visit in the dark with ill-lit streets, trying to identify landmarks, meant to Geoffrey Dowling.

> Ypres had claimed 400,000 Allied casualties: 54,896 bodies were never found. In spring and autumn ploughs still turn up their bones. The Germans, better trained and equipped, referred to it as *Kindermord*, the slaughter of the innocents.
>
> The Innocents, 'Our Boys', had a few weeks previously been polishing their buttons, learning to form fours and salute their officers. The staccato bark of drill-sergeants ricocheted across village greens and school playgrounds from Whitechapel to Cape Wrath. They were clerks, miners, parson's sons; a few, reared on G.A. Henty, longed to 'have a go at Jerry'; many simply because their pals had gone. They went to the line with scarcely enough rifles, fighting with picks and shovels, retrieving fire arms from fallen comrades. A handful of officers, believing it was ungentle-manly to bear arms, rallied their troops with walking sticks or hunting horns. Some never got as far as the front line. Blasted by shells from the approach duck boards, they drowned in a quagmire — for the water table in Flanders is very near ground level.
>
> The butchery became associated with one word along the Ypres salient: Passchendaele. Later it was said: 'We died in Hell — they called it Passchendaele.' With the passage of time — as crops grew again, and poppies, bright as the blood of the New Testament, flowered — Passchendaele symbolised the futility of war. But it didn't stop there, for tales of heroism and sacrifice came back down the line with survivors; so that in the end the futility was glorified! [Michael Watkins, *The Times*, 12 November 1988, p. 4.]

On 10 May in 1950, time pressed on Dowling and Tillman, and he could not respond further to that primitive impulse that makes people want to return to such scenes of their past. Some 45 years later the crew of the American Airforce B29 bomber *Enola Gay* returned to Hiroshima to see just where they had dropped the first atomic bomb.

But only people who were there can feel it. Would Dowling have wanted to ask Tillman to linger longer so that he could listen to the buglers sounding the 'Last Post' at the Menin Gate? Only he could say. For, as Alan Pryce-Jones wrote of his time at Oxford in the 1920s, 'We felt ourselves so bottled up by our elders, and bored to extremity by their tales of Passchendaele.'

Dowling retained almost no memorabilia of his war service years, but he had kept a postcard of himself on a horse which he sent to Mrs Harman at Sefton Place, Arundel, Sussex. She was a family friend of the Barrow-Dowlings and had undertaken to look after Geoffrey and Thomas during the war years at the request of their parents. Within a week of the Armistice declaration on 11 November 1918, Dr Barrow Dowling wrote to her to express his feelings:

18 November 1918

Dear Mrs Harman,

If my thanks and heartfelt gratitude to you for all you have done for my boys throughout these long years of war could ever be expressed in some tangible form, sure, the gift would be worth a King's Ransom. It is our great hope to meet you one day and say what we think personally of what you have done for us. Till then these few words must suffice. The relief that both the boys have been spared is very great and you can well imagine our feelings throughout this past week. There seems to be a vast amount to do in the meantime by the army of occupation, so we shall not expect Thomas for some time, and I am wondering whether or not he will remain in the army. It is a gentleman's profession and a good one, but this land is curious in the way it calls its sons back to it, so I expect Thomas will be wavering in his desires. I hope to get back to England next year as early as possible but I do not think it will be before June as we have two daughters to marry and settle — one this coming December and the other about March or April next year. After that we hope to be free — I can wish you every Christmas joy and happiness this year — Believe me.

Yours sincerely
T. Barrow Dowling

In 1919 Geoffrey was demobilized from military service and returned to Guy's Hospital to complete his training. Like many others the experience of military service in the war had some beneficial effect in concentrating his mind. He was now determined to work hard, being older and more mature. He qualified as a doctor with MRCS and LRCP of the Conjoint Board in January 1919. He passed the Final MB.BS examination of London University in May 1920, with Honours and Distinction in Medicine, the only one of 10 Guy's students who had passed. Amongst them was P.G. McEvedy, who became a lifelong friend. Geoffrey was successful in the MRCP examination in the same year and the MD a year later.

The Membership examination of the Royal College of Physicians was formidable in those days. It could not have been very different in 1920 from the event in 1933, so graphically described years later by Dr Alex Imrie of Glasgow:

> The standard for the conduct of higher medical examinations, particularly the Membership, has long been set by the Royal College of Physicians of London. Fifty years ago the examination was so different as to be almost unimaginable to the throngs of candidates of today. Then, about 100 candidates attended at each session, though quite a proportion were making their second, third or even tenth attempt.
>
> At 9 am on a hot morning in July 1933, about 100 of us assembled in the entrance hall of the old College in Trafalgar Square. The great majority were British males in their mid- or late twenties. There was a tiny leavening of ladies (six or seven), who tended to be slightly older and more mature than the men. There were also perhaps a dozen overseas graduates, all males and mainly from India. Candidates from the London teaching hospitals were recognisable by their morning coats, striped trousers and stand-up collars.
>
> Suddenly a uniformed servitor appeared on the staircase, bearing on a silver tray small envelopes, one for each of us. The envelopes contained a card requesting the recipient to attend a few days later for the clinical examination and giving the time and place. (All the clinicals were held in the London teaching hospitals, in my own case in Lord Horder's wards in St Bartholomew's). We were then summoned upstairs to the library where the written examination was set out. The invigilators were the Censors of the College. As the morning wore on it got hotter and hotter and signs of distress began to appear, notably

among the wearers of tails and high collars. Eventually we were graciously permitted to remove our jackets. The first session lasted from 9.30 to 12.30 and the second from 2 pm to 5 pm. The questions were all of the essay type and were surprisingly searching. In each paper there were two short passages for translation, Latin and French in one, Greek and German in the other. This section was optional but carried a few bonus marks and most candidates attempted at least two of the languages.

The clinical part of the examination took the form of one long case and several short ones. My own long case was one of meningovascular syphilis with flaccid paraplegia and dissociated anaesthesia. I had about 45 minutes to work up the case and was then examined by Lord Horder. The first 'short' case was an elderly man who, I learned later, was the last of the Spitalfields' weavers. As I approached his bed he informed me: 'Eart block's wots the matter wiv me, guv,' and indeed it was. He also remarked: 'The young gent yesterday giv me arf a crown,' so I took the hint. On this case and the other 'shorts' my examiner was R.A. Young of the Brompton, then the doyen of British and indeed of world chest physicians.

Next morning the candidates assembled in the College hall and the servitor again distributed an envelope to each one. The card inside thanked us politely for our attendance and either informed us that our presence would no longer be required or requested us to proceed to the next part of the examination. About 50 survived the 'cut' and went on to be examined in Pathology, and Principles of Medicine. These sections included X-rays, temperature charts, photographs of bizarre phenomena, bottled specimens, slides, urines and some rather primitive electrocardiograms. My examiners were G.P. Still, of Still's disease fame, and Hall of Sheffield, the world's leading authority on encephalitis lethargica. Next morning the same 50 candidates went through the same routine with notes. This time survivors, now numbering about 30, were requested to attend the final viva.

The final viva was held in the Censors' Room and was quite awe-inspiring. After waiting for some time in the library, we were admitted one at a time, the majority being asked to sit at the end of a table round which were ranged the Censors, with the President, Lord Dawson of Penn, at the head. They were then questioned on any aspect of medicine or indeed of anything else by any Censor who was so minded. A select few, having presumably reached a sufficiently high standard, were not subjected to questioning and passed rapidly through the room, shaking hands with Lord Dawson and the Censors on the way. A small number failed at the viva, leaving about 25 successful out of the original 100 candidates. As each successful candidate emerged, he was greeted by a gentleman who requested the entrance fee of £30, a lot of money in those days. This was excellent psychology on the part of the College; never was £30 parted with less reluctantly. There only remained the admission ceremony which took place a day or two later and culminated in a tea party in the College library. It was attended by the successful candidates, the Censors and a number of elderly, mostly retired, physicians, many of them of great distinction in their day. They were attired in an interesting variety of Edwardian styles, sponge-bag trousers, spats, elastic-sided boots, stocks, and monocles. College servants circulated bearing large silver teapots containing Indian and China tea.

We had been told that the MRCP examination was a test of basic medical principles conducted on a very high level. It certainly did test theoretical knowledge and clinical ability, but to the candidates it seemed also to be a check on their suitability for admission to the rather rarefied spheres of consulting medicine, not unlike an officer's selection board.

Dowling did indeed pass through this procedure. For the final viva he borrowed a morning-coat and striped trousers. They did not fit too well but they served their purpose. He had passed the exam.

For many medical students the immediate problem, after qualifying as a doctor and having one's name included in the Medical Register, was to find a job and earn some money. There were no student grants and no compulsory period of pre-registration work. The new doctor was licensed to treat patients immediately, and many did just that. But those who sought higher qualifications tried to find training posts in their own teaching hospital. In 1919 Geoffrey Dowling had been the Editor of the *Guy's Hospital Gazette*. This may have helped him to obtain posts as house physician and house surgeon at Guy's, where he also worked as a demonstrator in the department of pathology.

During these years after his return from the war Dowling shared a flat in Upper Brook Street with Robert Macintosh, who was six years younger. Macintosh was born in New Zealand but spent some of his childhood in South America. He came to Britain and joined the Royal Flying Corps in 1915 but was shot down behind German lines and spent two years as a prisoner of war. On being demobilized he became a medical student at Guy's and met Dowling, a fellow colonial. They remained lifelong friends.

They spent four years (1924–1928) together as part-time assistants in the venereology department. There were then only two reasons for working in this department — either to study for a higher examination or to earn money. Even junior hospital doctor posts were unsalaried or carried only a small honorarium. But the venereology department was different. It was funded directly from the Ministry of Health. Macintosh needed the time to study for the FRCS examination, and Dowling needed the money. The salary was £500 a year — handsome in those days. He never regretted this time spent on venereology, and always maintained it was essential experience for a competent dermatologist.

Macintosh turned from surgery to anaesthetics and built up a large and highly successful practice in London, before he accepted Lord Nuffield's invitation to the Oxford Chair to become the first Professor of Anaesthetics in England at the age of 40. He contributed enormously to his specialty with the development of apparatus (the Oxford vaporizer for ether and iron lungs), teaching and research and the organization of anaesthetists for the Royal Air Force as Consultant in the Second World War, for all of which he was knighted.

Robert Macintosh had great personal charm and an easy friend-liness which appealed to Dowling and made him very popular. He had a good sense of humour and was a tireless practical joker. Macintosh was the leader but Dowling was usually happy to go along with him. When going out with Macintosh, Dowling was the straight man. On one occasion Macintosh took him to a reception given by the Duke of Connaught. They were in a line of guests to be received. When they were a few paces away Macintosh turned round to Dowling and from the corner of his mouth said, 'I'll be Lenin, you be Trotsky.' Seconds later the toast-master announced 'Mr Lenin!' Macintosh went forward to shake hands and quickly passed on to take a glass of champagne from a waiter, at the same time glancing back over his shoulder and with the traces of a smirky grin on his face. Dowling flushed and his nerve failed him; 'Mr Trotsky', announced the toast-master, but Dowling corrected him and it was 'Doctor Dowling'.

On another occasion they went to an exhibition at the Queens Ice Skating Club, where Macintosh had seats in the Directors' Box. During the evening the manager came in and asked how they were enjoying the skating. Macintosh introduced Dowling and said his friend was a past free-style champion of Switzerland! The manager was delighted. The club would be extremely honoured if he would be willing to give a short exhibition for the guests. Dowling blushed and declined. He had never been on skates in his life, but could not let Macintosh down by revealing the truth. From then on he felt he must be more circumspect in accepting Macintosh's invitations.

They often had dinner together at small restaurants. One of their favourite dishes was curried lamb and rice for one shilling and ninepence! One evening they went to see a film at the Odeon Cinema at Marble Arch. In those days, at the end of the film performance just as in the theatres, the National Anthem was played and everyone was expected to stand up to attention and wait until it ended, although inevitably some people would leave early. On this occasion Macintosh and Dowling made first for the exit and stood there blocking it to prevent anyone leaving before 'God Save the King' was finished. As ex-servicemen they felt very proud.

Macintosh and Dowling were both keen golfers. Their handicap was 12. Once they had to play off in a match to send a representative to a national competition organized by the *Evening Standard* newspaper. Dowling just won — by one hole — and his name went forward, but alas no further.

It was his love of golf that started the sporting activities associated with the annual meetings of the British Association of Dermatology. His keenness was shared by Ivan McCaw, the consultant dermatologist at the Royal Victoria Hospital in Belfast, and together they donated a silver cup in 1950 for a golf competition of the members attending the Annual Meeting, which continues to this day — the Dowling–McCaw Cup. He won the cup himself in the first year (were the other competitors really trying?) and again in 1956, the year that he was President.

From 1919 to 1922 Dowling was a medical registrar (together with his friend J.J. Conybeare), and an assistant in the department of dermatology from 1920. He was appointed an assistant physician (dermatology) to Guy's Hospital in 1927. Dowling was a very popular medical registrar with the medical students because he was such a good teacher and took so much interest in their progress. He was the only registrar who used a special stethoscope with three or four attachments, so that the students could hear the heart and lung sounds on auscultation with him.

A good foundation of knowledge and experience in general medicine was necessary in his view to be a first-class dermatologist. Probably his first medical publication was while still a student — 'A case of Friedländer's bacillus septicaemia of sudden onset and rapidly fatal termination' — in the *Guy's Hospital Gazette* of 11 January 1919.

As a medical registrar he worked with Dr E.P. Poulton and published 'Study of a case of sino-auricular depression (S–A heart block) and its bearing on the genesis of the heart beat', in the *Guy's Hospital Reports* 1921, vol. 71, pp. 253–273. There is a footnote that the expenses of the investigation were defrayed by a government grant from the Royal Society. He wrote an article on syphilitic nephritis (*Guy's Hospital Reports* 1927, vol. 77, pp. 454–463), in which his characteristic clarity and literacy were already evident. Perhaps at the request of the editor, one of his lectures, 'Streptococcal infections of the skin', was published in the *Guy's Hospital Gazette* (1929, vol. 43, p. 30).

The skin department at Guy's Hospital had appointed H.W. Barber as its first full-time dermatologist in 1923, and it must have been Barber who influenced him to pursue a career in the subject. It is doubtful, however, whether Dowling had much in common with his chief. Barber had married a French lady, and was a fluent French speaker who knew the French dermatologists of his day very well. He was much concerned with attempts to explain many of the cutaneous disorders by the constitutional status (diathesis) and by the social, psychological and dietary habits of his patients. Of course, this led to theorizing and assumptions which would not be accepted nowadays because of lack of scientific proof. Dowling's approach was very much more critical, realistic and factual.

Louis Forman admitted that he was naïve enough then not to appreciate the differences in personalities and attitudes between these two outstanding men. Barber once told him at lunch in a peevish way that Dowling never did any work and was always away in Ireland.

Subsequently, after he had met Mrs Dowling, a 'very attractive, lively and intelligent lady', Forman considered that his absences in Ireland were understandable and commendable. One other obvious difference between Dowling and Barber was that Barber was rather aloof and not personally involved with other members of the consulting staff, while Dowling was essentially gregarious and liked mixing with his colleagues, particularly the younger ones. He appreciated their qualities, and yet at the same time he was capable of critical evaluation of their work and of their personalities.

Dowling's first senior appointment was in 1926 to the staff of St John's Hospital for Diseases of the Skin in Leicester Square. His abilities and reputation as an assistant in Barber's department at Guy's must have been recognized by the senior dermatologists of the day, because their method for appointments was casual in the extreme. The proposed candidate was asked to come to take tea with the staff at the hospital and engaged in general professional conversation. After he had departed, the senior physician would say, 'He seems a very nice sensible man. Is it agreed that we should invite him to join our staff?' The secretary was then asked to write to the candidate to invite him to join the staff. It scarcely justified the appellation of an interview or an appointment committee.

Other appointments soon followed — at the Miller General Hospital in Greenwich, where he opened a skin department ('the need for which has long been felt' by the Board of Management) in October 1927; at the West London Hospital in Hammersmith; and at the Ministry of Pensions. He resigned from these appointments when he was appointed to the permanent staff of Guy's Hospital. He remained at Guy's for five years as junior to H.W. Barber until he resigned in 1932.

In the early nineteen twenties there were relatively few full-time dermatologists in London or the rest of Great Britain. The number was largely determined by the amount of private practice available to support them, since all teaching hospital appointments were honorary and carried no salary. It was not surprising, therefore, to find that Dr Ernest Dore was physician for diseases of the skin to both St Thomas's Hospital and the Westminster Hospital.

In 1932 St Thomas's decided to appoint their own dermatologist. There were a number of applicants of the right age and experience available from other departments in London. But, when Geoffrey

Dowling applied, they realized that there was really no contest. They recognized his superior merit for the post. He was duly appointed and resigned from Guy's. It could not have been a decision taken lightly, for Dowling never lost his love and admiration of Guy's and always spoke of it with pride.

Thomas Hodgkin (of Hodgkin's disease) was probably the first physician to transplant from Guy's to St Thomas's, but was an example of the 'graft-versus-host' phenomenon. Hodgkin rejected the host in no uncertain terms in a letter to a friend, in which he wrote that he thought 'the Guy's staff to be the rudest and amongst the most unsociable of men, until he had been to St Thomas's, where the staff were almost bereft of all the social faculties of any corporation of men'. However, it was obvious that the Dowling graft was highly successful at St Thomas's (and never reacted against the host), where he developed to his full potential and attained the recognized position of a most outstanding dermatologist. He had justified the faith which his guide and master, Dr John Fawcett, had placed in him.

A detailed history called *Mr Guy's Hospital, from 1726 to 1948*, by H.C. Cameron, was published in 1954 and Dowling treasured it. Perhaps it was this which stimulated him to write an account of dermatology at Guy's Hospital (1850–1950), which was published in the *British Journal of Dermatology* in 1967. It makes fascinating reading.

> The first appointment in dermatology to be made at Guy's Hospital was that of Thomas Addison (1793–1860), who in 1850 became the Demonstrator of Cutaneous Diseases in the Medical School. At some later period the title became Physician for Diseases of the Skin. Addison retained this post until his retirement from the Hospital in 1860, sharing its duties from 1855 onwards with W.W. Gull.
>
> The foundations for a Department of Dermatology were, however, laid earlier. Addison came to London in 1815 having graduated MD at Edinburgh, to become first a pupil of Thomas Bateman and later Physician at the Public Dispensary in Carey Street, where Willan had done most of his work. In 1820 he entered Guy's Hospital as a pupil and in 1824, against vigorous opposition in the Court of Committees, he was appointed Lecturer and Assistant Physician through the powerful support

of Benjamin Harrison, the great Treasurer who ruled over Guy's Hospital for more than 50 years.

During the same period Joseph Towne, a youth of 17 from Royston, presented himself to Astley Cooper with a little model of the human skeleton which he had just completed. Deeply impressed with the beauty and accuracy of the work, Astley Cooper strongly recommended his services to the Treasurer and thenceforward Towne served the Hospital as modeller continuously for the next 50 years, now and again giving some time to sculpture with success. He made 200 anatomical models, over 250 pathological specimens and 560 of skin diseases. Most dermatological models were of cases in the wards selected by Addison though quite a number were added after Addison's time.

Addison was finally accepted at Guy's as a result of his researches. These, and his reputation as a magnificent and deeply admired teacher of students, contributed more than anything else to the great fame of Guy's in its early days as an independent medical school.* He outshone even his great contemporaries, Bright and Hodgkin, but recognition in the country generally

---

* It is known that Guy's Hospital was taking pupils in 1760, 35 years after its completion. By 1769 the new school and that of the ancient and illustrious Hospital of St Thomas across the road had agreed to pool their teaching resources. St Thomas's allotted itself the subjects of Anatomy and Surgery, leaving to Guy's 'Physic', for which there was very little popular demand at the time. The hospitals became known thenceforth as the United Hospitals of the Borough.

The termination of an uneasy partnership was precipitated in 1825 by a violent quarrel over the appointment of a successor to Astley Cooper, a Guy's man who held the lectureship in Anatomy and Surgery.

Astley Cooper nominated his nephew, Bransby Cooper, a much liked character but by no means as able as his uncle, and Harrison appointed him. The Grand Committee of St Thomas's responded by appointing a surgeon of their own, Mr South. Total separation was now inevitable and Guy's under the leadership of Harrison hurriedly built an anatomical department of their own.

An enduring offspring of the union exists in the shape of a dining club known as the United Boro Hospitals Club.

In 1948 Geoffrey Dowling was proposed for membership by James Wyatt (the obstetrician renowned for delivering Boo-Boo of her baby chimpanzee Jubilee), and he became a member in October of that year. The meetings were originally held four times a year, but more recently only twice. Dowling was a very regular attender, as one might expect from his strong feelings of friendships and conviviality. After the age of 60, members may become honorary members if they wish, and Dowling did this in 1959.

came late to Addison. He was painfully sensitive, hypercon-scientious and depressive, and sought no notice. The French, however, knew him well, and it was Trousseau who gave the name of *maladie d'Addison* to the disease, describing Addison as 'le doyen des professeurs du Guy's Hospital à Londres, et depuis longtemps connu parmi par les travaux dont il a enriché la Science'.

The successors to the Department often became very dis-tinguished. William Withey Gull (1816–1890) was a country boy living on the Guy's estate, in whom, on his periodical visits, Harrison had detected unusual ability.

Harrison put Gull to school in Bermondsey and in due course entered him as a pupil at Guy's. He was as brilliant as Harrison had thought and he was duly elected to the Staff at the age of 35, late for those days. In the meanwhile, Harrison had seen to it that he was provided with minor paid appointments, which enabled him both to gain experience and to live. This arrange-ment appears to have been the forerunner of the appointment of Registrar of subsequent times. He was one of the great Victorian physicians. Awarded a Baronetcy in 1872, he made a fortune.

Sir Samuel Wilks' (1824–1911) principal contributions to dermatology were the first description of striae cutis atrophicae and verruca necrogenica, 'caused by contact with fluids from the dead body'. Of this there are five models in the Museum, the patients having been two students and an assistant in the post-mortem room. He also published an account of the occurrence of 'Markings or Furrows on the Nails as the Result of Illness'. According to various sources, a whimsical sense of humour and a passion for truth are said to have combined to limit his prac-tice somewhat. When as President of the College of Physicians he gave annual appreciative notices on the departed Fellows for the year his remarks added notably to the terrors of death.

At the time of his appointment to the Staff, Philip Henry Pye Smith (1840–1914) was already regarded as a dermatologist of repute, having acquired considerable experience in the subject during a long period of study in Paris, Berlin and Vienna. He was a fluent French and German speaker, a Greek and Latin scholar, and altogether a brilliant person. Before being appointed to the staff, he had taught comparative anatomy in the Medical

School and subsequently he was elected a Fellow of the Royal Society for contributions to zoology.

From 1887, Edwin Cooper Perry (1856–1938), the last of the general physician dermatologists at Guy's Hospital, remained in charge of the department until his retirement in 1919. Perry's teaching sessions, both in the wards and in the skin department, were much enjoyed by students, but his major service to the Hospital and medical school were of an entirely different order.

Before entering the London Hospital as a first-year medical student, he had had a brilliant early career as Captain of Eton and as a classical scholar and Fellow of King's College, Cambridge. At first he had intended to enter the Church. He was appointed Assistant Physician to Guy's at a time when the Hospital and School were in dire need of a man of his special talents and character, and from the first he took charge. He became Dean and Warden of the College immediately and when within a few years the humble post of Superintendent fell vacant he volunteered to take it. He was a magnificent administrator and organiser and he served Guy's in a way that no one had been able to do since Harrison. Like others of great administrative capacity, he was also called upon to undertake outside work, as on the establishment of the Military Training College at Millbank, the College of Nursing and for the King Edward Fund. He was knighted in 1903 and created GCVO in 1935. After retirement, he served the University of London for 8 years as Principal Officer and Vice Chancellor.

Harold Wordsworth Barber (1886–1955) was the first Physician to Guy's Hospital to be appointed to the Department for Diseases of the Skin with no other duties. For about 70 years dermatology at Guy's had been in the hands of some of the outstanding physicians of a great era at the Hospital. Apart from Addison, whose stature appears not to have been fully appreciated at home during his lifetime, three had been Fellows of the Royal Society, two were Presidents of the Royal College of Physicians, four were Harveian Orators and others had gained honorary foreign degrees and recognition of various other kinds.

The Physicians had taken good care of dermatology and no doubt the students had been well instructed. Among their contemporaries elsewhere at home, Wilson, Hutchinson, Tilbury Fox and Radcliffe Crocker had contributed more to dermatology, but Guy's men were not primarily dermatologists and did not become so until Barber's day.

Throughout this long period, the dominant theme at Guy's had been the steady advance in knowledge of structural pathology. When Barber was appointed, this age was regarded as over and Wilks was spoken of as the last of the great morbid anatomists. Few physicians were now interested in dermatology and some claimed with both pride and ample justification to know nothing about it. The era of the major aetiological hypotheses was in full swing and, corresponding to developments in bacteriology, the concept of focal infection as the cause of much obscure disease held much attraction. Barber believed firmly in the validity of this, as well as of other general concepts which were on the way to development. His 100 contributions to dermatological literature were nearly all written in support of this outlook. In his final contribution, the Prosser White Oration for 1952, he summarised the observations that he had made during his life's work, and the conclusions that he believed could be drawn from them. He appreciated that a new era of advance in medicine by controlled experiment and statistical analysis had set in, but he expressed the fervent hope that the art of the great clinicians should not be allowed to wane.

It is impossible to judge at the present time how much of Barber's point of view is likely to survive. In his time he was the leader in dermatology in England. A fine clinician, a magnificent teacher and a gifted speaker and writer, he had a great following in whom he inspired both admiration and affection and by many of whom he was regarded as incomparable. His retirement from the Staff marked the end of a century of dermatology at Guy's Hospital.

Louis Forman first saw Dowling in the early nineteen twenties, probably in the second half of 1922, and remembered him as a medical registrar at Guy's Hospital. 'My recollection of him in the medical wards is his forward stance and his intent gaze and concentration, retained until the last. His contemporaries included Sir John Conybeare,

Physician to Guy's Hospital and an Air Vice Marshall, Consultant to the Royal Air Force. It is probably through this connection that Dowling later became Consultant to the Royal Air Force.'

When he first left Guy's in 1926, Louis Forman went to work at St Olave's Hospital in Kensington. Dowling visited as a consultant and Forman was again in contact with him. As he was in charge of the acute medical wards, he was privileged to be able to show Dowling patients whom he thought might interest him and on which he needed his help. This contact, no doubt, helped to determine Forman's deviation from general medicine to dermatology.

When he returned to Guy's in 1929 Forman found that Dowling was chief assistant in the skin department. Dowling would occasionally take him to the Miller Hospital in Greenwich. Although a small hospital, the Miller had an excellent staff and enjoyed a high reputation in medical circles. He remembered being driven down to Greenwich one afternoon in Dowling's large open American car. At the clinic, a woman patient came in with two large dusky granulomatous lesions on the shins, which he diagnosed immediately as bromoderma. In those days, bromide was the most commonly prescribed sedative; it was thought to enable the patient to sustain the burden of the environment and life situation as well as the irritation caused by skin disorders.

Forman's admiration for Dowling was reciprocated. Years later he told a medical friend that Louis Forman was the best house physician he had ever known — praise indeed. When Dowling resigned in 1932 to join the staff at St Thomas's Hospital, Louis Forman was appointed in his place.

Dowling was always generous and appreciative of his assistants, without being patronizing or over-praising them. Dr Charles G. Cassar of Valetta, Malta, GC, worked as a clinical assistant to Dowling at the West London Hospital in 1928–1929. Years later he recalled: 'This amiable and learned specialist. I assure you that one cannot grasp the interesting knowledge of skin ailments unless the master is imbued with as gentle and innate a capability to teach as he was. He used to listen to what the doctors around him suggested about the diagnosis of some of the difficult cases. He was an intelligent and practical specialist, and never tried to embarrass his listeners with far-fetched words and diagnoses. I have since found his teaching very practical in my practice here.' Dr Cassar probably did not spend more than a year attending the weekly skin clinics at the West London Hospital, but he received a typically generous testimonial (and possibly one of the first written by Dowling):

13 March 1929

Dr C.G. Cassar has acted as my Clinical Assistant at the West London Hospital during his period of postgraduate study in London.

I found his help most valuable and was much impressed by his knowledge of the subject of dermatology.

Dr Cassar has evidently made the best possible use of his period of study both in England and abroad.

G.B. Dowling
Assistant Physician to the Skin Department, Guy's Hospital
Dermatologist to the West London Hospital

Cassar never forgot those days and wrote to him from Malta more than 40 years later:

28 September 1971

Dear Dr Dowling,

Almighty God has today given me the chance to send you my sincere congratulations and good wishes on the occasion of your 80th birthday.

Kind individuals in this world are not numerous. You were one of them, when I was with you in 1929, in your teaching to me of my favourite line of medicine during my post graduate studies.

Much time has passed since then. I am now seventy.

May God bless you with many more years so that your kind heartedness and good teaching spread in many nations, will be further prolonged.

My kindest regards on my behalf and that of my wife.

Your sincere confrère
Charles G. Cassar

Chapter 7
The Patersons

MRS MARGARET Paterson lived for many years at 25 Weymouth Street, which crosses Harley and Wimpole Streets in the 'medical area' of central London. She had three sons and a daughter. One of the boys went to school at Dulwich College.

Margaret, always known as Maggie, Paterson was one of the 14 children of John and Anna Maria Agar. Most of the family were born in Glasgow and the rest in Northern Ireland, and their forebears were Scottish and Irish. John Agar was of Huguenot descent. They received the good general education of the nineteenth century in Glasgow, which fitted so many Scotsmen to take part in the industrial revolution and to organize and staff the financial and commercial institutions of the British Empire and elsewhere in the expanding world.

Maggie married William Morrison Paterson in Glasgow and came to London soon after the birth of their fourth child, Richard. The other three were called Anna Maria, James (known as Jay) and Agar. They lived for many years in a house on Wandsworth Common, later moving to Great Portland Street and finally to Weymouth Street. Their youngest son, Richard Agar Paterson, was adopted by Maggie's brother Richard and his wife, who had no children. His name was changed to Richard Paterson Agar and his adoptive parents sent him to school at Dulwich College. It was not uncommon then for childless couples to 'adopt' children of a fertile brother or sister. This custom is still current in Arab, African and Asian families — a less expensive solution, perhaps, than modern scientific techniques! However, in spite of this 'adoption', the Patersons spent most of their holidays together in one or other of the two houses.

From Exeter Cathedral School Geoffrey went to Dulwich College in 1906. It would have been during these years that Geoffrey first met the Paterson family.

After war broke out in 1914, the three Paterson boys joined up as soon as they were old enough to enlist. The two youngest served in different regiments and were both killed in action in France. Jay was invalided out of the army suffering from acute rheumatism and died soon afterwards. This was a shattering blow for the family and for Geoffrey, who was himself to survive the war as a trooper. But his association with the family continued and he often visited the Paterson household to see Mr and Mrs Paterson and their daughter.

Maggie Paterson loved Geoffrey and thought of him as a son. She was a very hospitable lady. Her flat in Weymouth Street, although not large, was often full of nephews and nieces, of whom she had many. They took the place of her family, the three sons she had lost in the war and her daughter, who was now married and living in the Argentine, but Geoffrey, although no relation, was a favourite visitor and he was a regular one. Mrs Paterson was a strong-willed Scotswoman. Many of her nephews and nieces felt intimidated by such a formidable character, but not Geoffrey. He himself had become strong and decisive and they seemed to understand one another; there was mutual respect.

In 1919 Anna Maria (or Pat as she was usually called) married Frank Gibson Lockwood, an English businessman who returned, after school and four years' war service with the Royal Artillery, to Buenos Aires. They lived at Hurlingham, a village near Buenos Aires, which is now part of its sprawling suburbs. They had three children: Agar and Margaret, who were born in the Argentine, and Jean, the youngest, who was born in London. The family came to London at frequent intervals and always stayed at 25 Weymouth Street. Agar went to school in England in 1929 and Margaret and Jean in 1937. Agar went to a preparatory school and then to Malvern College, and the girls went to Tolmers Park in Hertfordshire. The three children spent all their holidays with their grandmother, Mrs Paterson, in London.

Geoffrey never forgot the friendship and kindness of the Patersons, so he and his family knew the Lockwood children well. For many years, and especially during the Second World War, Geoffrey continued to visit Maggie regularly. At least once a week, he would spend some time with her or, if that were not possible, he would telephone her. She relied upon his friendship and advice and this kindly interest was a great comfort to her and therefore to her family. Maggie's husband died in 1930 and thereafter she rarely left London, where she remained throughout the war. In 1946 she went to the Argentine to live with her daughter Pat and she died there in 1947.

Margaret had eczema as a baby and was treated on many occasions by Geoffrey, who was now an established dermatologist. When she was about 16, she had some eczema round her eyes. An American lady who lived in London, a close friend of the family, saw her in this state and said that she could cure it with some ointment. Even today, there is no lack of medical and other advice from unqualified friends and relations for chronic ailments which prove recalcitrant to doctor's therapeutic efforts. This lady claimed that she could get any prescription that she wished made up for her by a pharmacist in Wigmore Street. She ordered a prescription and had it sent in a small parcel to Margaret at school. All parcels were normally opened by the matron, but this was evidently too small and was mistaken for a bulky letter. Margaret used the ointment on her eyelids before going to bed.

Next morning her whole face was extremely sore and her eyelids were completely closed by the swelling, so that she could not see. Jean remembers going into the sanatorium to where Margaret had been moved and cooling her hands on the iron bedstead and then holding them to her sister's hot and stinging face. The school doctor was baffled but Jean in some trepidation insisted that the headmistress should telephone her grandmother and 'Dr Dowling'. He immediately sent a chauffeur-driven car for Margaret and she was taken straight to his consulting rooms in Devonshire Place. She spent the next three weeks at home in bed at her grandmother's flat. Geoffrey explained to the frightened schoolgirl that she was not really blind and that her eyes were normal. He told her that she could not see out of them at present only because the lids were swollen and that when the swelling gradually subsided she would see as usual. Geoffrey had of course diagnosed an allergic contact dermatitis from the ointment recommended and supplied by the 'trying to be helpful' American friend. He thought the likely cause of the reaction was quinine, which was one of the constituents.

Many years later Margaret suffered the same reaction after drinking some 'bitter lemon'. Geoffrey wanted her to take legal action against the manufacturing company involved for not putting the quinine content on the label of the bottle, but she was reluctant to do so. They settled amicably without compensation when the company agreed to the amended labelling on its tonic and bitter lemon bottles. On three subsequent occasions Margaret has been offered drinks that she was assured contained no quinine. The same reaction recurred each time and after close enquiry it was conceded by the suppliers that the drinks did indeed contain quinine.

This quinine allergy was not her only frightening experience. In her garden in Peru she was once stung by a wasp and suffered an anaphylactic shock. Her doctor advised her to consult an allergy specialist in London, who might be able to desensitize her. With the help of the entomology department of the Natural History Museum in Kensington, the species of wasp was identified, but the specialist advised her that it would be too dangerous to begin a course of injections for the wasp.

Margaret had married David O. Duncan MC on 2 February 1946 at St James's Catholic Church in Spanish Place, London. Her two sons went to the Oratory School in Berkshire and her daughter to a school in Peru. At the time of her marriage her father was in the Argentine and so she was given away by Geoffrey. May Dowling insisted that her wedding reception be at their house in Porchester Terrace. May was always very kind to Margaret on her many visits to England. She saw quite a lot of her and, on one occasion at least, they went off to France together on a shopping spree on a supposedly 'no passport' visit. Unfortunately, they had not read the small print about identity papers and so failed even to get ashore at Cherbourg, but they enjoyed themselves none the less. May loved travelling, going whenever she was able to Paris, as a result of which she dressed with a panache which was not common in England in the post-war years.

Margaret decided to spend some months in England in 1960 and again in 1963 so that she could see more of her two sons, who were at boarding-school. She stayed with her parents Pat and Frank Lockwood, who were by this time living again in London. During these months she naturally saw a lot of Geoffrey and May, who were then living at 24 Wimpole Street. On one occasion she worked as Geoffrey's receptionist for three weeks. She remembers that he was very tolerant of her inexperience.

Geoffrey went to see the Lockwoods frequently after they returned to London in 1952. Frank had taught himself to be an excellent cook and Geoffrey paid him compliments on his expertise. They were more or less contemporaries and both fought in the First World War. Frank served at Gallipoli when he was a 20-year-old subaltern, and afterwards in France, where he was wounded twice. He was awarded the Military Cross in November 1916.

The two of them also shared an enthusiasm for Rugby football, often going to Twickenham together or further afield, complete with picnic basket and rugs. When Frank had retired from work in the

Argentine, the Lockwoods lived at 44 Hallam Street for about 20 years. They finally moved to Warwickshire, to be nearer their daughter Jean. Pat died there in 1974 and Frank died two years later.

Margaret lived in Chile for some years and since then has lived in Lima, Peru. She inherited the sun-sensitive Celtic skin but she has been most ably cared for by Dr Alejandro Morales, a dermatologist in Lima. Agar married and returned to the Argentine after his schooling and the war years spent in the Royal Artillery.

Jean Lockwood, on the advice of Geoffrey Dowling, trained as a nurse and a midwife from 1944 to 1951 at St Thomas's Hospital, where Geoffrey was the consultant dermatologist. One day early on in her career, she had a painful whitlow, an infection in one of her fingers. She was sent to the out-patients department to have it treated. She was surprised to find him there offering to treat it for her himself. When she was about to leave he said, 'Give my love to your Granny.' Jean answered, 'Yes, thank you and we both look forward to our dinner with you and Mrs Dowling next week.' In those days such familiarity between a consultant and a junior nurse was frowned upon and the sister in charge looked shocked and disapproving.

Jean married Richard Young, a brother of Professor J.Z. Young, and they have lived in Warwickshire ever since. Jean continued to see Geoffrey in London occasionally and she and her husband had lunch with him at his house in Ravenscourt Gardens.

Through Pat Lockwood, the children's mother, Geoffrey met her cousin Eileen Agar, the surrealist painter, who married Joseph Bard, a Hungarian writer. It is doubtful if he appreciated her paintings. In one of the letters to his children at school he wrote:

> I went to Eileen Agar's exhibition; she had one with Michael Rothenstein; I don't know who he is but he does the same thing but not quite so much. If you look at his pictures you can see that they bear some relation to the title, whereas Eileen Agar is I should say rather extreme in her art. However, Paul Nash says in a preface that she was one of the discoveries of the 1936 Surrealist Exhibition, and that there is poetry in her painting. Obviously he is a man who knows his business but I wish I could see daylight. When I see her next time I shall have to admit ignorance again.

Nevertheless, he enjoyed going to dinner with Eileen Agar and Joseph Bard, who was a good conversationalist and raconteur; he had grown up in the café society of Budapest, Vienna, Berlin and other continental capitals, where it was a normal way of life for writers, poets and other artists. They knew Dorothy Thompson, Ezra Pound, Paul Eluard and Sinclair Lewis, and they once spent a holiday at Mougins in the south of France with Picasso and his friends. Although Joseph decisively chose to make his home in England and found solace in the Royal Society of Literature, 'he felt there was great difficulty in preserving any expansiveness in this grey land'.

Eileen Agar published her autobiography, *A Look at My Life*, in 1988 when almost 90 years old. It paints a brilliant picture of the artist's world through most of this century.

Chapter 8
Huntercombe

HUNTERCOMBE Golf Club occupied a large part of Dowling's life over several decades. For four years while his children were growing up, he had a small country cottage with a small garden backing on to the sixteenth fairway, which provided escape from his busy life in London. It was there that he and his wife met and developed a long-lasting friendship with Viscount and Lady Nuffield.

The history of Huntercombe Golf Club, both before and after Dowling became a member, is interesting and has been chronicled by John Adams, to whom I am greatly indebted for much of the following account.

Jim Morris was born in Nuffield, near Henley, in Surrey on 24 September 1890. One day in 1900 he was playing with some other children outside the Crown Inn, when a nice gentleman, dressed in a light suit with a gold watch-chain by his left breast pocket and with a moustache, came up to him and said: 'Will you do a job for me?'

'Yes, sir'.

The gentleman took him over to the woodshed by the cottage and asked him his name. 'Morris', he said.

'That's a Scots name. We're going to make a golf course — you don't understand that, do you? You'll be able to caddie and earn some money.'

And this he did, as did all the other lads round about.

> There were some posts in the woodshed which were to be taken out to Nuffield Common, where the gentleman had got a little bit of gorse cut out where the greens and tees were going to be. When they had finished he said: 'There is a shilling for you, and you can say you were the first boy to take a shilling off the course.'
>
> But it was still Nuffield Common; it wasn't a golf course at all and it didn't shape like one either.

This encounter was vividly remembered by Jim Morris, who was caddie, green-keeper and professional for 43 years at Huntercombe.

The gentleman was Willie Park Junior, managing director of the Chiltern Estates Company, which on 9 April 1900 bought Huntercombe Manor, from which the future golf course and club were to draw their names.

Willie Park, the second son of Willie Park Senior, was one of the best-known and most respected professionals of his time. His father, who had won the first Open Championship in 1860 and again in 1863, 1866 and 1875, had established a club and bell-making business, Wm Park and Son, in his home town of Musselburgh in Scotland. From about 1897, however, he had become a very sick man and responsibility for the business fell increasingly on the shoulders of young Willie, who had won the Open in 1887 and again in 1889. Like his father, he had for several periods issued a challenge to anyone in the world to play him for £100 and had taken part in a number of such challenge matches, which aroused widespread interest — the galleries were sometimes numbered in thousands. Since about 1890 he had concentrated most of his energies on developing the business. He had experimented with new designs of club and ball, including his famous wry-necked putter and the bulger driver, and had established branches of the firm in Edinburgh, London, Manchester and New York. He had acquired a considerable reputation as a designer of golf courses and had visited America at least once, in 1895, to play exhibition matches, advise on the layout of courses and give instruction. On top of all this, he had published the first comprehensive book on golf by a professional, *The Game of Golf* (Longmans Green 1896), which deals with the types and manufacture of balls and clubs, the layout of courses and how to play, with a fluency and style which would do credit to a professional writer. He was still a formidable player; in 1898 he had been runner-up by one shot to Harry Vardon in the Open. Some time in 1889, probably in the latter part of the year, he had been commissioned by T.A. Roberts to design and supervise the construction of the old course at Sunningdale.

Willie was not only a man of great talent; he was evidently a man of sterling character. Contemporary writers go out of their way to praise his courage, temperance and hard work and the devotion with which he looked after his ailing father.

The Huntercombe estate included the manor, 724 acres of freehold farm land and woods, 113 acres of common and wasteland, three farms and a number of cottages, but not the Crown Inn, which had been sold to Wallingford Brewery in 1896. The price was £8000 — £3500 for the manor, buildings and land, and £4500 for the farming stock and other chattels. There was a mortgage on the manor for £6000; so the effective cost to Chiltern Estates was £14,000. In 1903 the Norwich Union Life Insurance Society advanced a mortgage of £15,000 on the property.

By acquiring the manor, Chiltern Estates became entitled to the manorial rights, which included being 'the person entitled to the soil of the Common'. A Commons Act had been passed in 1899, the main effect of which was to give district councils authority to make schemes and by-laws for the regulation of commons. Preparation of the golf course in 1900 and early 1901 evoked vigorous and even violent protest. The *Berks and Oxon Advertiser* of 29 March 1901 devoted nearly four columns to a report of the Annual Meeting of the Parish of Nuffield four days previously, at which there had been heated arguments between those who supported the promoters of the proposed golf links and some parishioners. Work was said to have been going on for about seven months on clearing and seeding the common, and £200 had been spent on seeds alone. The promoters had dug ditches along the sides of the roads to keep carts off the common, because they churned up the turf. The ditches were filled in by the promoters, after protest had been made by the villagers, and posts were erected instead. The posts had been torn down and turf had been dug up. Some of the more vocal parishioners at the meeting claimed that their rights were being invaded; they would soon not be able to walk on the common and it was all a plot to enclose it. One said that 'there used to be a rabbit or two on the common, but they had all gone now'. Mr J. Willis said that he and his father and grandfather had been agents for Huntercombe Manor for nearly two centuries. The only right the parishioners had was to the firing they could pick up and carry on their backs; even the rabbits belonged to the lord of the manor. Most people now had kitchen ranges and preferred to buy coal rather than cut fuel on the common. This opposition was, he said, the result of outside agitation by people who had no interest in the parish.

The Editor of *Golf Illustrated* wrote a lyrical account of a visit to Willie at Easter, six weeks before the course was to be opened.

> On arriving at Henley, which will shortly be reached by the Great Western express trains in an hour or less, we found the Huntercombe motor car waiting for us, a fine Daimler seating nine persons comfortably . . . the farmhouse beautifully furnished and fitted up as a temporary residential club . . . an all-round

panorama of endless distance immediately suggested the scenery of the Lothians ... the fresh strong air ... the immemorial turf, again strongly reminiscent of Gullane ... the putting greens of great beauty and extent ... the long and sporting course laid out with such art that nothing but all-round excellence will carry the golfer round without serious mishap ... we should judge, when all is in order, that anything under 85 will mean first class play ... Those who know Willie Park will wish him all success in his new enterprise. There is probably no professional golfer who commands so much respect and even the affection of all classes. He is the embodiment of all that is thorough and upright and a venture of which he is the guiding spirit is assured from the start and it is pleasing to learn that he is daily receiving the names of intending members ... on Mr Park's estate there is ample room for two other courses of equal extent and possibilities and he intends when the present one is fairly started to lay them out also. Part of the immediate scheme is to build a large hotel with 100 bedrooms, which will be situated by the first hole of the three completed courses.

The golf course was ready for the opening challenge match on Whit Sunday, 25 March 1901. It was the venue for the last 36 holes of one of the 72-hole challenge matches, which were such a feature of the professional game at that time. The stake was £50 a side. After the first half, played on the Royal Mid-Surrey course, J.H. Taylor, who was the reigning Open Champion, was six up. Jack White, who was to be the Open Champion in 1904, had chosen Huntercombe for the second half; after the first 11 holes he had reduced Taylor's lead to one hole. So it turned out to be an exciting match, though Taylor drew away again and finally won by four and three.

The Editor of *Golf Illustrated*, who refereed the challenge match and described it in detail in the issue of 31 May 1901, commented:

In spite of the dry weather Willie Park had got the course into excellent order, and it is evident that in Huntercombe he has provided a course that is destined to take rank as one of the best first-class courses ... The long game of both men was superb; indeed, we have never seen more phenomenally long shots played in a match both off the tee and through the green. Taylor quite excelled himself in this direction and ascribed his added force to the bracing quality of the Huntercombe air.

...There are few greens so near to London where such a complete change of climatic environment...can be had; and the jaded suburban golfer, who toils with difficulty round 18 holes of redeemed plough land and artificial bunkers, will experience no fatigue after 36 or even more holes over the Huntercombe sward. Indeed, we heard of one enthusiastic sportsman after his third round on Whit Monday vigilantly seeking an opponent with whom to contest a fourth.

This formal opening of the course was evidently a great local event. The *Henley and South Oxfordshire Standard* of 31 May reported:

There was a rushing and tearing of motor cars through Henley on Saturday, their destination being Nuffield, where the second half of the match between J.H. Taylor (the Open Champion) and Jack White was played on the links of the recently formed Huntercombe Golf Club. About 200 ladies and gentlemen (many of whom are well-known in golf circles) followed the players and the greatest interest was evinced in the match, which proved a very close one. Half a dozen policemen (under Sgt Longshaw) were present, but they really had nothing to do, as everyone behaved in a sportsmanlike manner and gave the players plenty of room. Everyone seemed to be delighted with the links, which out and home cover about four and a half miles and are 500 yards in excess of the famous St Andrew's links. There is no doubt that Huntercombe links will soon be known among the best in England. Willie Park is to be heartily congratulated upon the way in which the long course has been laid out and planned.

Mr Lardner of the Bull, Nettlebed, is credited with providing lunch for 200, which must have been a considerable achievement. Reports in the newspapers and journals all speak of a gallery ranging from 200 to 400; but contemporary photographs of the match do not seem to show such numbers.

An article in *Golf Illustrated* on 16 August 1901, which accompanied a plan and photographs of the course, praised the way in which the natural resources of fine turf, the varied character of the ground and numerous hazards had been used and how on a site of only 120 acres 'the fairway of each hole is of ample width and is separated from its nearest neighbours by broad belts of whins...Huntercombe is undoubtedly the most up-to-date course in the kingdom — an erratic full stroke or approach rarely goes unpunished, and a good stroke meets its just reward'.

But the most remarkable tribute to the then very new courses was paid in November 1901 by Mr Walter Travis, the winner of the American Amateur Championship in 1900 and 1901. He played at Huntercombe on Sunday 11 August during a visit to a large number of the great British courses. *Golf Illustrated* in its issue of 16 August records that 'he gave it unqualified approval and said it was the finest inland course and one of the best tests of golf he had seen'. When he returned home, Mr Travis contributed to *Golf Illustrated* his observations on the tour, with interesting comparisons between the US and Britain on courses, standards of play, caddies and attitudes to the game, in which he wrote:

> I consider that Huntercombe is easily the best laid out links that I have ever played over anywhere. There, in order to negotiate the round properly, you must be a master in the art of both scientific slicing and pulling, and be able to get the full measure of every conceivable stroke that occurs in the game, or else be subject to some penalty — in short, every shot has to be played for all it is worth. That is GOLF.

A full-page advertisement, which appeared in *Golf Illustrated* on 30 August 1901 and was repeated in the next five weeks, stated:

> This magnificent course is now open for play and is in splendid condition. Neither trouble nor money have been spared in taking full advantage of the wonderful natural features of the course, which is now admitted by all who have seen it to be as perfect a golf course as can be desired. The length of the course is 6503 yards. There is a good Club-house and the catering is looked after by a competent Steward. Sleeping accommodation for members has also been provided in the Club-house. The Club has now been organised and members will be admitted (the first 50 without ballot and thereafter on election) at the following rates: Entrance fee £5.5s; Annual Subscription £5.5s; Life Membership, transferable during Holder's lifetime, 50

Guineas ... Motor Cars meet the 9.5 am and the 6.30 pm
from Paddington, at Henley Station. Players can return to
London by the 8.50 am or the 5.30 pm trains from Henley
to Paddington ... An hourly service of Motor Cars is in course
of arrangement. Playable all the year round. A perfect seaside
course inland. Grand old turf, gravel and sand subsoil, health-
giving breezes. An ideal course for London Golfers. Intending
members are invited to seek further information and permission
to play over the course from the Honorary Secretary or from
Willie Park.

The number of men members grew steadily from 109 in 1901/2
to 236 in 1904 and then fell away to 162 in 1906/7. Only three lady
members are recorded as being elected in this period, but perhaps wives
and daughters playing on a revocable annual ticket were not listed as
members.

Two main discontents which were said to be discouraging potential
members from joining were the need for a more adequate clubhouse
and the unreliability of the cars which transported members to and
from Henley station. As early as its second meeting, the committee was
evidently thinking about a new clubhouse, nearer to the first tee and
with rooms to put up more members. The manor was about 300 yards
from the first tee; for the first autumn meeting in 1903 it was decided to
erect a tent for luncheon and tea closer to the course, to save members
the walk back to the clubhouse. Only about six people could get beds in
the manor; a few more could be put up in Willie Park's cottage near the
Crown Inn and in Bleak Villa next door, which was a cyclist's rest, as a
notice on the main road advertised.

In the early years of the century provision of motor cars to ferry
members from and to the station, and sometimes between the manor
and the other houses where members stayed, must have seemed an
imaginative and enterprising service. The original cars were under-
powered and not very reliable. Jim Morris recalls:

They were three old Daimlers with solid tyres — one with red
wheels, one with blue and one with yellow; they had an iron step
at the back and two to get up by the driver. The drivers were
Stephen, Sweet and Brown. The carters at the Manor used to
chant a little ditty:

*'Why does Stephen, Sweet and Brown
Every morning go to town?'*

Sometimes it was the yellow one that went out; that was supposed to be the best . . . sometimes it got to Henley; sometimes it
didn't. Then the red or the blue went to pick up the people and
the other had to go and tow back the yellow and that was
always happening.

In October 1903 it had been recorded that negotiations were pro-
ceeding for the purchase of two new higher-powered cars which would
make the journey from Henley within half an hour. In the mean while,
it was reported in February 1904 that one of the old cars had been
thoroughly overhauled and put into good running condition, a second
was at present at Coventry being thoroughly overhauled, and the third
would be sent there as soon as this one came back.

In November 1905, however, Willie Park, answering a complaint
about the non-arrival of new cars, said that three new cars had been
ordered and the makers had promised delivery of the first that week.
On 17 November 1905 *Golf Illustrated* recorded with a photograph
that:

> On the occasion of the Autumn Meeting Willie Park had his
> new car out for the first time. It made the journey from London
> the same morning and then did its run from Henley to the
> clubhouse in twenty two minutes, which is very much faster
> than the old cars are capable of. The latter are only nine horse-
> power . . . the new car is 24 horse-power and is a very business-
> like and elegant piece of work, being made to accommodate nine
> passengers.

The Autumn Meeting in 1905 received great publicity in one of the
weekly glossies, called *The King, His Navy and Army — A Weekly
Illustrated Journal For Society, the Salon and the Services*. In its section
'On the links' of the issue of 25 November there are a substantial report
and eight photographs illustrating various members in action on holes
from the first to the eighteenth. It also shows the girl caddies, 'a feature
of the course', and Mr Lester Palmer with his famous caddie dog — a
black retriever.

Not all members were happy with their fellows or their guests.
In October 1904 a member complained to the committee about the

language used by another in reference to himself and his partner, but a letter of apology was sent to the two aggrieved parties and to the committee and was accepted by all concerned. At the same meeting several complaints were received about the 'class of visitor introduced by a certain member'. There was a proposal that a rule should be passed reserving to the committee the right of withdrawing from members the privilege of introducing guests, but this was deferred to the next meeting and nothing more is heard of it.

It was not only the members and the professionals who were playing. It must have been about the turn of the century that Jim Morris, who caddied and then worked on the course when he left school, remembers his first efforts at club-making and play.

> I was only knocking about with a lump of wood and a stick cut out of the hedge. I used to get a block of beech, cut it up with a billhook until it got dangerous for the hand and finish it off with a knife — cornet shape was the best — and get Francis in the blacksmith's shop to put a hole in it and then I would go out and get as straight a stick as I could, put it in with a little wire nail and then get a bit of glass as a scraper and scrape it off, and then get a bit of sandpaper from the back of the shop and some chair varnish. Of course, using the gutty ball, you couldn't get the damned ball off the ground. There were sand boxes, so you could have a good high tee, but when you got on the fairway the only hope was to find a divot. There weren't too many of them, because you had to put them back, or else the player did, so you carried this divot with you, put it into your pocket and stuck the ball up on it until you knocked the divot to pieces. If I was near the bushes, I used to nip off a little bit of gorse; that made a lovely tee. Lewellyn Davies, Mrs May-Smith's father, gave me my first club — an old Willie Park cleek. I was very well away then. I used to be able to get the old gutty ball over the bunkers — this cut shot which has now gone off; the experts don't do it now, but it had to be done with the gutty ball. Then a man named Weigall gave me a wooden club. Eventually I got some irons. Different people gave them to me. I used to play with some of the members.

Caddies came from Nuffield, Nettlebed, Ewelme, Watlington and other places round about. Some were women and girls, and very elegant they looked in the long coats of the time, as the photographs in *The King* showed. Jim and Tom Streak recall:

> A new caddie had to have three pieces of emery cloth in his pocket — a new piece, a piece that had been worn and a very fine piece for a lovely set of clubs which you didn't have to scratch, and very often a gentleman would arrive, especially if he had been abroad, with the sea air on his clubs and say: 'See if you can get the rust off, caddie, while I am changing.' Then you had to clean them again after the round and it was no good putting the cover over them because they wanted to see whether you had cleaned them or not — you didn't get any tips if you hadn't.

1925 – 1963

Early in 1925 it was understood that the Norwich Union Society was anxious to dispose of its interest in the club. Mr W.R. Morris told his private secretary, Wilfred Hobbs, to go and buy the clubhouse and the course. When Hobbs asked what he should pay, Morris is reputed to have replied, 'I expect you to get it at the best price you can.' From an abstract of the conveyance attached to the deeds now in the possession of the club, it is known that the price was £32,500 for 967 acres, including the three commons and Hayden, Huntercombe and Timbers farms.

Various stories have been put about concerning the purchase by W.R. Morris. It is palpably untrue that he bought it to get into the club. He had been a member for five years. Though he grew up in Cowley, he may well have been thinking of living in the country outside Oxford. He was already a man of great wealth. He counted many of the members of the club among his personal friends. What more natural than that he should seek to safeguard the club and preserve the amenities of a beautiful piece of the country, when there was danger that the Norwich Union might dispose of it to someone less interested in the locality? He and Mrs Morris evidently had a great affection for Huntercombe; he may even have bought it partly for her. He preserved the club for many years and contributed generously to it in many ways.

W.R. Morris succeeded Earl Howe as president of the club. In 1929 he became Sir William Morris Bt., in 1934 Baron Nuffield and in 1938

Viscount Nuffield. Lord Nuffield took a keen interest in golf and at one time had a nominal handicap of 12. He once said to Jim Morris:

'If you can teach me how to play as well as you, I will set you up for life.'

'Yes, my Lord, and how long will you give me?' asked Jim.

'One month.'

'Oh, it will take longer than that,' said Jim.

'Well,' replied Nuffield, 'If I had to make my living at this game, I wouldn't eat more than bread and lard.'

'No more would I', replied Jim, 'if I were to try making motor cars.'

On one occasion, Jim recalls, Nuffield found in the changing room a tall, willowy, pale, almost frail-looking stranger, who did not look much like a player and had not fixed up a match. Nuffield suggested a game and declared his handicap. The stranger then said, 'I suggest I give you a half.' Nuffield was somewhat taken aback but he was eight down at the twelfth. His opponent was the Hon. W.G. Browlow, whom Bobby Jones once described as one of the finest amateurs he had ever met.

As sole proprietor, Nuffield took the final decisions in matters great and small, with that mixture of great generosity and some parsimony which has characterized the actions of some other men of great wealth. He ran the club through his personal staff and the secretaries, whom he appointed and dismissed. From 1926 until 1953 there were no captains and effectively no committee.

The finances of the club were his private affair until 1963. He decided who would become members. Even until the late fifties he was frequently in the clubhouse. Philip Brownrigg, whose father had been headmaster of Magdalen College School, remembers that, when he came to live in Checkendon in 1946 and went to see about joining, only Nuffield and the secretary, Kennerley Rumford, were in the clubhouse. He spoke to Kennerley Rumford and Nuffield said, 'Did you say Brownrigg? Not the son of Charles Brownrigg? I made a bicycle for him with my own hands in 1896. I'll propose you and Kennerley will second you and you're elected.'

Dr E.O. Seward, then a member of Sunningdale, used to play at Huntercombe with the golfers from Guy's Hospital, in whom Nuffield took a particular interest. He had therefore met Nuffield on a number of occasions when he was put up for membership in the late nineteen-thirties. Nuffield's comment was: 'Another bloody doctor!' There are various ways in which an autocrat signifies assent.

In 1930 R. Kennerley Rumford, a member since 1920 and a close friend of Lord Nuffield, became club secretary. He and his wife, Dame Clara Butt, used to bring a number of distinguished people from the musical world to the clubhouse. Some older members remember him as a courtly figure who used to preside over the dining room from a place where he could see the glass entrance door, which he rose to open for any lady he saw about to enter the room. In 1945/6 Arthur Aman, Lord Nuffield's stockbroker, ran the club for about a year, believing that he could do it on a profitable basis, but without success. Nuffield always said that Huntercombe was the only venture he had undertaken which never made a profit.

Shortly after he bought the property, Nuffield made extensions to Chestnut Cottage, the house on the right of the fourteenth fairway. He also built a new changing room and above it a private flat on the north front of the clubhouse and a second floor above the ladies' room on the south front. In 1927 alone, he spent more than £4100 on these additions. In 1933 the Nuffields bought Merrow Mount, which was renamed Nuffield Place. In the early thirties Nuffield built on the south side of the clubhouse two indoor wood-floored, covered tennis-courts, a badminton-court and two squash-courts. This munificent development must have provided one of the finest centres for those sports in the country outside London. Over the years, the tennis-courts were also used for practice by the British Davis Cup team, and matches between teams of leading players and the Oxford University Lawn Tennis Club were arranged.

During the Second World War the tennis-courts were requisitioned for military purposes and suffered considerable damage, but they were reopened after the war with exhibition matches, in which Jean Borotra, H.G.N. Cooper and other leading players took part. There was, however, trouble with leaks in the roof and Lord Nuffield was not willing to spend the substantial sums necessary to have the damage put right. The tennis side of the club was also said to be costing the club a deficit of about £150 per year. So they gradually deteriorated. In April 1958 they were closed and subsequently dismantled. The badminton- and squash-courts were included in a house and exercise centre which S.C. Rand, the distinguished sculler, and his former wife, Mrs Mary Bignell Rand, the Olympic athlete, built on an adjacent site. In the late fifties and early sixties Mary Rand was often to be seen training on the common.

Ian Fleming, the author, who was a grandson of Mrs Robert

Fleming, the formidable lady member 40 years previously, was a member from 1932 until his untimely death in 1964, with a short break in the early forties, and played regularly. Devotees of James Bond will remember that, when fixing his match with Goldfinger, Bond declared that his handicap was nine at Huntercombe, on the grounds that it was an easier course than Sunningdale, where he was also a nine, and so less likely to arouse the suspicions of his formidable opponent.

Nuffield liked to walk round the course with his friends or good players. In the forties and fifties he often walked round with Ian Fleming and Philip Brownrigg, who recalls one such occasion. At one point, Ian remarked, 'Mr President, you ought to do something about the chrome on your recent models.' Nuffield turned on his heel, walked back to the clubhouse, looked at Ian's car in the car-park and ordered that the chrome parts were to be redone immediately. Alan Hartley had a letter of 1962 in which Ian suggested assigning the copyright in one of his short stories to the club, which would no doubt have eased its persistent financial problems, but — alas — he died before following it through. Philip Brownrigg also says that Stephen Potter worked out some of his gamesmanship ploys during a round with Ian Fleming and himself. His book on *Gamesmanship* was illustrated by the late Col. Frankie Wilson, whose wife, Judy, was one of the leading players among the ladies in the fifties.

Alan Hartley, as captain and chairman of the standing committee, used to have regular meetings with Lord Nuffield about the affairs of the club. At one of these meetings, in April 1961, Nuffield indicated that for some time he had been worried about the future of the club and offered to give the Crown Inn outright to the club. Some negotiations followed, but then Nuffield decided that for the time being he would continue to run the club as before.

In June 1962 the committee was informed that Lord Nuffield was no longer willing to subsidize the club. He realized that time must be allowed for alternative arrangements to be made and was willing to let the club have the use of the clubhouse for a nominal rental for the rest of his life. He offered to give the course and the clubhouse to the members, but it had to be pointed out to him that, if he were to die within three years, there would be a duty of 80% of the value of the gift. He generously agreed to sell to the club, at the lowest price which would be accepted by the Inland Revenue, the clubhouse and the club, his rights on the common, the course maintenance equipment and the part of the course he owned which was not on the common.

The standing committee continued to operate until 3 February 1963, on which date it held its last meeting and the board of directors of the Huntercombe Golf Club Limited its first. The first directors of the company were the same as the members of the committee, which ensured continuity. Lord Nuffield was invited to continue as president.

With Nuffield's death in August 1963, the club lost a benevolent friend, though his heirs, Nuffield College, Oxford, were helpful and friendly.

In 1964 Jim Morris intimated that he wished to retire when the new clubhouse came into being. He was then 73 and had been a professional for 32 years. Before he became professional, he had worked on the course as a caddie and green-keeper since he was a boy. He was a natural golfer and remained so even at 92. Once he said to Selby Armitage, 'Huntercombe's been the same for me since I was a caddie. Pleased to say I've enjoyed every year of it. Couldn't wish for a better set of members.'

He died on 4 March 1984, at the age of 93.

Nuffield had been a member of Huntercombe Golf Club since 1920. And it was there that he met a number of golfing members on the staff of Guy's Hospital — Robert Macintosh (anaesthetist), William Hale-White (physician), Herbert Eason (ophthalmologist), Geoffrey Dowling, Nils Eckoff (surgeon), John Conybeare (physician), W.B. Doherty (genito-urinary surgeon) and T.B. Johnson (professor of anatomy). He was on Christian name terms with them, but they always referred to him as 'W.R.' (W.R. Morris).

Lord Nuffield had no children but he liked the company and social life of the golf club. The group of Guy's doctors would spend perhaps 30 weekends a year there, for several years, going down on Friday evening and returning on Sunday evening, often with their wives. They generally sat at a large communal table and were often joined by the Morrises (later Nuffields). Dinner-jackets and long dresses were worn. They all had dinner together on a Saturday evening, around the large dining-room table, usually with just a few maids in attendance. Nothing could be more informal. After dinner they would play cards, billiards or snooker together. Under these circumstances friendships deepened and remained lifelong.

It was there, in the 1930s, that the possibilities for a clinical school of medicine attached to Oxford University, with its already eminent preclinical school, were discussed. Nuffield was persuaded, and offered to fund it with an initial sum of £1 million (which was later raised to £2 million). He naturally wanted the staff of such a school to be of the highest academic quality. There can be little doubt that he trusted the men round the dinner-table at Huntercombe to give him the right advice on the senior appointments, which included Professor L.J. Witts (medicine), Professor J. Chassar Moir (obstetrics and gynaecology) and Professor Hugh Cairns (neurosurgery).

Later, an academic department of anaesthetics was planned and Robert Macintosh was asked to head it as professor. Nuffield had already had some personal experience of anaesthetics himself. It was well known to anaesthetists that, before the days of curare and muscle relaxant drugs, some patients required much more ether or chloroform than others, to achieve adequate relaxation for surgeons, even in patients of the same weight. Nuffield was one such. He had once had a dental extraction by a dentist, who gave the anaesthetic himself, and the experience was evidently not a pleasant one. Many years later, Robert Macintosh was asked to give Nuffield an anaesthetic for a particular operation. Macintosh used the intravenous drug Evipan. When Nuffield woke up his first words were: 'Why has my operation been put off?' It had already been completed! There were no further problems in the support for an academic department of anaesthetics.

Nuffield was not a great reader. He rarely read a book but he was a good listener and had a very perceptive mind. He could detect the bogus and the charlatan in medicine and probably in many other activities. On one occasion he consulted a chiropractitioner or an osteopath for some troublesome complaint. He received the verdict that the cause was weakness of his abdominal musculature. But Nuffield was a man who had the capacity to so tense his abdominal muscles that he could receive punches on them with impunity. Needless to say, he never returned to the osteopath for treatment.

Nuffield was fortunate in having such first-class advisers at the dinner-table at Huntercombe for the appointment of staff at Oxford, many of whom headed the first academic departments for these subjects in the country — Pomfret Kilner in plastic surgery and J. Trueta in orthopaedic trauma surgery.

Nuffield knew the value of publicity and public relations. After the pleasant surprise of his anaesthetic with Evipan, he saw that it received a big write-up. Robert Macintosh had designed an iron lung in the form of a wooden box for the victims of poliomyelitis or other causes of chest paralysis. He demonstrated it at an Open Day Exhibition in Oxford a year later and Nuffield was naturally invited. It was a piece of machinery which he understood. In 1938 there was a newspaper report that a patient had died because one of the few iron lungs in the country arrived at the hospital two hours too late. Nuffield was shocked. He ordered 5000 iron lungs to be manufactured and one to be supplied to every hospital in the country. Furthermore, he arranged for one of his staff to make a visit and inspect every one of them once a year to see that it was always kept in working order.

Dowling undoubtedly enjoyed the golfing and hospitality weekends at Huntercombe as much as anyone. He was an excellent listener and very gregarious. Most, if not all, of the doctors there received financial support for their departments from Nuffield when they needed it. But Dowling never received or asked for any. One wonders why. Was he ever offered an academic department at the Oxford Medical School? Probably not, but he would almost certainly not have accepted such a position while the consultant dermatologist there was the charming Alice Carleton, for whom he had very considerable respect.

Chapter 9
St Thomas's Hospital

IN THE 1920s Geoffrey was busy learning dermatology under the tutelage of H.W. Barber, at Guy's Hospital. During that time he probably undertook the lesser teaching commitments, such as lectures to nurses, junior students and so on. Most of the teaching of medical students would have been done by Barber, who was a much more extrovert character.

When Geoffrey moved to St Thomas's Hospital in 1932, he was the only dermatologist there. Hence, he was responsible for all the teaching activities. At the beginning of the thirties, dermatology was overshadowed by the venereology department, which was headed by Dr Anwyl Davies. Each year Davies gave a course of racy lectures, which ensured a good attendance from the students. In contrast the teaching of dermatology was almost non-existent. The housing of the department in the basement of the old hospital was a reflection of the neglect of the subject by both management and students. Student attendance at the out-patients' clinic was not mandatory.

It must have been a depressing prospect. But within a decade Dowling had changed all that. One can only guess at the thoughts and plans which must have gone through his mind. He produced no programme of lectures to excite the interest of the medical students. In fact he did not like formal lecturing. One student of the time recalls only one lecture on dermatology, and that was given by a 'German refugee on skin histology' (he must have been Walter Freudenthal from Vienna). It excited little interest, for skin histology, apart from the differentiation of basal from squamous cell cancer, was not then part of the pathologist's curriculum.

Hugh Wallace first met Geoffrey Dowling about 1933 when a student. His initial reaction was that he was very, very old, although Dowling was then in his early forties. He got to know him better when he was appointed a house physician. At the time Dowling was allocated two beds (one male, one female) for skin patients in the hospital.

In those days he had a reputation for being more liberal in his political views than many of his contemporary colleagues on the staff at St Thomas's Hospital, possibly because he agreed with Herbert Morrison's decision to take over the London Underground Railway. Wallace recalled that when he mentioned to Dr Joseph Bamforth that he was thinking of taking up dermatology, he was told, 'Beware of that man Dowling. He's a bloody red!' It is interesting that Bamforth later became one of Dowling's greatest admirers.

As a teacher of undergraduates Dowling was practically a non-starter. He was so anxious not to appear patronizing that he gave them credit for knowledge which they did not in the least possess. And, by the time the information got lost with Dowling's far from perfect diction, regular attendance at his out-patient clinic was almost non-existent. Wallace admitted that he himself only called twice at the out-patient clinic when a medical student. At the time, Dowling was recognized as a 'character' and was very popular with those who came to know him well, particularly in the Hospital Choral Society, which he ran with Dykes Bower, brother of the distinguished organist. On one occasion, after a rather exhausting performance, at least three of the choir had to be admitted to hospital (and possibly Dowling should have gone with them) as a result of alcohol excess.

Wallace did not get to know Dowling really well until he became clinical assistant in the department along with John (later Sir John) Richardson. Geoffrey was always very kind to Hugh and his doctor wife Norah. He used to take them out to dinner at Genaro's restaurant in Frith Street, Soho, where he always seemed to have a large female following. Some five or six handsome ladies would arrive and greet him. He would explain that they were all his cousins!

When Hugh Wallace and Edward Prosser Thomas were registrars together after the war, they would sometimes take difficult cases into his room at the out-patient clinic for help in diagnosis or treatment. After a short time a remark such as 'obviously pityriasis rosea' followed. The students looked at them with hardly hidden disgust, after which they changed their tactic, and would take in a patient to him saying 'I thought this would be a very good case to show the students', and waited for the diagnosis to be revealed — a technique not infrequently used by later generations of registrars.

The medical students were often amused by his habit of looking at the patient, feeling their skin eruption, and then stroking his face in his characteristic way, washing being almost unheard of in those days!

Wallace was appointed consultant to the department in 1946. He always realized how fortunate he was to be selected as Geoffrey's partner and successor, and the two became very close friends in spite of, or perhaps because of, so many differences. Whenever he put forward another opinion or opposed him in any way, Dowling obviously did not care for such opposition, but always contained himself, much more, one suspects, than most others would have been able to achieve at his age. Nevertheless, the two became very close friends. They had entirely complementary personalities, and worked incredibly well together.

K.M. Tomlinson qualified from St Thomas's Hospital in 1940 and, incredible as it may seem against this background of indifference, decided to apply for the post of clinical assistant to the department of dermatology. To this day, he can find no explanation for making such a decision. There was no other applicant and he was appointed.

The out-patient department was a large room below floor level with inadequate lighting. There were two tables, one for Dr Dowling and one for Dr Prosser Thomas. They were placed six feet apart, but consultation between the two was a rare event. Advice and instructions from Dr Dowling were not given unless requested. It soon became apparent to Tomlinson that Dowling was particularly interested in one disease, lupus vulgaris (tuberculosis of the skin). At that time all these patients were being treated with a type of vitamin D (calciferol) in large doses. Each patient had to be seen at their follow-up appointment by Dowling himself as well as the clinical assistants, to whom the reason was not readily apparent, since their appointments in the department only lasted for six months.

Nevertheless, this experience engendered in Tomlinson a special interest in lupus vulgaris. After the war ended in 1945 he was appointed as registrar in the dermatology department in Coventry, mainly as a result of Dowling's support. At that time there was a wealth of untapped clinical material in Warwickshire. Clinics of over 100 patients per session were commonplace. There were many with lupus vulgaris, and so Tomlinson began treating them with high-dosage calciferol. He took biopsies from the areas of healed lupus and normal skin. The specimens were micro-incinerated and the calcium content estimated. The healed lupus tissue always contained a higher calcium content than unaffected skin. Tomlinson sent his results to Dowling in London, who encouraged him to continue the work and eventually arranged for him to present it at an International Conference of Physicians in 1948. This encouragement was a tremendous boost for Tomlinson's morale.

In 1948 Dowling persuaded Tomlinson to take an appointment in the venereology department at St Thomas's Hospital and to spend half his time in the dermatology department. It had always been Dowling's wish to foster a liaison between the two departments. He wanted the wealth of clinical material from the venereology department to be available for him in his teaching of dermatology. It then became Tomlinson's task to pick out cases with skin manifestations of venereal disease and take them over to Dowling in the dermatology department. It proved to be a very successful and valuable exercise.

After some 18 months Tomlinson began to feel the pressures of a young wife and children. He met Dowling one day in a hospital corridor and asked him: 'How long will it be before I could be sure of an annual income to support a family?'

Dowling stopped and eased himself on to one of the wall radiators, rubbed his face in his characteristic fashion and after a long time said, 'Four years . . . at least!'

That night Tomlinson decided to leave London and become a general practitioner in the country. He settled on Newent, a delightful village in Gloucestershire. When Dowling heard this, he supplied the information to the local dermatologist, and within six months Tomlinson was appointed as a general practitioner assistant in dermatology at the local hospital, a post which he held for 30 years. This appointment enabled Tomlinson to maintain his connection with the dermatological community, particularly through meetings of the West of England and Wales Dermatological Society and the George Club.

Whenever there was a dermatology meeting in Gloucester, Dowling would stay with the Tomlinsons, sometimes accompanied by May Dowling. If they had time he would accompany Tomlinson on his round of home visits to his patients. On one occasion Tomlinson explained how the country people treated ringworm of the scalp (before the introduction of griseofulvin) by massaging bacon fat from their home-cured pigs into the lesions. Dowling ridiculed the magical powers of bacon fat, but he did take some home with him. He later told Tomlinson that he had actually grown the ringworm fungus on the bacon fat! So much for country tales. Perhaps the reported beneficial effect was due to the high salt content of the fat producing a non-specific inflammatory (kerion) effect.

John Simpson was a medical student at St Bartholomew's Hospital, where the senior dermatologist was A.C. Roxburgh, an inspiring under-

graduate teacher who had written one of the most popular textbooks of
dermatology. Simpson was very impressed by Roxburgh's teaching and
liked the subject so much that he decided on his own initiative in 1937
to go to some of the evening lectures advertised at St John's Hospital
for Diseases of the Skin, and also attended an evening out-patient clinic
run by Dr Isaac Muende. In those days some patients could not afford
to lose time from work during the day and would only go to a hospital
clinic in the evening. It was usually crowded, but in the decades
after the Second World War the pressures at work had changed,
and eventually the evening clinic was discontinued because of lack of
demand. Simpson remembers hearing Dowling lecture there but was
much less impressed by him than by many other lecturers. Dowling's
style of imparting knowledge was not well suited to the student mind,
all eager for lists, causes and classifications.

Simpson subsequently worked as a house physician to the skin
and venereology departments at St Bartholomew's Hospital before
joining the Royal Air Force in November 1940. Although he worked
as a general physician at RAF hospitals at St Athan in South Wales
and Halton in Buckinghamshire, he took on the dermatology work
unofficially, there being no Air Force specialist at the time apart from a
civilian consultant. In 1943 Dowling replaced Sir Archibald Gray as
the civilian consultant. Simpson recalls a twinge of disappointment
when he learnt this and was then deputed to attend the RAF Central
Medical Establishment building in London once a week to see selected
Air Force patients who had been referred to the civilian consultant.

But his opinion of Dowling was changed completely within half an
hour of starting the first of these weekly sessions. He left the Central
Medical Establishment building that evening feeling absolutely delighted
by his good fortune, and the opportunity to work with such a remarkable man. He had already had some postgraduate experience of dermatology, so he had some idea of what the problems were in the subject.
But he was surprised that Dowling could 'tell you more in a few words
than some could say in an hour's lecture. If you knew enough to ask the
right questions and understand the terse and pithy answers, he was a
mine of information. He readily forgave honest ignorance but expected
and gave nothing but the truth. He was never afraid to say when he did
not know the answer to a question.' Simpson began to look forward
eagerly to the weekly session, which was later extended when Dowling
invited him to go along with him to the regular histology sessions given

by Walter Freudenthal at University College Hospital, before returning to the RAF Hospital at Halton.

After the war ended, to Simpson's great satisfaction Dowling asked him if he would care to join his department at St Thomas's Hospital when he was demobilized. He finally left the Royal Air Force in May 1946, and started work as a supernumerary registrar at the hospital. These salaried supernumerary posts were created to provide training, occupation and 'rehabilitation' for ex-service doctors.

At St Thomas's Hospital he entered a very novel atmosphere. He found himself one of a band of very enthusiastic registrars and clinical assistants, amongst whom the rivalry was keen but amazingly kind and good-natured. He was the only outsider, being a Bart's man, but was at once accepted and made to feel at home. He realized that this 'atmosphere' in the department was created by Dowling, who set them all such a marvellous example, not just in medicine and dermatology but in life itself. He enjoyed everything as it came along and made the most of it. He particularly enjoyed the company of young people, with whom he managed to join in as an equal and yet hold his own. He never stood on his dignity but was held in great respect.

Dowling took great pains to look after the general welfare and progress of all the registrars in his department. He used his influence to see that their supernumerary registrar appointments were extended as long as possible. When Simpson's was coming to an end, he told Dowling that he must now find a permanent appointment, and expressed a wish to work in a country town. He was interested in a post advertised in Exeter, and wondered if he was experienced enough yet to apply for it. Dowling was doubtful, but simply said, 'You know enough to teach yourself the rest'. Dowling was well aware of the financial and other pressures on ex-service registrars at the time. He had satisfied himself by repeated enquiry that Simpson really did want to leave London.

His confidence was, of course, justified and his support at the time presumably helped when the appointment was made in 1947, because competition was strong in the early post-war years. Meetings of the West of England and Wales Dermatological Society were held in Exeter at regular intervals and Dowling attended them all. On at least four of these occasions Dowling stayed with John and Mary Simpson in their house.

As with so many others they remained lifelong friends. Simpson

found him such a marvellous companion. He took Dowling to a test
match at Lord's Cricket Ground one day when not a ball was bowled
because of rain. They sat there all day until afternoon when the
announcement came that play was abandoned. They chatted happily
together all the time, and the hours passed almost too quickly. On
another occasion at a supper picnic party after a dermatology meeting
at Exeter in 1950, Dowling insisted on driving a golf ball from the hill
where they were sitting into a wild valley, where it was irretrievably lost
— and he didn't call 'Fore!'

Renwick Vickers qualified in Sheffield in 1934 and soon after began
his career in dermatology with Dr Rupert Hallam, one of a number
of general physicians who conducted the dermatology clinics in their
hospitals, being more or less entirely self-taught. Hallam was a rather
reserved man of high principles who was much ahead of his time, and
firmly believed that for the advancement of dermatology it should
remain a branch of general medicine. He advised the young Vickers to
pursue his training in London and Copenhagen. He gave him an introduction to Geoffrey Dowling, relatively 'unknown' in 1939 compared
with Barber, Roxburgh, MacCormac, O'Donovan, Gray and Goldsmith.
These were the best dermatological feet at which to sit.

Vickers arrived at the age of 27 from a small provincial medical
school (there were only 14 students in his year at Sheffield), and
regarded the London teaching hospitals with great awe. He presented
his letter of introduction and was pleased to find that Dowling and
Hallam had a high regard for each other. The warmth of his reception
made an enormous impression on Vickers. He was welcomed to the
department and invited to attend the special Wednesday morning
sessions, when Dowling with his assistants Prosser Thomas and Wallace
and the rest of his staff presented and discussed various problem cases
of the week. One can imagine his surprise when Dowling asked Vickers
for his opinion on particular patients, and even for his comments on the
draft of a paper he was writing with Walter Freudenthal on the muscle
changes in systemic sclerosis. This was one of his many great qualities,
the ability to encourage young doctors and instruct them with patient
understanding, and yet without any trace of a deferential or patronizing
attitude.

Vickers was appointed to the honorary consultant staff of the
Sheffield Royal Infirmary in August 1939. He had joined the Royal
Naval Volunteer Reserve when a medical student, and was at once

mobilized when the war started in September 1939. There were no dermatologists in the Royal Naval Medical Service at that time and skin patients were looked after by general physicians. In 1940 Vickers was such a physician at the Royal Naval Hospital at Haslar, Portsmouth. He made a diagnosis of leprosy in a long-serving English naval officer. The Navy authorities must have been very alarmed when the news reached them, and as a result dermatology specialists were appointed to the naval hospitals at Haslar, Chatham and Plymouth. As one of them, Vickers was able to attend the regular meetings of the Dermatology Section of the Royal Society of Medicine where, of course, he had the opportunity to meet Dowling again and maintain contact.

This was valuable because it enabled him to ask advice on decisions in his own career. At one time he had considered applying for an appointment at a major London teaching hospital. One of the attractions was that Geoffrey had invited him to share his consulting-rooms at 24 Wimpole Street. As usual there was no criticism but only understanding when Vickers withdrew his London application and decided to stay in Sheffield. Dowling had given his approval when Vickers chose Ian Sneddon as a colleague, and must have derived much pleasure from the way they built up the department in Sheffield with its outstanding reputation for undergraduate education, culminating in the publication of the best-selling students' book *Diseases of the Skin* by Sneddon and Church.

The George Club met in Sheffield in 1956 and Vickers obtained a block booking for a concert given by the Hallé Orchestra conducted by Sir John Barbirolli. This was when he first became aware of Dowling's love and knowledge of music.

Dowling was not entirely happy when Vickers decided to move from Sheffield to Oxford, but did nothing to dissuade him. There was then and still is in Britain a surprising disapproval of an established consultant moving from one centre to another. However, Dowling later admitted that such moves could sometimes be a good thing. At the Radcliffe Infirmary (now extended to the new John Radcliffe Hospital) Vickers succeeded Alice Carleton, who was a long-time personal friend of Dowling and a very remarkable lady.

After moving to Oxford Vickers was able to see a lot more of Dowling, who often accompanied him to concerts given by the Oxford Bach Choir, in which he (Vickers) sang. Dowling revelled in the sound of such works as the B Minor Mass and Verdi's Requiem. It must have revived childhood memories (which he presumably kept to himself) of his life in Cape Town with his parents at St George's Cathedral and of Exeter Choir School. Vickers became a Fellow of Magdalen College and Dowling greatly enjoyed the opportunities to put on a dinner-jacket for dinner at the high table on Sunday evenings after sitting behind the choir at evensong.

Dr Stephen Wight was one of the original group of registrars at St Thomas's Hospital who made up the Journal Club at the George Inn in 1947. He was an undergraduate at the hospital, but his memories of Dowling during his student days were dim and rather off-putting. There were a number of reasons for this.

> It was wartime, and the medical school was fragmented. Most of what I learnt of dermatology came from Hugh Wallace. He, of course, had much more charisma and zest for teaching than Dowling ever had, and it was he who came to our Sector Hospitals in Guildford, Woking and Chertsey. Dowling remained in London, and on the few occasions that we went to his clinics there we found the teaching from him both dull and unrewarding.

Like so many others Stephen was soon afterwards called up for war service, and went out to India with the Royal Army Medical Corps. There he met Wolf Tillman, whose enthusiasm and guidance led him into dermatology and to become an Army specialist.

It was in 1949 that things changed so completely and dramatically. Hugh Wallace arranged for him to join Dowling's team as a junior registrar. The other members of the group were Arthur Rook, Douglas Sweet, Eric Waddington and Darrell Wilkinson, who always referred to Dowling as 'the Headmaster'.

They were happy and rewarding days, and during this time he came to know and love 'the old man' as he never had before:

> I was impressed by his immense knowledge not only about skins, but about medicine in general, and by his modesty which at times amounted to humility. He had, too, a lovely boyish sense of fun. He was always very kind to me, and took a fatherly interest in me and my doings and aspirations.

Wight recalled that they:

used to meet as a group, about once a month for an evening's session of beer and sandwiches at the George Inn in Southwark, and read learned papers, and have good fun. The Headmaster was always the life and soul of these happy little parties.

Two small incidents come to mind which are typical of this wonderful man. In one of my out-patient sessions a patient arrived with peculiar lesions on his feet, the like of which I had never seen before. I asked Eric Waddington and Arthur Rook for their opinion, and they were equally baffled; many weird diagnoses were put forward.

The patient returned a week later to see the Headmaster. He pondered long and hard, and then said, 'I think it's lichen planus.' He added that there had better be a biopsy to make quite sure, but 'in his humble opinion' that was the diagnosis.

Later that afternoon at tea, and not in Dowling's presence, we were wondering about his diagnosis. Could he really be right? Might it not also be possible that he was wrong, and that in suggesting such a 'simple' diagnosis he was showing his age, and beginning to 'lose his grip'? But the biopsy proved he was right, and all of us bright young boys were confounded!

The other incident occurred many years later. I was married and had a young family. With finances getting low, I had to change course and go into general practice in Derby: a decision which I never regretted. Dowling and I parted at the conclusion of one of his clinics at the end of November 1949. We did not meet again for nearly fifteen years. I was at the Hospital, and met him by chance in the Central Hall. He was obviously as pleased to see me as I was to see him. He knew my name, and knew that I was a general practitioner in Derbyshire! I regret that I never saw him again.

Though Dowling had left Guy's by the time Wolf Tillman got into the wards, his name was well known, but they were not to meet until after the war. It was early in 1948 that he had a phone call from Stephen Wight, who had been with him in India, inviting him to a meeting of the George Club. Apart from his host, he recognized only Hugh Wallace, whom he had met four years earlier as the Medical Superintendent of Woking Hospital. He was, however, introduced to Dowling and remained forever grateful to Steve Wight.

When Dowling took over the dermatology patients at Goldie Leigh Hospital from Sir Archibald Gray, Tillman used to meet him there during his weekly visit, which usually coincided with his own travelling from a hospital morning to an afternoon clinic. He very much enjoyed sitting in the clinic with Dowling and seeing something of chronic skin diseases in children.

When Paul Naylor had completed his army service, where he had been involved in some experimental work with skin, an appointment as Research Fellow at the Institute of Dermatology in 1951 enabled him to continue with this work. There were no suitable laboratory facilities at the Institute and having previously worked in the department of medicine at St Thomas's Hospital he was provided with bench space there. It was necessary that he should learn some clinical dermatology, and to start this process he 'sat in' with a number of dermatologists at St John's Hospital and with Dowling at St Thomas's. During this period Paul had a most interesting opportunity to compare Dowling's characteristics with those of other senior dermatological figures in London.

Perhaps his most striking characteristic was that when involved with work he spoke very little. Paul later found that this contrasted markedly with his social behaviour, when he chattered on in an extremely animated way, was warm and friendly, and showed a very lively sense of humour. His apparent unwillingness to express his views very freely on clinical matters unfortunately often extended into his lectures and he was an extremely bad lecturer. This was in sharp contrast to his writing ability, for he wrote most beautifully.

During his out-patient clinics he always worked at the same pace, no matter how many patients were waiting to see him, and he was clearly oblivious of everything except the problem in front of him. He was usually the last to finish the clinic, often to the annoyance of the nursing staff. He seemed to have no feelings of self-importance, in spite of his considerable reputation, nor did he display any tricks of showmanship. On occasions when perhaps some reassurance to the patient or a white lie might have been indicated, this rarely appeared. On one such occasion the mother of a senior member of staff at St Thomas's Hospital was ushered in for his opinion about her excessive hair fall from the scalp. When the examination was finished, there followed a very long silence, Dowling sitting with his head forward and one hand over his forehead and eyes, the patient meantime showing signs of mounting anxiety and agitation. Finally, Dowling said that he didn't know why the hair was falling out but, apparently to soften this blow, went on to express the hope that she wouldn't lose all her hair! That was the end of the consultation! On other occasions, however, he was able to express intense sympathy with patients who were seriously ill, and this he sometimes did by resting a hand upon them as he spoke. Physical contact with patients is not infrequently practised by very experienced physicians under such circumstances, but with Dowling it was more notable as it was in such sharp contrast with his more usual behaviour.

His long silences were studied with interest by his registrars, and at one time several of them took to timing the length of these with a stop-watch to try and establish a record. The general consensus was that the silences were an important component of his armamentarium, as they sometimes provoked patients or colleagues into unguarded remarks; when this happened Dowling could deliver a terrible broadside. On one occasion which Paul remembers vividly, after examining a patient there followed the usual period of silent thought and finally the patient said, 'Well, what is it, or don't you know?'

The silence went on for another minute or so, when Dowling took his hand away from his forehead and eyes and raised his head, turned to Paul and said, 'Damned cheek, don't you think?'

Nor was he any more tactful with senior colleagues when he was called upon to give an opinion, and would often contradict their views flatly. One subject which could always be relied upon to produce an interesting response would be the suggestion that urticaria was psychogenic or 'due to the nerves'. On another occasion, a dermatological colleague produced a patient with Kyrle's disease and asked Dowling what he considered to be the background to such lesions. There followed a long silence and finally the colleague was driven to saying, 'I have always regarded these lesions as metabolic in origin.'

'I would have thought they were degenerative.'

The colleague somewhat unwisely replied, 'Well, degenerative—metabolic.'

No reply at all from Dowling as he wandered away.

If these anecdotes give the impression of an aloof character, this is quite incorrect. He loved parties and, after he stopped driving, which he hated and at which he was extremely bad, a colleague would not infrequently call at his house to pick him up and drive him to the current party. On such occasions, he was always ready hours before the appointed time with his overcoat on and ready for a quick departure. He was frequently the first to arrive and the last to leave and would talk endlessly with other guests.

Dowling was always extremely active in attracting into dermatology people who, although only on the fringe of the subject, could, because of specialized skills or knowledge, make a real contribution to its advancement. In doing this, he would often cut right across the conventional aspects of recruitment. How he would have disliked the present system with its rigidity and associated self-important hierarchy.

One such person was Dr Ian Whimster. In the late nineteen-forties he was a lecturer in Professor Barnard's department of pathology. He became interested in the histopathology of skin biopsies from the dermatologists because they were always so interested in his report. The association with Whimster gradually built up and Dowling encouraged it.

At that time there were two special skin pathology problems which intrigued the dermatology registrars. One was molluscum sebaceum. This was a button-like lump on the skin which had always been thought to be an early type of squamous cancer until about 1938 when Macormac (a dermatologist) and Scarff (a pathologist) at the Middlesex Hospital claimed at a meeting of the Royal Society of Medicine that it was not a cancer at all, and would often resolve without treatment. They were derided. Almost no one in the room believed them. But Dowling did, and he remembered. When he had registrars with time after 1945, he set them to collect such patients to prove the point. They soon did, with the help of Ian Whimster doing all the careful pathology. It is now accepted that molluscum sebaceum, now called kerato-acanthoma, is a benign lesion.

The other was pemphigus. This is a very serious skin disease, which in those days was almost universally fatal. But some patients here and there were known to survive. Was there any reason for this? The first visit abroad on which Dowling took his newly founded George Club was to Paris. There they listened to a demonstration by Achille Civatte at the Hôpital Saint Louis of the distinctive histology of pemphigus. This was found in all the patients who died, but those who survived had a different histology, and it is a different disease, called pemphigoid. When they returned to London, one of the registrars, Arthur Rook, asked Whimster to look at the histopathology of all their patients with pemphigus. They were surprised to find that the results exactly paralleled the Paris experience. The difference between pemphigus and pemphigoid could be exactly defined. Arthur Rook wrote his MD thesis on this work.

From then on Whimster became closely integrated with the dermatology department. He did all the skin pathology, including that for the plastic surgeons, and his laboratory soon became a major reference centre for many dermatologists in the country.

Whimster was utterly dedicated. He developed a laboratory for experimental work and kept small reptiles there for his studies of their pigmentation and spots. He received support from his professor of pathology, on whom Dowling almost certainly had some influence (in his quiet and unobtrusive way). He soon responded to a request from the registrars to hold a histopathology teaching session once a week, to which everyone came, including the consultants, Dowling and Wallace.

In the late nineteen forties and early fifties, there were so many extra or supernumerary (ex-service) registrars that it became the largest staffed department in London. There were George Wells, Robert Bowers, Arthur Rook, Hugh Calvert, Martin Beare, Douglas Sweet, John Simpson and Darrell Wilkinson, as well as visitors from Australia and other countries. As time went by, all of them went on to consultant posts in the south and west of England.

There was no doubt that the centre of gravity of London dermatology was firmly anchored to Geoffrey Dowling at St Thomas's Hospital. And so it remained for many years — until the years after 1951 when he became Director of the Institute of Dermatology at St John's Hospital. He quickly realized the enormous potential of the hospital, with its large out-patient attendance. And there the centre of gravity of London dermatology remained until 1990, when the hospital in Lisle Street, Leicester Square, closed to be re-established as the Saint John's Dermatology Centre within the area of St Thomas's Hospital. One cannot but feel he would be quietly pleased at the merging of the two hospitals to which he had contributed so much.

In 1946 Dowling began a long association with the Lord Mayor Treloar Hospital at Alton in Hampshire. This hospital was built in 1901 for sick and wounded soldiers returning from the Boer War in South Africa. The land was provided by Sir Alfred Harmsworth (later Lord Northcliffe), the money being provided by public subscription and donations from the *Daily Mail* newspaper. It was called the Princess Louise Hospital, but was not completed until after the Boer War ended in 1902, when it was handed over to the government. It was used briefly by the Royal Army Medical Corps, and then left empty before being taken over by Sir William Pardie Treloar in 1907. He was Lord Mayor of London in 1905.

Treloar had no children of his own, but was passionately interested in the fate of poor children in London. When Lord Mayor he launched the 'Lord Mayor's Little Cripple Fund'. He had support from the royal family and his fund exceeded its target. He arranged to buy the derelict hospital with 70 acres of land at Alton and to convert it into the Lord Mayor Treloar Cripples Hospital and College. It was opened in 1908 with 18 patients.

They needed a resident medical officer. An advertisement for the post with a salary of £200 per annum brought no response. So Treloar decided to take the matter into his own hands. He was an ex-officio Governor of St Bartholomew's Hospital and on one of his regular visits asked advice from one of the consultant surgeons while talking in 'the Square'. Could he recommend a suitable young doctor for the post, which would provide a stipend and plenty of time to study for a higher examination in medicine or surgery. Just at that moment, and quite by chance, a 29-year-old Doctor Henry Gauvain was walking across 'the Square' (courtyard in the hospital). He was waylaid and the offer put to him. But he said he had opted for a lectureship in gynaecology at McGill University in Canada, and politely declined.

But then Treloar turned on his charm and asked Gauvain to think over the needs of the new hospital for crippled children and its future. Soon afterwards Treloar took him to lunch at de Keyser's restaurant and he accepted. Next day Gauvain received a letter confirming his appointment to the lectureship in Canada. He wrote his apologies that he was unable to accept the appointment, but never told Treloar.

Gauvain started his career at Alton, where he was known as 'the Earl', in August 1908, eventually became an international figure, and was knighted in 1920 at the age of 41. From the first day, he insisted that the resident medical officer must have complete autonomy, accept all responsibility and be 'dedicated to his work'. He set the objectives of the hospital as care and treatment of the highest standards. It was to aim for cure of the patients and not to be just a care institution or convalescent home. The medical board were amazed that he did not plan to study for a higher examination and leave after a year. He intended to stay.

The hospital was designed to care for and treat children with tuberculosis of the bones and joints. The treatment consisted of good food, fresh air, sunshine (natural and artificial) and appropriate surgical and orthopaedic procedures. But there is no doubt that Gauvain's drive, energy and ambition made a big contribution, and he firmly believed that making the children happy was of major importance. A hospital school was added to provide education. The hospital had workshops to make everything that was needed. Recurrent appeals for funds were made and the response was generous. Royal patronage came with visits from Queen Alexandra and Queen Amelia of Portugal in 1914, and later from Princess Alice, the Duke and Duchess of York (now Queen Elizabeth), the Queen Mother, the Duke of Kent (later King George VI), and Princess Alexandra of Kent in 1956.

Sir William Treloar died in 1923 at the age of 80. Sir Henry Gauvain developed a paralytic condition of his legs and died in 1945 at the age of 66.

Gauvain had qualified at St Bartholomew's Hospital and married one of the nurses there. She was his constant support at Treloar Hospital, and operated the X-ray machine in the early years. They had one daughter, Suzette, who qualified as a doctor in 1943, and soon after became the resident medical officer. She married Dr Ronald Murray in 1940, when he was in the Royal Army Medical Corps. After the war he became registrar in radiology at Treloar Hospital and later a consultant at the Royal National Orthopaedic Hospital at Ascot. In 1954 they went together to join the staff of the American University of Beirut Hospital in the Lebanon for four years.

Ronald Murray first met Dr Hugh Wallace and Geoffrey Dowling, who were working at St Thomas's Hospital, in 1946. His wife Suzette had inherited her father's private hospital, Morland Hall, which catered for non-pulmonary cases of tuberculosis above the age of 16 years, when they could no longer remain at Treloar Hospital. It had 100 beds and patients came from a wide area. Among the patients at Morland Hall were 20 with tuberculosis of the skin (lupus vulgaris), who were being treated by heliotherapy. When Geoffrey Dowling heard about this from Ronald Murray, he was extremely interested. So Ronald Murray and Suzette invited him to see all the patients with lupus vulgaris at Morland Hall and Treloar Hospital, with a view to using his newly discovered treatment with calciferol (vitamin D). This gave him a wonderful opportunity to test the effects in a large group of patients. With his usual generosity, Geoffrey published his results with Mr D.E. Macrae, the resident surgical officer at Treloar Hospital.

Thus began a long inter-family friendship. Geoffrey was invited to become a consultant to both establishments. Because his week was so busy, he visited them on a Sunday morning once a month. This was followed by lunch at Morland Hall, and then a round of golf with Ronald at various courses. Ronald was a member of the club at Rye and introduced Geoffrey there.

In 1957 Ronald Murray established a consultant radiology practice with Dr John Sutcliffe at 25 Wimpole Street, just next door to Dowling at number 24. Geoffrey was very impressed when he sent them a patient for an X-ray of the skull, and they sent him back with the correct diagnosis of tuberous sclerosis.

The Murrays had a son and two daughters. Geoffrey was godfather to their younger daughter, Virginia, who is now a doctor in occupational medicine and a consultant in the poisons unit at Guy's Hospital. Her brother Nigel was about the same age as Geoffrey's youngest son Simon; while at school May and Geoffrey took the two boys on a holiday together by ship to the Canary Islands.

Chapter 10
St John's Hospital for
Diseases of the Skin

DR JOHN Laws Milton gained his medical qualifications in 1843 and practised in London as a surgeon. Like Sir Jonathan Hutchinson, FRS, FRCS, the famous surgeon, he became particularly interested in diseases of the skin, and

> . . . was struck with the misery which those diseases entailed. With the co-operation of several friends he took and furnished a small place in Westminster. The subscription list did not cover more than a quarter's rent; yet, from that time to the present, St John's Hospital has continued, and had gained the confidence of the thinking portion of the public to an unexampled extent until at present, it has a list of supporters second, perhaps, to none of our charitable institutions. For 10 years Mr Milton has continued to give his services as a professional man to the Hospital and in addition, as I well know, devoted all his spare time and much from his private practice to promoting its influence. That London shall soon have a proper Skin Diseases Hospital is the one idea of his life.
>
> In the ten years of its existence, St John's Hospital has had 20,000 patients. These have been attended to by Mr Milton and his colleagues who are unsalaried, in a quite unostentatious way — their reward resting entirely on the consciousness that they were relieving those who but for them would be uncared for. (Charles Mercier, *The Echo*, 25 April 1873)

For most of the first half of the twentieth century aspiring dermatologists regarded St John's Hospital as a starting-point or adjunct to their training before obtaining a position at an undergraduate hospital, where the skin departments developed and grew dominant in the specialty, presumably as a result of their role in teaching medical students. For postgraduate education there was no alternative but to go to one of the leading European university departments in France, Switzerland, Germany and Austria.

At the end of the Second World War, demobilized doctors who

requested postgraduate education were provided with grants and positions as supernumerary registrars. Many of them were attached to the undergraduate hospitals and St John's Hospital. In 1946 there were courses of lectures, but most of the teaching was on out-patients, and on an apprenticeship basis. This was later extended to histopathology, clinical pathology, mycology and biochemistry, before a professorial unit was created in 1961.

In the immediate post-war years, conditions in the hospital were somewhat primitive, due to lack of space and the considerably increased numbers of patients and doctors wanting to learn. Clinics were held every morning and afternoon, and there were extra clinics on Monday and Tuesday evenings to accommodate patients who could not take time off during the day.

One of the consultants would work with three or four assistants in one large room each at a desk with a chair for the patient, and only a portable screen to separate one patient from another and provide minimal privacy for undressing. There were no couches. The consultant's desk was surrounded by a group of chairs for the trainees, and all would move from one desk to another to see a patient of special interest. But enthusiasm and morale were surprisingly high, and there were lighter moments. One day in 1943 a young soldier in uniform came to the clinic and sat down in the chair next to the consultant's desk. With no service cap on, he had obvious lesions of secondary syphilis on the face.

Consultant: 'Good afternoon. What have you been doing, young man?'

Soldier: 'I have been on Combined Operations, sir.'

Consultant: 'Yes, I can see that!'

There was little time for discussion. One had to learn as best one could, and talk about the cases with the other registrars over a glass of beer in a public house (the Imperial) in Leicester Street for half an hour or so at the end of the clinic before going home.

The registrars, both at St John's and at several of the undergraduate hospitals, were so keen that they soon made an arrangement to bring their patients of special interest back to a special session on Friday evenings at 6.30 pm and discuss them until 7.30, before retiring to the Imperial or going home to waiting wives. The ancillary staff were wholly co-operative in this, especially the senior nurse, Enid Kelly, and the head porter, Albert (Pellett). One of the senior registrars kept the list of patients in a book, and after the meeting wrote a few notes on each patient. The Friday evening registrars' meeting soon became a major event in education, run entirely by the registrars for the registrars, at which the juniors learnt from the seniors.

An equally important person in the hospital for the registrars was a (largely self-taught) technician, Reg Syms, who spent all his working life at St John's Hospital. It was Syms who taught the registrars how to find the acarus of scabies and fungus in skin scrapings. He was an enthusiast and a tireless teacher, who devoted his whole life to St John's Hospital and to its Dermatological Society.

The method of election to the staff of St John's Hospital, prior to the National Health Service in 1948, was similar to that of a London club. At a staff meeting a member would suggest the name of a suitable person. If there were no adverse comments, the nominee was invited to take tea in the boardroom with the medical staff, the chairman of the governors and the secretary-treasurer, some weeks later. After he had left, again if there were no adverse comments, the secretary was asked to write a letter to the nominee inviting him to become a member of the staff. Almost too simple, but one should remember that in those days the number of dermatologists in London was small. It is also possible that character and personality were qualifications of importance, as well as dermatological knowledge and ability.

Geoffrey Dowling was appointed to the consultant staff in 1926, presumably after the informal introduction over tea in the boardroom. He simply did an out-patient clinic on a Monday morning and spent the rest of his time at St Thomas's and other hospitals. He saw a lot of patients, and being relatively untalkative made little impression on the various assistants. Several other consultants were more extrovert and more voluble and attracted a larger following.

Dowling focused his training of registrars mainly at St Thomas's Hospital, which in the immediate post-war years came to be considered one of the best training centres, along with Harold Barber at Guy's and A.C. Roxburgh at St Bartholomew's Hospital. But very gradually the situation underwent an important change. The impetus was the start of the National Health Service in 1948.

In contrast to most of his colleagues, Dowling saw this as a great opportunity for dermatology. He was senior enough to exert some influence in appropriate places on the qualifications required to be a consultant. For so many years he had watched dermatologists, along with a number of other specialist physicians, relegated to Division II in the medical hierarchy, most of them holding positions as assistant physician rather than that of physician to a hospital. He was also aware that there may have been some justification for this. Many of them were self-taught and amateurs for whom dermatology was something of a hobby. And many were primarily general practitioners without a great deal of hospital training and with no higher qualifications.

Dowling foresaw that the way to change this situation was to make the Membership of the Royal College of Physicians (MRCP) examination an essential qualification for the position of consultant dermatologist in the National Health Service. And he succeeded. He would not accept a registrar for training unless he had already passed the examination, or did so within about a year.

No other country in Europe or America had such a system or adopted it; there it was not considered that two or three years' training in general (internal) medicine was a necessary or useful requirement for training in dermatology. Years later, dermatologists have voiced the opinion that such a study of neurology, psychiatry, cardiology and so on will only diminish the trainee's time, energy and enthusiasm which should be devoted to dermatology. In the United States and most European countries, dermatology training is normally started no more than one or two years after medical qualification.

But the reason was that the situation in Great Britain was different. In European universities and hospitals, the dermatologist already had equal status with physicians. In Britain they did not. The purpose of the MRCP qualification was to give the National Health Service dermatologist equal status in every way with the physician. And none will doubt that this policy was successful. Dermatologists are now given their own beds and departments in hospitals, and have achieved positions as chairmen of medical staff committees and deans of medical schools.

Now that medicine has become more specialized and subdivided, it will be asked again if the MRCP examination is really a necessary prerequisite to training. Fortunately, the Royal College of Physicians has changed, and the examination is no longer a qualification to practise as a consultant physician; rather is it a qualification for suitability for training as a physician. Much detailed knowledge of neurology, endocrinology and cardiology is no longer required, and most dermatologists in Britain now accept that the period spent on internal medicine to acquire the qualification prior to training in dermatology is an advantage. This is especially true when the practice of medicine and therapeutics has become so advanced and complex, and the interrelationships between dermatology and internal medicine have become much more widely recognized.

The Postgraduate Medical Federation of the University of London was formed in 1945 as the administrative centre for the 12 academic institutes attached to the special disease hospitals, as well as the postgraduate medical school at Hammersmith Hospital, and was responsible for the funds for them provided by the university. Initially, the Institute of Dermatology's staff consisted only of a part-time dean (Dr J.E.M. Wigley) and secretarial staff. Sir Archibald Gray was a trusted guide and friend, in helping the Institute to establish its place in the federation, and obtain a share of the university funds.

But in 1951 its most important decision was made. Dr G.B. Dowling was invited and appointed to be the first director of the Institute, on a part-time basis (four sessions or half-days per week). It was this appointment (at the age of 60) which gave him the opportunity to exert his maximum influence on British dermatology, although few of his contemporaries realized it at the time. Like Winston Churchill, his call to assume the leadership came late in life. In most branches of medicine, this would be a disadvantage, but in dermatology, which was largely a clinical subject at the time, the greatest asset was experience, and of that Geoffrey Dowling had an abundance. He had seen an enormous number of patients and worked in many different hospitals in London and the surrounding counties, and he had a prodigious memory.

None of the rest of the staff foresaw how he would use his position as director of the Institute of Dermatology — he had no love of administration or committees — but Dr J.E.M. Wigley as dean was entirely willing to continue with these commitments.

Dowling held his usual out-patient clinic once a week on a Monday morning, with the class of postgraduate students in attendance, but he was never very vocal, and it is doubtful if he had much effect on them. His clinical assistants and registrars, who were seeing the rest of the patients in his clinic, soon recognized his special way. When one took a problem case in to see him for advice on diagnosis or management, he would listen carefully and thoroughly, and perhaps ask an additional question or two. He would be wrapped in thought for a minute or so and would then turn to the registrar and say, 'Yes, it is difficult. What do you think about it?'

Only after the registrar had had his chance to shine would Dowling

either agree with him (if possible) or put forward an alternative suggestion in an apparently tentative manner, such as:

'Do you think it could be . . . ?' or

'Is there any possibility that it may be . . . disease?' or

'Do you think it is worth taking a biopsy, or looking for . . .
disease?'

Never was the registrar allowed to feel humiliated or deficient, and
the patient was always returned to the care of the registrar. At the end
of the morning, he always went to have lunch in the hospital canteen,
and the wise registrars went with him. He lingered over lunch, talking
dermatology with any of the registrars who wanted to stay, and almost
always the group at his table were the last to leave. He was never in a
hurry. It was the registrars who had to leave first, often after a third
telephone call from Sister Kelly in the clinic, demanding their presence
to return to work. Only then did Dowling leave to go to 21 Wimpole
Street to start his afternoon of private practice.

There was no formal plan for the training of registrars at St John's.
The consultants worked only one half-day per week, while the five
registrars were employed full-time by the hospital. It was entirely an
apprenticeship system. They simply got on with their work, and only
sought help from the consultant when they felt they needed it. For some
this was a rare event; self-confidence among registrars is a variable
commodity, but, since most of the senior registrars stayed there for
three or four years, there developed a camaraderie among them and the
juniors would frequently seek help from the more senior registrars.

Dowling's position as Director of the Institute provided him with
time, and he used it to make himself available, so that all the registrars
should have the opportunity to appreciate what he had to offer them.
And it was not only the registrars. Several of the non-medical staff also
recognized what was happening and saw the effect he was having. It
raised the prestige of the hospital, of which they felt proud. This was
especially true of Sister Kelly, in charge of the out-patient clinic, and
Albert Pellett, the head porter. Without being pressed they were willing
to do anything required of them. Dowling never gave an order or even
made any requests. All his wishes were indirectly transmitted through
the registrars.

One day, in August 1928, St John's Hospital acquired one of its
greatest assets and best investments. For it was in that year that Albert
Pellett joined the staff as head porter, and he retained the same position

throughout all the changing circumstances of the hospital until he died following a coronary occlusion in November 1965.

He rarely talked about his early years before, during and after the First World War, but they could not have been easy. He knew his way around Covent Garden market and all the tricks of the fruit and vegetable trade, and in addition made several valuable friends amongst the salesmen there. He also acquired an extensive knowledge of the catering trade when a waiter at the Holborn Restaurant, which was in its heyday in the twenties. This made him something of a connoisseur of food and wine, which in later years enabled him to give helpful advice to visiting doctors in their choice of restaurant for lunch or dinner. But these years included a period of unemployment, which, as in so many other instances, had a deep and lasting effect on Albert. When he first became head porter (at an unmentionable wage), he made a promise to himself, that he would never give any employer any possible reason or justification for firing him. And, of course, he never did. Instead he became the major-domo, the factotum of the hospital and, at the same time, the friend, confidant and Good Samaritan of all who worked in it, whether they be cleaners or consultants, secretaries or students. For Albert developed as great an affection for St John's as St John's developed for him. The hospital and the Institute will never have a more loyal fan and supporter, be its fortunes up or down. He lived through a period of great change, having served three different secretaries to the hospital and four deans of the Institute. He witnessed with pleasure the growth of the Institute and the establishment of new departments, as well as the increasing role of the hospital as the major meeting place and Alma Mater for successive generations of registrars. Albert knew the junior medical staff by their Christian names and followed their careers with a paternalistic interest, whether they be in London, in other parts of Britain or as far away as the Antipodes. Generations of ex-registrars sent him Christmas cards and never failed to call in to say 'hello' to Albert if they were in London.

Possibly because of the hardships of his own early years, he was all for youth. He was full of encouragement and help to the young and ambitious registrars, whom he appropriated as 'his boys', and would most tactfully give them paternal advice on such things as clothes, behaviour and hair-styles! The trust in him which was engendered in this way must have been gratifying. It was said that everyone had borrowed money from Albert (he always had it) but he never had a

single bad debt. There was indeed no limit to his generosity of spirit —
such as the time when the police were making a sweep down Lisle Street
(before the 1959 Act) against the 'ladies of easy virtue', and Albert gave
them all refuge in the basement of the hospital until the emergency was
over; or when a group of senior visitors came to inspect the vaccines
and sera in a refrigerator and a frozen turkey fell out!

Albert loved children, whether his own or anyone else's. Scores of
doctors entrusted their children (and sometimes their wives) to his care
while they were working, but few things gave him more pleasure in
later years than his own wonderful grandchildren. For, in spite of being
home only at the weekends, Albert was a strong family man.

It is not possible to record more than a few of Albert's numerous
activities 'beyond the call of duty', but he could and did perform any
emergency task. He willingly attended lectures and operated the pro-
jector; he served at the tea and coffee breaks at all the Institute's
courses; he frequently ran the staff canteen and on at least one occasion
he cooked and served a complete Christmas lunch for the whole staff.
But perhaps his best remembered activity was the excellent social
tea which he served before every meeting of our own Dermatological
Society.

Less well known to the staff were his relations with patients and the
Soho community. The patients were always a first priority with him.
Not surprisingly, he acquired a considerable knowledge of dermatology
and its largely empirical treatments — to such an extent that he is said
to have had one of the largest private practices in the area! But he knew
equally well when he or his patient needed a 'second opinion'. He was,
of course, very well known to all the shopkeepers, residents and other
people who lived or worked around the hospital. He lived in the
hospital basement throughout the whole of the Second World War and
was always a member of the local Fire Guard. His friendship with the
shopkeepers always enabled him to obtain goods in short supply, even
though he took the added precaution of keeping his own chickens in the
yard outside the dispensary.

Albert's strong qualities were his loyalty, his humility and his innate
common sense and cheerfulness, which latter characteristic was only
seen to be dimmed when he became seriously ill. He had never missed
a day at work through illness for more than 35 years, a fact that
merited special mention in the *London Evening Standard* when he was

admitted to the Middlesex Hospital. The society was fortunate indeed to have been served for a lifetime by Albert Pellett.

In 1952 St John's Hospital was able to open an in-patient department again, in part of the Eastern Fever Hospital at Homerton Grove in East London, nine miles from Leicester Square. They began with 16 beds, but gradually increased the number to 69 in four wards. The first research laboratories were opened there as well, with Arthur Tickner in biochemistry and Ian Magnus in photobiology.

Dowling went there for a ward round every Friday morning, accompanied by one of the senior registrars and a house physician. Again, his technique for a ward round was distinctive. He never stood at the front, as it were, as the group came to each bed. Imperceptibly, the senior registrar found himself at the front reciting the history of a new patient or giving a progress report on another. Dowling would examine some features pointed out to him or if he was asked his opinion on diagnosis or treatment or some other aspect of the case. It was all done to let the senior registrar feel that he and not Dowling was responsible for the patient's care. Never once did he give any instructions to the nurses about treatment or write anything in the patient's notes or on their treatment card. But he would ask the senior registrar how he was treating the patient. When told he simply nodded approval or, if he felt the patient would benefit appreciably from different medication, he would put out a suggestion in the form of a tentative enquiry such as:

'Have you ever found ... useful in patients like this?' or

'Do you think it would be of any value to add ... to his treatment?' or

'Would it be worth trying ... here?' or

'I have seen this condition improve with ... Have you ever used it?'

The suggestion was of course taken up and the treatment prescribed by the senior registrar, who would often be awarded the credit by the patient the following week.

The ward round of only 16 beds at Homerton did not, of course, fill the whole of Friday mornings. But Dowling was never in a hurry to rush off. The group would retire to the nurses' office for coffee and embark on dermatological talk for another hour or more. At these times Dowling never led the conversation, but he had an uncanny way of making others talk. He was such a good listener and appeared intensely interested in the opinions of the registrars, who were always keen to tell him about some unusual case they had seen, or their success in diagnosis or treatment, or of some important paper they had read in a journal. It must have been very similar to children coming home from school and telling their father or mother about the things they had done in class during the day, or of some experience they had had, or discoveries made, or jokes and stories heard (which they had themselves heard years before). It seems entirely natural now that in those years he was known as 'Daddy Dowling' among the registrars. It was not long before all the registrars at the hospital realized the benefits of these Friday mornings. So they arranged that only one of their number would remain in the out-patient clinic at Leicester Square, while the others went to spend the morning at Homerton.

It was about this time also that Dowling took over the care of patients at Goldie Leigh Hospital near Woolwich in South London. This hospital had been established in the nineteenth century for children with ringworm of the scalp. Scalp ringworm was regarded as a public health problem and a visible manifestation of the inadequacy of local government authorities to control infectious disease. There was no reliable treatment for the condition, but it was thought to remit spontaneously at the time of puberty. In Paris a residential hospital and school, the Hôpital et Ecole Lailler, was built to provide isolation and education for children with ringworm of the scalp up to the supposed time of remission at puberty. The Goldie Leigh Hospital was similar.

With the introduction of X-ray epilation, thallium and then griseofulvin treatment, in addition to public health measures, the number of patients steadily diminished. Instead of closure, the hospital was kept open and admitted children with severe chronic skin diseases for long-term care, such as epidermolysis bullosa, ichthyosiform erythroderma and severe eczema. Some of the children had been there for years.

Dowling visited the hospital every Thursday morning. One day he casually asked one of the senior registrars if he would be interested in seeing the children there with him. He offered a lift in his car because he was driving there from Wimpole Street. The registrar accepted and asked if he could come again next week.

'Yes, certainly, if you would find it interesting.'

And so it became a regular habit, a fixture. Few realized that this was Dowling's insidious way of making a registrar interested. The first such registrar was Robert Meara, who later succeeded Dowling as the consultant in charge of the patients at the Goldie Leigh Hospital. His interest was stimulated and his investigations under Dowling's guidance resulted in several publications, including papers on the relevance of skin tests in infantile eczema and the description of a special type of epidermolysis bullosa, now known as the Dowling–Meara type.

But most of the senior registrars had such an opportunity during their time at St John's Hospital, and the benefit was not only the chance to study the patients there. It was the unique advantage to travel by car alone with Dowling and spend the morning with him, talking dermatology, or on any other subject of his own choice. And there was also a long coffee break with Dr S. Cochrane Shanks, the radiologist and radiotherapist who had treated over 7000 children by X-ray epilation for ringworm of the scalp. Such mornings were more valuable and educative than any textbook.

Dowling's greatest influence on St John's Hospital, and the dozens of registrars and clinical assistants who attended it, must surely have been on Saturday mornings. In 1946 the registrars spent an hour from 6.30 to 7.30 pm on Friday evenings discussing a small number of special patients. It was the registrars' clinic, run by the registrars for the registrars. When he became director in 1951, Dowling suggested that it might be easier for them if the time was changed to 10.00 am on Saturday morning, and asked if they could arrange it with the hospital staff. Morale was high in the hospital, and the senior registrars had no difficulty in obtaining the co-operation of the nurses and of the porters to open the hospital. The name of the clinic changed imperceptibly from the registrars' meeting to the Saturday morning clinic, and so it continued up to the Lisle Street closure in 1990. Dowling had, of course, been invited (as the only consultant), having said that he merely wanted to be an observer. Although in the front row, he did not often speak. It was not his nature to assume any dominant role. He was always a man of few words. But, when he did speak, his words were always totally relevant and helpful in any problem. He was never inhibited from saying, 'I don't know,' and he never missed a single meeting.

His presence did, of course, change and enhance the status of the Saturday morning clinic. Gradually, most of the registrars from the other university departments in London attended whenever they were able, and, more importantly, they brought patients from their own hospitals for demonstration or for diagnostic and clinical help. As senior registrars became consultants, many continued to attend, encouraged by Dr Dowling, although the character of the clinic was never allowed to change from that of a registrars' meeting. Visitors from abroad sometimes attended; some were puzzled. Their comments afterwards would vary between extremes:

'Who is that old man who has nothing to say?'

'That man has more dermatology in his little finger than all the others in the room put together.'

When Dowling retired from the consultant staff in 1956, his attendance at the out-patient clinic, at the in-patient department at Homerton and at the Goldie Leigh Hospital all ceased. But he continued to come to every Saturday morning clinic for nearly 20 years.

One advantage of the change from Friday evenings to Saturday mornings was the opportunity to extend the discussion of patients. Several registrars would retire after the meeting to have coffee in a well-known coffee shop in Gerrard Street behind the hospital. It had been there since before the Second World War and, in the post-war years, was run by a Belgian manageress. It was mostly patronized by film and television people from Wardour Street (the London centre of the film world) and by the junior staff of St John's Hospital. Dowling always came over for coffee (often picking up the bill), where he stimulated further discussion of the patients. At these sessions he would also introduce further comment about interesting cases presented at the monthly meetings of the Royal Society of Medicine and the St John's Hospital Dermatological Society. Whatever the clock said, he was never other than the last to leave. Although everyone else was busy or pressed by the family and recreational demands of Saturday afternoons, he seemed to have all the time in the world to discuss dermatology.

The 25 years from 1951 to 1976 gave the trainee dermatologists in London who were able to make use of these opportunities the best possible clinical education. He shaped their ideas at a very formative stage in their careers, and his influence was the dominant one for an entire generation. It was an influence which persisted throughout their years as consultant dermatologists all over the country.

Dermatology like every other speciality was affected by the changes from clinical medicine to scientific medicine separated by the Second World War. It is not easy for present-day doctors to understand what it was like to practise medicine before the start of the so-called antibiotic– steroid era following the discoveries of penicillin in Britain and cortisone in America. The Institute of Dermatology naturally wanted to respond to the changes.

There was much discussion among the staff as to which spheres would be the most likely to benefit dermatology and should be developed at the Institute. The decision in committee was made to promote biochemistry and psychiatry. Whether Dowling supported this choice is uncertain. None of the staff had any special knowledge in these spheres, so it was something of a step in the dark, and none appeared to have any conception of the difficulties. But money was provided and appointments made. The experiment lasted perhaps 10 years, and the departments eventually closed.

About the same time, however, one of the consultants, Dr Arthur Porter, wanted to study skin diseases due to sunlight exposure. Dr Ian Magnus joined him and pursued the subject single-mindedly. With the help of a physicist, a monochromator instrument was built and proved most successful. An early reward was the discovery of a new but not uncommon disease, erythropoietic porphyria. Magnus developed this field relentlessly and established the department of photobiology, which soon attracted world-wide interest, and the subject is now a recognized subspeciality of dermatology.

Concurrently, Calnan and Meara, as senior registrars, became interested in allergic contact dermatitis and established a patch-testing clinic in 1953 on the lines of the clinic founded by Poul Bonnevie at the Finsen Institute in Copenhagen. It grew into the department of contact dermatitis and occupational dermatology, which also became a recognized subspecialty of dermatology. Both departments were encouraged to continue by the support of Geoffrey Dowling.

Quite separately, R.W. Riddell, a pathologist at the Brompton Hospital for Chest Diseases, started a mycology department, which has since flourished and grown in importance, partly as a result of the therapeutic advances in antibiotic, corticosteroid and immunosuppressive drugs.

But the most important development was histopathology. Walter Freudenthal came to London in 1939 as a refugee from Vienna. He was welcomed by Sir Archibald Gray and provided with a laboratory at University College Hospital. He started small teaching sessions in skin histology and Dowling was one of the first students. He realized its importance.

At St John's Hospital, H.M. Macleod and Isaac Muende were in charge of the small pathology laboratory and they had written a book on *Pathology of the Skin*, but it was on a small scale. Muende continued to supervise the hospital's histopathology until the introduction of the National Health Service in July 1948, when Dr John Oliver was appointed a full-time clinical pathologist. The hospital was fortunate to have the help of a clinical assistant, Dr Henry Haber.

Haber died tragically in Edinburgh during the annual meeting of the British Association of Dermatologists. His colleagues were bereft and stunned by their inability to foresee it, none more so than Geoffrey Dowling. At the funeral in London a few days later, the emotion was still intense and a numbed silence pervaded the atmosphere. The feeling was expressed in a letter from Dowling to Charles Calnan.

13 July 1962

Dear Charles,

I am glad you did not speak to me on Wednesday. I have never been so shaken at a funeral. Why was it so infinitely pathetic? I believe most of us tend to feel that if only we had known what was happening we might have done something helpful, but I believe that is quite wrong. There is something wickedly cruel about mental disorder. The victim is so utterly helpless and so is everyone.

I agree of course that Henry's name and work ought to be perpetuated, but I can't for the moment think of anything practical. Meanwhile Lunnon has taken a first rate picture of him, of which I borrowed a copy for the BMJ, and an enlarged copy in a big frame like Bloch's picture at Zurich would look well on the premises, at least I would think so. Wolf is thinking about how to perpetuate Henry.

Yours
GBD

Haber had started a weekly teaching session for the registrars on Friday evenings, and soon Dowling joined them, bringing with him his own registrars from St Thomas's Hospital. These sessions were followed by retirement for a beer to the Imperial public house in Leicester Street for further discussion, and Dowling was happy to remain at the bar as long as anyone wanted him to stay.

With Haber's sudden death in 1962, the role was soon filled

by Edward Wilson Jones, who built up the department and developed all the newer techniques of histochemistry (started by Dr George
Wells who had worked for three years with the great Stephen Rothman
in Chicago), immunopathology, electron microscopy and cytochem-
istry. Dermatopathology is now another recognized subspecialty of
dermatology.

In 1960 a major change took place when the University of London
decided to establish an academic department of dermatology at the
Institute, headed by a professor. This was only a short time after
the Ministry of Health had persuaded Dr J.T. Ingram to retire from
the General Infirmary at Leeds and become a full-time professor at
Newcastle upon Tyne, and to prepare the ground for an academic
university department there.

When the London University chair was advertised in *The Times*, the
consultant staff had great difficulty in making a choice. It had long been
felt that George Wells, after three years of intense academic life with
Stephen Rothman, was the most able and the best trained candidate. He
was a consultant at St Thomas's and St John's Hospitals and had his
own histochemistry laboratory, as well as being universally popular and
highly respected. Dowling had by then retired and had no influence. But
George Wells made it known at once that he had no wish to apply or
accept the position. He was the choice of the younger staff consultants,
Gold, Samman, Meara and Calnan. They conspired to take him to
dinner in the Cabin Room at Manzi's restaurant opposite the hospital,
and persuade him that it was his duty to accept for the sake of the
hospital and British dermatology. At the end of a long evening, Wells
relented and agreed to accept nomination if they wanted him to apply.
But long before dawn next day the 'conspirators' were individually
beset with remorse at having pressurized Wells against his will. One of
their number was deputed to express their apologies and release George
Wells from his undertaking, but they must have felt some shame in their
mistaken action.

In due time Charles Calnan was appointed to the chair. He had
recently returned from America, where he had worked with A.M.
Kligman at the Duhring Laboratories in Philadelphia. It was a major
research centre for dermatology, headed by Donald Pillsbury, Walter
Shelley and Albert Kligman. Calnan was able to familiarize himself with
the structure and needs of an academic department. He was fortunate
in appointing Dr Sam Shuster as his chief assistant. Shuster at once

embarked enthusiastically on experimental projects on acne, sweating, skin ageing, thermoregulation and cutaneous metabolism. The research laboratories developed rapidly and soon attracted registrars from Britain and abroad. Shuster's progress was meteoric and after three years he was appointed to succeed Professor John Ingram in the chair at Newcastle.

But by this time John Turk had arrived to build up a Medical Research Council-funded unit to study the pathology of cell-mediated immunity in skin diseases. He had been trained at the MRC laboratories at Mill Hill, where Professor Peter Medawar had established the basis of transplantation immunity, which was to win him and his colleagues a Nobel Prize.

Concurrently, Ian Magnus was expanding the photobiology and biochemistry departments. The achievements and publications from the basic science departments attracted much more attention and recognition than the Institute had ever had before. The American Specialty Board in Dermatology approved St John's Hospital as a suitable place for training for American residents in dermatology. By this time, there were full-time departments of genetics (R.S. Wells), mycology (Y.M. Clayton), microbiology (W.C. Noble), histopathology (E. Wilson Jones), photobiology and biochemistry (I.A. Magnus) and immunology (J.L. Turk), in addition to the laboratories of the professorial unit.

The establishment of such an academic unit was important in obtaining adequate financial support from public and private sources. In this regard, Dr Louis Forman was especially helpful; his friendship with the late Sir Herbert Dunhill and his daughter Mary Lane and their family was the initiative for the provision of research grants on many occasions. Through them a Herbert E. Dunhill Laboratory for electron-microscopy was opened; and the professorial unit was able to initiate research into microcirculation in the skin (T.J. Ryan) and hair and nail pathology (R.W.P. Dawber). This expansion of the academic environment inevitably brought a continuous stream of dermatologists for sabbatical leave, researchers for training in special fields, and even undergraduate medical students for elective periods of study. They included doctors from Japan, the United States, Central and South America, Eastern and Western Europe, the Middle East, India and Africa. An active vibrant community was maintained and morale was high.

Dermatology in London was no longer a Cinderella.

ST JOHN'S HOSPITAL
DERMATOLOGICAL SOCIETY

The following account was written by Mr R.C. Syms and was published in the *Transactions of the St John's Hospital Dermatological Society* (vol. 58, p. 139, 1972).

On 16 January 1912 the first meeting of the London Dermatological Society (later to become the St John's Hospital Dermatological Society) was held at St John's Hospital, which at that time was situated on the west side of Leicester Square.

The birth of the society was conceived out of a strongly felt need for such an institution or, perhaps more accurately, a need to replace a lost institution, for there had been two 'dermatological societies' meeting in London prior to this. The Dermatological Society of London, founded in 1882, was a small select body of some 20–30 members who met at the Medical Society of London and counted among its members such giants of the day as Radcliffe-Crocker and Colcott Fox. Also in existence at about this time was the Dermatological Society of Great Britain and Ireland, meeting at St John's Hospital. A far less selective body, it catered not only for specialists but for all those in general practice interested in dermatology.

At this time there were relatively few specialists who devoted themselves entirely to dermatology, and even they included venereology with their practice. Some of the consultants at St John's Hospital continued to a limited extent in general medicine, while registrars and clinical assistants were drawn from those in general practice as late as the 1930s. The senior registrar at St John's Hospital was paid a salary of £50 a year and was expected to rely on other sources of income. This was usually general practice, but among the clinical assistants in the 1930s were to be found a barrister, a deputy coroner and an army medical officer.

In 1907 the two existing societies merged to form the Section of Dermatology at the Royal Society of Medicine. This loss of the clinical meetings at St John's Hospital was not sufficiently compensated for by the section meetings and in the years that followed the wish to re-establish a society at the hospital grew in strength. The movement was sponsored principally by Drs

Morgan Dockerell, William Griffith and Knowsley Sibley, supported by other colleagues on the consultant staff of the hospital.

However, it was not until 5 December 1911 that those concerned met formally as a council to elect officers and formulate rules of a new society, which was to be called the London Dermatological Society. There were 56 prospective founder members and at this meeting Dr Morgan Dockerell was elected as the first president, Dr Griffith as the honorary secretary and Dr Knowsley Sibley as the honorary treasurer, an office he held until December 1937. The annual subscription for Fellows was to be 10 shillings, and 5 shillings for Associate Members, while Life Fellowship could be obtained for an initial payment of £5. Among several curiosities in the original rules was one that entitles Fellows to 'the use of the pathology facilities and prior claim on out-patient treatment and admission to the in-patient department for their patients'.

At the first meeting of the newly elected council on 9 January 1912, it was announced that the Earl of Chesterfield had agreed to become the Society's patron. A programme and arrangements for the first clinical meeting to be held on Tuesday, 16 January, were agreed: it is interesting to note that at this meeting the honorary treasurer announced that the funds amounted to £13.15s.0d. Twenty-six Fellows and seven visitors met for this first clinical meeting and were invited to inspect the X-ray department and the pathology laboratory. The first case to be shown on that day was one of dermatitis herpetiformis, and among others were smallpox scars treated by X-ray, alopecia treated by vaccine and superfluous hair treated by X-ray.

The social side of the society was apparently of some importance in these early years, for two items that got some priority in the council's discussions were the provision of refreshments at meetings and the holding of a dinner. In fact, the first dinner was held as early as 3 July 1912, at the Trocadero restaurant, and until 1927 three or four dinners were held each year!

Towards the end of 1912 there was a proposal that the Society should publish an annual report to include proceedings and in which to publish papers. It was agreed to proceed with this and at the April meeting in 1913 a draft copy of the first *Annual Report and Transactions of the London Dermatological Society* was placed before the council, together with an estimated cost of £18 for 200 copies. There was some further delay while the possibility of carrying advertisements was explored, and eventually 1000 copies were printed at a cost of £28.15s.od, the revenue from advertisements being £21. It is interesting to note that several members of the council promised to buy 20 or even 50 copies to enable the larger number to be printed.

One of the earlier Fellows of the society was Dr R. Prosser White, who, although in general practice, was profoundly interested in industrial diseases and had just founded the first skin department at the Royal Infirmary, Wigan. He was one of the earlier presidents of the Society (1920–1923) and in 1921 founded and endowed an annual oration.

In 1924 the Society changed its name to the St John's Hospital Dermatological Society and, although legally it was a new Society, all rules, procedures and activities continued unaltered. These included the endowed annual oration, which, upon the death of Dr Prosser White in 1934, was to become the Prosser White Annual Oration. The first of these in 1935 was held at the Royal Society of Medicine in the West Hall, and the president and members of the Section of Dermatology were invited.

By the early 1930s the Society was increasing rapidly both in membership and popularity, some 50–60 Fellows gathering at the hospital each month for the clinical meetings, and they were often hosts to distinguished personalities from abroad as visitors or as annual orators. Among the orators of those times were such names as Prof. Oppenheim from Vienna, Prof. Haxthausen from Copenhagen, Dr Allen Pusey from Chicago and from the United Kingdom Sir Humphrey Rolleston, Lord Horder and Prof. Sir Leonard Hill.

The clinical meetings were held in the large consulting-room at the hospital in Leicester Square and the procedure at these meetings is worth mentioning. The 50 or so Fellows were seated along three sides of the square room, while the president occupied a table in the centre of the fourth side. Each case would be brought in by the out-patient sister and deposited on a centrally placed chair. Whoever was showing the patient would give a brief introduction to his 'exhibit' and the president would leave his chair and carry out his own examination of the patient. His return to his chair was a signal for a rather undignified stampede by those seated on the other three sides. The patient disappeared in a seething mass of Fellows grateful for obtaining even a few square inches of the patient to look upon, touch or palpate. At a signal from the president there would be a rather reluctant retreat, the slower and less agile Fellows having probably seen very little of the patient. Sister would then collect the often very hot-and-bothered patient, together with any odd garments lost in the affray, and the discussion of the case would then take place.

When in 1936 the hospital moved to Lisle Street, the procedure at meetings went through a radical change. Instead of one large consulting-room, there were three smaller ones, none of which was large enough to house the meetings. The pathologist, Dr I. Muende, had been elected honorary secretary in 1934 and, with his co-operation, the patients were exhibited in the main clinical laboratory, either singly or in groups of two or three behind screens, and in the cubicles and biopsy room. Based on the procedure used at the Royal Society of Medicine Section meeting, patients could be examined more leisurely, and at 5 pm the Fellows gathered in the adjacent lecture room for the discussion and for the reading of papers. This new arrangement was welcomed by all concerned, not least of whom to benefit was the patient!

At the St John's Society meetings, junior medical staff were encouraged to show cases on behalf of their chiefs and to take part in discussion, both of which they were reluctant to do in the more formal atmosphere at the Royal Society of Medicine meetings. Towards the end of the 1930s, all seemed set fair for a rosy future. The new arrangements attracted a greater and more enthusiastic attendance, finances were improving and the status of the Society was being accepted all round. This might well be illustrated by a Council minute of that time: 'that the Hospital Board of Management be asked to change the day of its monthly meetings as they clashed with the Society's meeting days'!

However, the war came in 1939 and on 25 October of that year the council met and suspended all activities until further notice. But for a brief meeting of the council in June 1940 to deal with financial matters, no further meetings were held until 1947.

On Wednesday, 26 March 1947, the council met to make arrangements for the resumption of meetings. It was agreed that the same arrangements for meetings would continue, but that they would take place on the first Thursday of each month and that the council would meet immediately prior to each ordinary meeting. Within a few months, the pre-war popularity of the clinical meetings had returned and by 1949 the congestion in the pathology laboratory, together with the increase in the work of that department, made it impossible to continue showing the patients there. Several alternative arrangements were tried but in 1950 the demonstration of clinical cases returned, perhaps quite naturally, to the out-patient clinic. Patients continued to be shown separately in cubicles and behind screens and, when later the new enlarged out-patient department, was built much more room was available and the meetings took the form in which they are conducted today.

The number of Fellows both at home and overseas had steadily increased year by year and the attendance at the clinical meetings is now such that the areas in which they are held are at times uncomfortably overcrowded.

When St John's Hospital in Lisle Street, Leicester Square, closed in 1990 and reopened as the Saint John's Dermatology Centre in St Thomas's Hospital, the regular meetings of the Society continued as before on the first Thursday of the month. The 510th meeting of the society was held in June 1991. There is now an annual symposium held in April, in addition to the Prosser White Oration followed by a dinner. The total membership of the Society in 1991 is more than 200.

The Society originally published its *Transactions* once a year. In 1954 it became biannual, when Charles Calnan took over the editorship from Stephen Gold, and the size of the journal was greatly expanded. With support from American dermatologists and pharmaceutical companies, the circulation rose to more than 2000. In 1974 Calnan handed over the editorship to Martin Black. Two years later the *Transactions* were incorporated into a new journal, *Clinical and Experimental Dermatology*, which is published six times a year, with a large circulation.

In 1991 the Society inaugurated a prize, to perpetuate the memory of Dr Louis Forman (Dowling's first registrar and his successor at Guy's Hospital). He was an outstanding dermatologist and continued the great tradition of Guy's as a leading educational and research centre. Following the work of E.J. Moynihan and R.S. Wells, it now has its first full-time professor, R.J. Hay, whose special interest is in mycology and microbiology of skin diseases. The Louis Forman Prizes are for the best published work by a senior registrar and a registrar, with an initial value of £500 and £250.

G.B. Dowling was president of the Society in 1951, when Professor Holger Haxthausen gave the oration, entitled 'How are dermatological diagnoses made?' It was a brilliant exposition of the morphologist's art and the use of the 'dermatological eye'. Surely, every dermatologist should read this at an early stage in his training.

In 1971 Dr Dowling celebrated his eightieth birthday. The *Transactions of the St John's Hospital Dermatological Society* published a Festschrift for the event. This special volume of the *Transactions* carried the following introductory editorial:

> If anyone feels he would like to make friends and influence people, he could be given no better advice than to get to know Dr Geoffrey Dowling; for he has made more friends and influenced more people in dermatology in Britain than any of his predecessors, perhaps ever since Willan founded the subject as a specialty here.
>
> Like Winston Churchill Dr Dowling received his call from the country relatively late in life. He was over sixty when he was asked to take on the part-time Directorship of the newly formed Institute of Dermatology, and to assume responsibility for charting a new course in dermatological teaching and research for Britain. Perhaps his age and experience were an advantage. He could clearly see what needed to be done. All he required was the will and the energy to do it. And fortunately for all of us he was not found lacking in either of these attributes. The task was not an easy one. He saw the introduction of the National Health Service as a help and not a hindrance to his plans, for in an unexpected way it provided the time as well as the facilities for postgraduate education. But the ingredient in shortest supply then, as it still is more than twenty years later, was the

consultant's time. Time is our most expensive commodity. Of his own time Dr Dowling could not have given more lavishly. Generation after generation of registrars, now scattered over Canada, Australia, New Zealand and South Africa as well as all over Britain took liberal helpings of his time while at St John's Hospital. In return they gave him their most valuable commodity, namely, their friendship; and now, on his eightieth birthday this will surely be the possession which he prizes most.

This birthday volume of the *Transactions* is dedicated to our man — Our Man for All Seasons — not only by the contributors to it but by the St John's Hospital Dermatological Society, of which he has been such a staunch supporter, and all its members both at home and overseas. We offer him our very best wishes on a festive occasion and sincerely hope that we shall continue to see him at all our Meetings for many years to come.

The *British Journal of Dermatology* also published a commemorative Festscrift for the occasion. It was arranged and edited by Dr George Findlay of Pretoria, and all the papers contributed came from departments in South Africa.

APPENDIX I
THE ROYAL SOCIETY OF MEDICINE DOWLING ENDOWMENT FUND

Regulations for its administration

1   The fund shall be known as the Dowling Endowment Fund of the Royal Society of Medicine. It shall be formed by the investment in Trustee Securities, which may include the Charities Official Investment Fund, of the sum of £1000 given to the Society in 1970, together with such other funds as may be added to it from time to time by the Council of the Society on the recommendation of the Council of the Section of Dermatology, or by appeal, or from other sources. All expenses necessarily incurred in establishing or augmenting the Fund shall be a first charge upon the capital of the Fund.

2   The object of the Fund shall be advancement of the science of dermatology.

3   It shall be incumbent on the Council of the Section of Dermatology to make such recommendations for any awards to be provided from the income of the fund, which shall require the approval of the Council of the Society, as will, in their opinion, act as an incentive to the production of, and the dissemination of information about, original work in dermatology, and to the constructive

interchange of knowledge both at home and abroad. The two Councils shall also give effect to the founders' wish that the income of the Fund shall be used at least in part for the encouragement of young practitioners and research workers in the field.

4   The income of the Fund shall be applied in the following manner:

(a)   A sum not exceeding 10% of the total may be used by the Society to cover the administrative cost of the Fund.

(b)   When the income is sufficient, a minimum sum of £50 per annum shall be set aside to provide an honorarium for a lecturer, the Dowling lecturer, to be appointed from time to time to deliver a lecture on a dermatological subject, or a subject related to dermatology. The lecture may be given in the Society's house or elsewhere.

(c)   On the advice of the Council of the Section of Dermatology and at the discretion of the Honorary Treasurers, a grant may be made to the lecturer for travelling expenses.

(d)   When the accumulated income allows, awards may be made from time to time to British dermatologists for travelling expenses for visits in this country or abroad, with the intention of furthering the study or advancement of dermatology.

(e)   Any income surplus to the foregoing may be applied by the Council of the Society upon the recommendation of the Council of the Section of Dermatology in any manner consistent with the object of the Dowling Endowment Fund which may include adding all or part of such surplus income to the capital of the Fund.

5   All lecturers shall be appointed, and all travelling expenses awarded, by the Council of the Society on the recommendation of the Council of the Section of Dermatology.

6   There will be a Committee of five, all elected annually, two of whom shall be appointed by the Council of the Society, two by the Council of the Section of Dermatology, and the President of the Section of Dermatology ex officio. They shall have the power to co-opt, and shall meet in November or December of each year to receive a statement about the financial state of the Fund, and to make such recommendations to the Council of the Section as will enable them to take action required in 4(b), (c), (d) and (e) above.

Additional meetings of the Committee may be held to consider applications for travelling expenses accumulating during the year, and to make supplementary recommendations to the Council of the Section.

Dowling Endowment Awards

1976	Dr D.M. MacDonald	St John's Hospital for Diseases of the Skin
1977	Dr R.J.G. Rycroft	St John's Hospital for Diseases of the Skin

1978	Dr D.J. Atherton	Guy's Hospital
1979	Dr R.D.R. Camp	St John's Hospital for Diseases of the Skin
1980	Dr S.M. Breathnach	St John's Hospital for Diseases of the Skin
1981	Dr R. Holmes	St Thomas's Hospital
1982	Dr R. Graham-Brown	Royal Free Hospital
1983	Dr R.H. Meyrick Thomas	St Bartholomew's Hospital
1984	Dr J.J. Horton	Guy's Hospital
1985	Dr M. Muhlemann	Charing Cross Hospital
	Dr S. White	Western Infirmary, Glasgow
1986	Dr R. Lever	Western Infirmary, Glasgow
1987	Dr M. Rademaker	Royal Infirmary, Glasgow
1988	Dr P.D.L. Maurice	Charing Cross Hospital
1989	Dr B. Bittner	Royal Hallamshire Hospital, Sheffield

APPENDIX II
THE DOWLING TRAVELLING FELLOWSHIP

At a meeting of the Executive Committee of the British Association of Dermatologists on 16 January 1964, the treasurer, Professor J.T. Ingram, proposed that the association should award a Fellowship every three years to enable a junior consultant, senior registrar or registrar to spend a period of time in study and/or research abroad.

The proposal was accepted and it was to be known as the Dowling Fellowship, in honour of Dr Geoffrey Barrow Dowling. The Fellow is elected by a subcommittee consisting of the president, secretary, two members of the association and a non-dermatological assessor.

Regulations for the Fellowship were drawn up and the first holder was appointed in 1965. The value of the Fellowship has been gradually increased by the association and is now £10,000. Later it was awarded every two years, and now annually.

The past holders of the Dowling Fellowship have been:

1965	Dr E. Wilson Jones	1985	Dr P.S. Friedman
1968	No award	1986	Dr C.B. Archer
1971	Dr M.M. Black	1987	Dr C.E.M. Griffiths
1974	Dr E. Abell	1988	Dr J. Barker
1977	Dr R.J.G. Rycroft	1989	No award
1980	Dr S.M. Breathnach	1990	Dr N. Reynolds
1983	Dr C.A. Holden		

Chapter 11
The Dowling Club

THE FOLLOWING account of the Dowling Club up to 1970 was written by Hugh Wallace and published in the *Transactions of the Saint John's Hospital Dermatological Society* in 1971. It was compiled from the notes handwritten on 23 pages of airmail paper by Dowling himself — his memory was evidently better than Wallace's! These notes contained a number of additional brief and cryptic comments.

In the years immediately following the Second World War there gathered at St Thomas's Hospital a group of enthusiastic embryo dermatologists, later to take their place among the leaders of dermatology in the United Kingdom. They included Martin Beare, Hugh Calvert, Geoffrey Hodgson, Arthur Rook, John Simpson, Douglas Sweet, Darrell Wilkinson, Eric Waddington and George Wells; and they were soon joined by Geoffrey Beck, Robert Bowers, Kenneth Crow, Oliver Scott and Ian Whimster. The magnet was Geoffrey Dowling, soon to become known affectionately as the Headmaster, whose clarity of thought and critical faculty, particularly in questioning long-held dermatological shibboleths, was equalled by his kindness, his inestimable enthusiasm and his perennial youth.

Amongst such a group the formation of a journal club was probably inevitable and, although it came into being by apparently spontaneous generation, its true parenthood was never in doubt. The first meeting was held in October 1946 in the surgical out-patient department at St Thomas's Hospital. The club soon decided to meet monthly and gladly accepted a suggestion from Dr Dowling, who had in mind the then flourishing journal club of Guy's Hospital, that discussion of the journals should be preceded by a simple dinner. Over the next few months we dined at various hostelries, amongst which the Antelope in Eaton Terrace figured prominently, afterwards repairing for discussion of the journals to St Thomas's where, through the kindness of the resident assistant surgeon, we were soon able to exchange the rather unsalubrious surroundings of the surgical out-patient department for a room in the residents' quarters. The disadvantages of this spatial dichotomy between refreshment of the body and of the mind were obvious, and in the spring of 1947, and again prompted by the founder's connection with Guy's, the club moved to the historic, and at that time unsophisticated, George Inn at Southwark. Here, for a time, the dining-room sufficed for dinner and the discussion of journals, the latter occasionally arousing slight but well-disciplined interest amongst the few other lay diners. The club owes much to the proprietors of the George Inn for their help on so many occasions, not least in the early days, when excellent meals were provided in spite of strict food rationing. Here the club continued to meet at monthly intervals from October to June.

For centuries London Bridge was the only crossing point of the Thames into the City of London, and Southwark, which grew up at the southern end of the bridge, owed much of its importance to its strategic position. Its High Street was also the main thoroughfare into London from the southern counties and the Continent. Southwark was both a suburb of the City and a market town in its own right, and for much of its history there was conflict between the City and the local authorities. One frequent bone of contention was the question of who had the right to license the town's inns and alehouses.

Much of Southwark's prosperity depended on the goods and travellers using the highway. Many carriers and country folk bringing provisions to London found it more convenient and economic to transact their business in Southwark. Travellers to and from the City frequently found it convenient to stay overnight in Southwark.

Outside the tight control of City jurisdiction, it was also a refuge for anyone in trouble with the law and a magnet for the pleasure seeker, who could enjoy the Bankside theatres, such as the Globe and the Rose, the brothels, shady inns or alehouses. The market and annual fair, though vital to the prosperity of Southwark, only added to the town's reputation for unruly goings-on.

The George Inn was already well established in the reign of

Henry VIII. The stage-coach service from the George Inn — from London to Brighton — was started in 1732, but its role deteriorated with the growth of the railways when London Bridge station opened in 1844.

As a child Charles Dickens walked from Camden Town to Southwark every Sunday to visit his father in Marshalsea Prison. He mentioned it in *Little Dorrit* when young 'Tip goes into the George to write begging letters'. His descriptions in *Pickwick Papers* of the tap, bedrooms and inn yard could well apply to the George, and coachmen not so different from Sam Weller frequented the George.

Among the clubs and societies that met there were the Selbourne Society, the Cult of London, the Shakespeare Society, the Dickensian Fellowship and the Ballam Antiquities and National History Society. The Tabard Players and other groups used the courtyard for open-air plays, and several eminent people enjoyed a visit, among them Winston Churchill, who brought his own port, only to be charged 1s/6d corkage.

In 1937 the George was taken over by the National Trust, and the lease was given to the Flowers brewery of Stratford-upon-Avon. In 1962 Flowers brewery was taken over by Whitbread brewery, who are the present owners and will maintain its historic tradition.

Dowling's dermatology group soon became known as the George Club, whose fame spread rapidly. It was characteristic of its parenthood that it should be open to all young bona fide dermatologists, preferably below the rank of consultant. Another characteristic of its parenthood was that it was devoid of any form of organization and, although with the increased membership some minor rules had to be introduced, it still retains an informal and relaxed atmosphere.

The dinners at the George Inn were important. Dowling knew innately that people who eat together work together. He never missed a single meeting. It was no accident that, whatever the pressure of work, he was always the first to arrive and was at the bar with a glass of beer in his hand to welcome the registrars as they came in. Initially the cost of the dinner was five shillings (or 25 new pence), but prices escalated gradually with inflation. In the early years the waitresses (in their attractive Dickensian dress) simply cleared the tables when dinner was finished, and the discussion of journals began. In later years a refurbished panelled dining-room upstairs was made available. It provided space for the larger numbers and some privacy from other diners at the inn. As the economic climate for the registrars improved, wine would replace beer at dinner; and later still, almost unnoticed, two decanters of port appeared on the table after dinner, with scarcely anyone realizing that this was not included in the price of the dinner, but had been unobtrusively settled by Dowling at the bar.

The first to arrive, he always seemed the last to leave. He remained as long as any of the registrars wanted to talk to him.

In retrospect it again seems obvious that the club would sooner or later wish to visit dermatological centres abroad, and particularly the famous clinics on the continent of Europe. Time occasionally lays its hand on memory but the writer vividly recalls how he was privileged to take part in the conception, gestation and delivery of this now famous travelling club, all accomplished within two minutes in the staffroom lavatory at St Thomas's Hospital. The difficulties were formidable. Most Continental clinics had suffered grievously during the war and contact with many had been lost for some years. Equally formidable was the problem of monetary exchange control. Nevertheless, in 1948 the Club, which for fiscal reasons had given itself the temporary eponym of the London Dermatological Travelling Club, was able to make its first visit abroad to the famous Hôpital Saint Louis in Paris. The Club may well count itself fortunate to have begun its travels in such happy circumstances, and to be invited on a second occasion in 1952 at the time of the Franco-British reunion.

In 1949 Professors Haxthausen and Lomholt invited us to Copenhagen. Both were world figures in dermatology, Lomholt for his great contribution to the Finsen Institute and Haxthausen for being one of the earliest and certainly among the most distinguished exponents of the experimental method in the investigation of skin disorders. His monograph on *Cold in relation to the Skin* has long been a dermatological classic. In Copenhagen as in many other Continental clinics the ample space allotted to dermatology in contrast to its paucity in the

United Kingdom was striking and for many a considerable stimulus. The professional and social hospitality was incomparable. For the writer and his friends the outstanding social recollection was a dinner given by Professor and Mrs Haxthausen, after which Dr Dowling demonstrated the incomparable breadth of his inspiring talent as well as his sheer joy of being in good company by drinking a glass of beer whilst standing on his head. This was followed by Professor Haxthausen giving his equally famous impersonation of an anxious seal and later his piano recital of the overture from Tannhauser, accomplished solely by dextrous movement of a hairbrush on the keyboard. We were privileged to receive another invitation to visit Copenhagen in 1970, to be entertained with equal friendliness, hospitality and professional distinction by Professors Asboe Hansen, Holger Brodthagen and Niels Hjorth.

1950 was memorable for a visit to Belgium, there to be regaled by Professor (then Dr) Dupont at Namur and Professor Lapière at Liège, together with their colleagues, including Professor (then Dr) Pierard. We were also invited to participate in a meeting of the Belgian Dermatological Society and many lasting friendships were made. In the following year we received an invitation to the Netherlands and were cordially entertained by Professors Praaken, Siemens and Zoon in Amsterdam, Leiden and Utrecht. We were impressed by the high professional standard in all these clinics and the visit was also notable for the common interests discovered between ourselves and our hosts, particularly between Dr Dowling and Professor Zoon. Many of our journeys abroad have become cherished memories for incidents not immediately relevant to the purpose of the visit, and so it was in Holland where some members openly expressed a wish to remain indefinitely in the beautiful city of Leiden. The Club was privileged to be invited again to the Netherlands in 1964 where we received an equally warm welcome. Our hosts on this occasion were Professors Praaken, Jansen and Mali in Amsterdam, Utrecht and Nijmegen and Professor Craps in Brussels. We were again impressed with the continuing high standards of clinical care, which were now matched by an equal enthusiasm and skill in experimental studies.

West Germany was visited in 1952 at the invitation of Professor Alfred Marchionini at Munich and Professor Oscar Gans at Frankfurt. In 1953 a very enjoyable expedition to Italy included visits to Milan, Pavia and Venice (including a wonderfully elegant dinner at the Hotel Bauer Grünwald) where the beauty of the environment was a great distraction for the dermatologically less industrious. We were generously entertained professionally and socially by Professors Crosti, Falchi and Flarer and Professor (then Dr) Serri, all of whom were most generous to us in their clinics and in social hospitality. One of the highlights of this visit was a joint meeting with dermatologists of northern Italy under the admirable and memorable chairmanship of Professor Serri.

In 1955 we were invited to Lyon, France, there to be welcomed by Professor Gaté with inimitable enthusiasm and charm, admirably supported by his family and colleagues. The excellent clinical fare and the guided tours of this historic city were surpassed only by the Lyonnaise cuisine so generously provided. The weather was beautiful and the high spot was a banquet, where the menu held the British housewives enraptured with admiration and envy. Not for the first time the Lyonnais were determined to show that they had few equals in the field of gastronomy, and would yield nothing to Paris or Strasbourg. This visit was also notable for the eccentric method of transport and equally eccentric dress adopted by a young member, now a world-famous dermatologist. In the following year we journeyed to Basle at the invitation of Professor Schuppli and to Zurich at the invitation of Professors Miescher and Burckhardt. We greatly admired the high standard and industry achieved in their magnificent clinics. Social hospitality was of the highest order, marred for the writer only by the wilful ignorance of some of his colleagues in misinterpreting the message conveyed by the charming flags displayed on Professor Burckhardt's lakeside house.

We did not go abroad in 1957 owing to the International Congress at Stockholm. In 1958 the Club was invited to join the reunion of the French and British Dermatology Association in Nantes. Professor Bureau's enthusiasm and friendliness, the excellence of the clinical presentations, the social expeditions and the cuisine made this a highly successful visit.

In 1959 we visited Vienna and Zagreb. In Vienna we were
generously entertained by Professor Tappeiner and Dr Riehl, and
were accorded a reception by the Lord Mayor. Zagreb afforded
the privilege of meeting one of the greatest dermatologists of his
generation, Professor Kogoj. His kindness and modesty made
us all captive, and it is pleasant to record that although he
has retired from his professional duties his researches continue
unabated.

An invitation in 1960 to Barcelona appeared to some motoring
members to call for a Monte Carlo rally, but happily all arrived
safely. The high clinical standard and the enthusiasm, friendliness and hospitality of Professor Xavier Vilanova, his family
and colleagues remain an abiding memory. His early death was a
great loss to his many friends. Our subsequent visits to Poland
and East and West Berlin in 1961, to Hungary in 1963, to
Sweden in 1965 and to South Africa in 1969 have been so
admirably described in the *Transactions of the St John's Hospital
Dermatological Society* (vols 47, p. 108; 50, p. 166; 52, p. 283;
55, p. 229) that no detailed comment is required. All these visits
proved memorable and in all we were most generously received.

We were delighted to receive another invitation to Sweden
in 1970 during our visit to Denmark, on this occasion to visit
Lund and Malmo at the invitation of Professors Hagerman
and Magnusson, who, with their colleagues, received us most
generously. We were very impressed with the clinical and experimental work in both centres. At Malmo we were privileged to
hear a paper by Dr Waldenstrom on the mechanism of flushing.
He gave further pleasure by expressing his admiration for
Dr Dowling, whose clinic at St Thomas's he had visited before
the war.

The visit in 1969 to South Africa, with a short stop at
Kampala, Uganda, merits special attention since this was the
first time the Club had journeyed outside Europe, and incidently
the first time in which the latent broadcasting talent of some
members declared itself so admirably. Dr Dowling was born and
spent his childhood in South Africa, and this was but his second
visit since his early days. That he should have made this journey
at the head of his Club seemed particularly fitting.

We have journeyed far and wide and a detailed description

of all we have experienced would fill a complete journal. Our indebtedness to our hosts in many lands is beyond compare, and here the writer particularly craves forgiveness for defects in memory and muse in this short account. For successive generations of younger members of the Club, appointment to consultant status has usually meant an end to their monthly visits to the George Inn and for these and for a few other highly privileged consultants the travelling activities have afforded a very popular reunion. What have we gained from our travels and what have we been able to contribute? Recollections there are plenty whenever past journeys are discussed, whether they be of Dr Dowling's fantastic mental and physical stamina; or of a young member, now eminent, braving the nightclubs of Copenhagen and returning with a present for his wife; or of the equally unhappy and undernourished member who, on the first visit to France, had to leave a sumptuous dinner prematurely, suffering from a surfeit of delicious food and not, as some of his unkind colleagues suggested, from an excess of the equally delicious wines.

Professionally our gains have been so great and so numerous that any selection is arbitrary. For some the highlights may have been the privilege of meeting such brilliant and contrasting figures as Gougerot and Haxthausen, Civatte and Lomholt, Tzanck and Zoon, or of experiencing the contrasting styles in brilliant exposition of Degos at the Hôpital St Louis, or of Kogoj at Zagreb. For others it may have been the recent and very successful development of experimental techniques, particularly in the Netherlands and Scandinavia. The relative incidence of skin disease in different countries has engaged our attention and we have been able to acquaint ourselves with disorders that are seldom, if ever, found in the United Kingdom. Our biggest gain, however, has unquestionably been the acquisition of so many and lasting friendships. We cannot hope to repay more than a fraction of our indebtedness to our hosts in many lands and are proud that many have consented to become honorary members of the Club. We have been able to entertain all too few in the United Kingdom and look forward to entertaining others for whom a visit to our country has not yet been possible.

In 1953 Dr Alice Carleton invited the Club to Oxford and so began a continuing series of visits to centres in the United

Kingdom, which have included Belfast, Birmingham, Brighton, Bristol, Cambridge, Cardiff, Coventry, Dartford, Derby, Edinburgh, Gloucester, Guildford, High Wycombe, Ipswich, Kingston upon Thames, Lincoln, Manchester, Newcastle upon Tyne, Northampton, Plymouth, Reading, Rochester, Rhyl, Sheffield, Southampton, Stoke-on-Trent, Truro and Winchester, together with a visit in 1968 to Eire at the invitation of our old friend Dr Donal Buckley in Cork. With increasing membership of the Club, these visits became almost an invasion, and the Club owes much to our hosts, who have never failed to provide us with excellent professional and social fare.

1956 was a very significant year in the history of the Club. In that year, to honour our founder and to mark his alleged partial retirement, the George Club was renamed the Dowling Club and an annual oration followed by a dinner was established. Without exception these orations and dinners have been of the highest order. Most of the orations have been concerned with original observations and have acquired an international reputation. Many still remain as standard references in print.

The monthly dinner and discussions of journals have continued to flourish and have long been an integral part of the professional and social life of dermatological registrars working in the Greater London area, including several from overseas. By its various activities, the Club has become an integral part of dermatology in the United Kingdom. Happily, it continues to prosper and expand and now has a membership of over 130, including members from most European countries, North and South America, Australia and New Zealand. What has been the secret of the Club's continued success? First and foremost there has been the never failing encouragement of Dr Dowling. To this must be added the zeal of successive presidents and secretaries, to whom the Club is deeply indebted, and last but not least the enthusiasm of its members. What of the future? This year (1970) we hope to visit Beirut in May at the invitation of Professor Amal Kurban, and later in the year to visit Liverpool and Belfast.

Success and an increasing membership are not without their difficulties, and here the essential tenet of the Club, so diligently advocated on all occasions by Dr Dowling continues to be sustained, namely that the interests of the younger members must always be paramount. Thus on visits abroad the most generous hosts could not entertain more than a fifth of the Club's 130 members, and priority is rightly given to our younger colleagues. Thanks to the initiative of a recent president of the Club, Dr R.S. Wells, a highly successful Dowling Fund has been formed, to which the members of the Club have contributed very generously. The income from the fund will ensure the perpetuation of an annual Dowling Lecture and it is hoped to use any unexpected income to facilitate exchange visits for young dermatologists in this country and abroad.

Generations of dermatologists have wondered about the origins of the Dowling Club, and whether they were any different from those of many other journal clubs. They certainly were, but few people realized it.

Dowling's childhood and young adult years were responsible for impregnating his mind with very strong feelings on friendship and personal relationships. He had known loneliness and valued friends intensely. He enjoyed almost all forms of social intercourse, and had the facility to be at ease with almost anyone.

When he moved from Guy's to St Thomas's Hospital he was surprised by the thinly veiled, deprecating attitude, if not hostility, from his new colleagues in other specialities. There was no senior colleague like Harold Barber to defend dermatology at St Thomas's. He was on his own. He had to represent his subject of dermatology before his hospital colleagues. In addition, over the next few years, as a young consultant he became aware of divisions in the medical profession between different groups in particular specialities. There still existed subgroups within each specialty, usually based on a particular university or academic centre, often led by a professor or chief with a powerful and dominant personality. Medicine at the time was not in a stage of great scientific progress, and most medical education came 'ex cathedra' from leading teachers of the day. Such teachers naturally collected acolytes around them, who became disciples and propagated their professors' ideas on the particular specialty.

Although such a system might be seen to make for a healthy atmosphere of rivalry and competition, it could also result in envy, jealousy and hostility. This would be exacerbated by the fact that doctors in training rarely went from one centre to another. Such a pattern is still the norm in much of Europe and some other countries, where it is not easy to move from one university centre to another. Dowling was thus very conscious of rivalries among groups and pupils of dermatologists in the various teaching centres in Britain, just as he saw it in other specialities. In his view it was a harmful trend.

He found his remedy in the journal club. His idea was to copy the Guy's Hospital journal meetings, which were very successful in the years around 1945–1946. They were held initially at the Cheshire Cheese public house in Crutched Friars, and later at others. But they gradually lapsed, possibly because they included physicians, surgeons and pathologists — with interests which were too disparate. But it gave Dowling the idea, and he started monthly meetings with five or six registrars in dermatology.

By 1946 he foresaw the advent of the National Health Service and there were many young doctors being demobilized from the armed services who were keen to train in dermatology. He quickly made it clear that entry to the journal club was limited to registrars. In 1951 when he became director of the Institute of Dermatology he had contact with many more registrars. Being such an astute observer of human nature he soon got to know their names and assessed their abilities; and in turn they found he was approachable and receptive to requests for help.

His obsessional fear of power made him determine the rules of the club. There were to be none. At meetings he never took the chair himself. There were always a new president and secretary elected annually. The election of these 'officers' and new members was also uniquely Dowlingesque. Towards the end of his year the president would ask Dowling who should be the next President.

'Who do you suggest?' he always replied.

'Well I think Doctor Z at . . . Hospital would be very good.'

'Fine. Why don't you ask him and see if he would be willing to do it?'

And of course 'he' always was willing. It was the same with the selection of new members. In the early years it was almost always a result of Dowling chatting with some members and the president and secretary in the bar at a pub. He would say:

'Doctor Y, in the department at . . . Hospital seems a keen chap. He showed a very good case at the Royal Society of Medicine last month.

What do you think of him? Do you think he would like to come to our meetings?'

'Yes, he is very good. I know him quite well.'

'Good. Would you like to invite him then and see if he would be interested in joining us?'

And he did! There was never any voting at the meetings or formal election. In this way, slowly but gradually, the numbers increased, so that all the serious and career registrars in dermatology were incorporated, and, because each new member was known to be Dowling's choice, any reluctance or unfavourable opinion from the members was overcome. On a few occasions, if he detected any coolness about his suggestion, he would say:

'Well, he (Doctor X) only recently started in dermatology. Perhaps we should wait a little.'

But after a few months he would bring up the name again and make some favourable comment on Doctor X. And this time he would find agreement.

No members ever resigned or were asked to resign. As the senior registrars moved on to consultant appointments in London or other parts of the country, they would find it difficult to attend the monthly meetings, and so there was room for new members. In this way he slowly but surely achieved his unspoken plan to incorporate all the registrars at the hospitals in London. Trainees and research workers from European and overseas countries were treated in the same way, and introduced into the dermatological community.

When the members of the Club were invited to a dermatological meeting at a department outside London, Dowling would propose that the dermatologists at that centre be invited to become members. But the invitation would always come from the president, not Dowling himself. In this way the Dowling Club became a national organization, and each new member gained acceptance by the group. Rivalries and animosities never really surfaced, or were rapidly defused. Thus Dowling had achieved one part of his personal master plan. How pleased he would have been if he could read the *Dowling Club Newsletter* of spring 1990, with an item announcing 'pleasure in welcoming 31 new members'; and the notice to its current members: 'Please ensure that all of those new to dermatology are aware of the Dowling Club and encourage them to join.' No other established medical society or group would conceivably issue such an invitation, unless it was in desperate straits from loss of support or facing bankruptcy. But those words could have been written by Dowling himself. It was the way he always wanted it to be.

This feature of welcome and hospitality gained appreciation from numerous temporary trainee dermatologists in London, although few had much chance to record it. An exception was Dr Hiroshi Shimizu from Keio University in Japan. He spent two years as a research worker at the Institute of Dermatology from 1987 to 1989. He was invited to reflect and comment on his experiences in London. In a 'Letter from Japan' he wrote:

> For most of my two years in London I was the only Japanese dermatologist working long-term in the UK.
>
> One British dermatological institution I should desperately like to import to Japan is the Dowling Club. It is an excellent forum for meeting and exchanging views with professional colleagues. I have met many people through the Dowling Club meetings, and I particularly enjoyed the overseas trip to Jordan in 1989 during which I made many good friends. What an excellent experience for foreign doctors to join a fantastic tour composed of friendly dermatologists from various parts of Britain.

It was 20 years earlier that W.J. (Bill) Green from Austin, Texas, was a registrar and first met Dr Dowling at St John's Hospital. He recalled:

> As octogenarians, most physicians have totally retired from dermatology, yet he assiduously attended conferences and played a very active role. The conference room became quiet when he spoke; as we all realised a revered physician was in our midst. His smiling informal manner cut across all age, cultural and social barriers. He had that unique ability of making the most junior person feel important. He was always youthful and never showed the crabbiness of old age.
>
> Personally, I feel his greatest achievement was in founding the Dowling Club and my fondest memories were of its meetings at the George Inn. On several occasions he and I arrived early and had time for private conversation. He was particularly interested in my boyhood home amid the large ranch areas of West Texas. I remember his excitement when I assured him that cowboys

(minus the six-guns) were still an integral part of ranching. We also discussed his boyhood in South Africa at length. More than anything else, the Dowling Club has fostered fraternalism among dermatologists and, in its travels, has shown the excellence of British dermatology. Recently, I was honoured to be a host when the Club visited Texas.

Renewing old friendships from early Dowling Club days has been one of life's blessings. The ongoing activity of this Club will forever be a monument to his genius.

Perhaps because he was such a personally private person, few people were allowed to see into Dowling's mind. And scarcely anyone ever discussed with him his vision or thoughts on the specialty.

The other part of his personal and private plan concerned the status of British dermatology in the world. He had always been aware of its low standing in relation to the renowned departments in Europe. He was once asked, 'Who were the outstanding dermatologists in Britain during the two decades between the world wars?'

In his characteristic way he paused in thought for several minutes, and answered with another one-liner, 'There weren't any!'

And after a further long pause, with that slight twinkle in his eye, he turned and said, 'Only me!'

He was indeed well aware of his own high standing, both in Britain and abroad.

Through correspondence, meetings at international conferences and visitors to London, he felt he had established a connection with many of the leading dermatologists in European centres. He planned to exploit this for the benefit of succeeding generations. Early on in its activities he suggested that the members of his journal club (the George Club) should make a visit to Paris. One of the early members was Dr James Marshall, who had spent time in Paris during and just after the end of the Second World War. He had married a French lady and studied at the Hôpital Saint Louis, where he came to know Garnier, Gougerot, Degos and Touraine. So James Marshall made the contact and the George Club group visited Paris in the spring of 1948.

It was a big event. Dowling had primed his group of young registrars not to talk too much but to listen and learn, which they did to good effect. Arthur Rook was particularly impressed by the work of Civatte and Tzanck in recognizing histological differences between pemphigus and other bullous diseases. After the visit Rook went back to Paris for three months to study with them. On his return to London he analysed the patients at St Thomas's Hospital and found they agreed perfectly with the French findings. He made this work the basis of his MD thesis.

Touraine was especially enthusiastic to bring British dermatology into touch with France and, after further discussions during the Tenth International Congress of Dermatology in London in 1952, he and Dowling initiated a regular Franco-British reunion, to be held every two years, alternately in France and Britain. As a result many individual personal relationships were established between the young British and the young French dermatologists, often familiar friendships which continued for life. How delighted Dowling would now be to know that in later years a small group of young British and French dermatologists have arranged annual meetings, alternatively in each country. At these meetings the French present their papers in English and the British in French. These have been so successful that they have been succeeded by a yet more junior (in age) group of French and English dermatologists arranging their own meetings. For some years now, at the annual March meetings of the French Dermatological Society at the Hôpital Saint Louis in Paris, British dermatologists have been regular contributors — and in reasonable French.

But Dowling was not content with Paris alone. In subsequent years he would take his George Club group on an annual visit to other European centres — in Belgium, Holland, Denmark, Sweden, Switzerland, Germany and Italy. It became the overseas visit of the club, but each time the invitation came through Dowling. He made the introduction but the arrangements were put into motion by the president and secretary. In each country personal friendships were fostered and cemented. His low profile always allowed others to shine, but he was ever present.

The meeting in Copenhagen was a great success, where Sven Lomholt and Holger Haxthausen were world figures. Gradually, after each visit, Dowling encouraged the club to invite a group of young dermatologists to make a return visit to London, so that they came to know their opposite numbers in England, and they came to learn of the progress of dermatology in Britain.

The German visit to Munich and Frankfurt-on-Main in the spring of 1952 was of special significance. In the years immediately following the end of the Second World War, fraternization with Germany was discouraged. But Dowling wanted to overcome this. He sought approval for the visit from the British Foreign Office for what would be the first official scientific visit. In Munich Professor Alfred Marchionini had returned from wartime exile in Ankara, Turkey, and in Frankfurt Professor Oscar Gans had returned from exile in Bombay, India. Both had chosen exile from the Nazi government.

The departments in Munich and Frankfurt were enormous to British eyes, and the work being done was of a very high standard. The British learnt a lot and made many new friends, especially Hans Götz, who had been a submarine officer in the war and had been captured in the Atlantic, spending the rest of his time as a prisoner of war in the United States.

At the time of the London International Congress in 1952, all the dermatologists from the various countries visited were invited to a George Club party, which was a great success and helped further international friendship and co-operation. The idea for holding such a party came from Dr Dowling, but it did not meet with universal approval or acceptance so soon after the end of the European war. Nevertheless, Dowling was very insistent that Britain should be seen to be encouraging friendly social contacts among the young post-war generation of dermatologists in Europe. He had heard so much of the past rivalries and acrimonious disputes between the leading derma-tologists in Paris, Vienna, Breslau, Budapest, Hamburg and so on. He deserves much credit for breaking down these rivalries. How pleased he would have been to see the inauguration and development of the European Academy of Dermatology in 1988 and so many other European specialist groups over the past decade.

Dowling himself had never studied abroad, but on the club's visits to various European centres he was constantly surprised by the size of departments of dermatology, with their large number of beds, extensive laboratories and other facilities, as well as their large staffs and the high status of the professor. Their origin is to be found in the different development of dermatovenereology in Europe and Britain. In the nineteenth century, when syphilis was rife and uncontrolled, govern-ment authorities were conscious of the national shame of widespread venereal disease. When effective treatment became available through Paul Ehrlich's discovery of the therapeutic efficacy of arsphenamine (Salvarsan), those governments were keen that it should be widely used. The doctors who cared for syphilis patients and treated them were the dermatologists, and they knew how to use the new drug. So the governments were only too eager to provide them with all the facilities they sought. They were given professional status and large departments with plenty of beds. They had equal status with professors of medicine, surgery and gynaecology. And they retain such a position today, even though syphilis has been largely conquered with antibiotics.

In Britain it was different. British governments did not have the same attitude to venereology, either before or after the discovery of Salvarsan in Germany. Most universities in Britain do not yet have a professor of dermatology or the extensive facilities available to their European colleagues. In spite of the handicap, and only since 1945, British dermatology has been striving towards equality with Europe, and has at last gained recognition for its efforts. With the decline of venereal disease, as a result of antibiotic therapy, and other major therapeutic advances, the need for large numbers of beds has gradually diminished, although the power and influence of university professors of dermatology in European departments remain.

When Geoffrey Dowling died in 1976, many silent thoughts pondered on the future. Would the club die with him? Few of the older members appreciated at the time the strength of the bond between members of the younger dermatological community. Louis Forman (Dowling's first registrar), though retired from the active staff at Guy's Hospital, quietly slipped into the vacant 'chair'.

Like Dowling he never missed a meeting and was universally popular. But it was largely due to the efforts of Martin Black and Charles Wells that the future course was plotted. They foresaw that the most important role for the club was now not so much social as educational. These activities gradually expanded and sponsorship funding was obtained from pharmaceutical companies. The George Inn was soon too small for the numbers wishing to partake in the monthly dinner meetings, and the venue was eventually arranged at the Institute of Directors or the Reform Club in Pall Mall. Generous sponsorship funds made it possible for the costs to be maintained at a low level, which ensured that the most junior registrars would be able to attend.

The club was accepted by the Inland Revenue as a charity with a small annual subscription. Office space was provided by the British Association of Dermatologists in Regent's Park, and the membership has grown to more than 400, spread over the whole of Britain. It is a truly national institution. Clinical meetings are held, by invitation, in various dermatological centres all over the country.

An educational or study weekend has become a regular event. The annual overseas visits have ranged far beyond Europe — to the United States, Israel, South Africa, India, Thailand, Kenya and Egypt — always by invitation from dermatologists, who have usually spent some time in England.

The Dowling Club has become a kind of British version of the American Academy of Dermatology. It is interesting that the American Academy had very similar beginnings. That also was the brainchild of one man, Dr Earl Osborne, who was a 'down-town' dermatologist from Buffalo in upstate New York. He felt that there was a need to provide an educational forum for dermatologists like himself, who were separated from university departments and who needed an annual update. The American Academy exists for the primary purpose of education and reunion, and its officers continue to adhere to the ideals of its founder. While Osborne was alive and the programme was being discussed, the organizing members always agreed, 'If Earl wants it, then we include it.'

At the annual meetings of the American Academy of Dermatology, there are numerous cocktail parties for the alumni of various university departments. One of the biggest is now the Dowling Club Reunion there, generously organized by James Roller from Missouri, who had spent a year as a registrar at St John's Hospital in London. All the Dowling Club members visiting the academy, as well as the American members, receive an invitation.

As part of these educational activities, the Club is now able to offer 15 training fellowships in Britain and abroad, sponsored by pharmaceutical companies; and most recently the successes of the Dowling Club can take some credit for inspiring the foundation of the European Academy of Dermatology, which held its first meeting in Milan in 1989.

Apart from the regular journal club meetings each month, the most important date in the Club's calendar is the annual Dowling Oration, followed by a dinner. It began in 1956 and was linked to the week-long Refresher Meeting for Consultants held at St John's Hospital, but more recently it has become incorporated into the Club's educational weekend, held in various places around the country.

In 1971 there was a special event to celebrate Dowling's eightieth birthday. Wolf Tillman, with whom he shared a birthday, was the prime mover in organizing the evening at Greenwich District Hospital. Dowling was overwhelmed by the vast number of friends who attended the dinner, despite the fact that it was in the middle of the holiday period. The Tillman family, with whom the Dowlings had often stayed, had prepared a 'This is Your Life' presentation book, which he later treasured, and the evening was rounded off with a recital given by the Philip Jones Brass Ensemble to mark his lifelong interest in music and the arts. Geoffrey was deeply moved by the whole evening. It was ultimate happiness for him.

APPENDIX I
MUSICAL PROGRAMME AT
DOWLING'S EIGHTIETH BIRTHDAY

Fanfare
Music for brass from the Renaissance to the 20th Century
played by
The Philip Jones Brass Ensemble

Philip Jones, trumpet; Elgar Howarth, trumpet
Ifor James, horn; John Iveson, trombone
John Fletcher, tuba

PROGRAMME

Fanfare	Richard Rodney Bennett *b.* 1936
Music of 16th century (Italy)	
Toccata from *L'Orfero*	Monteverdi 1567–1643
Canzon *La Seraphina*	Lappi ?–1630
Ricercare	Palestrina 1525–1594
Canzon a 4	G. Gabrieli 1557–1612
Music of 17th century (Germany)	
Battle Suite	Samuel Scheidt 1587–1654
Music of 19th century	
Three Pieces	Ludwig Maurer 1789–1878
Music of 20th century	
Petite Suite	Jan Koetsier *b.* 1911
Quintet for Brass	Malcolm Arnold *b.* 1921

APPENDIX II
THE DOWLING CLUB

Past presidents and secretaries

Year	President	Secretary
1947–48	Dr H.J. Wallace	Dr G.C. Wells
1948–49	Dr G.C. Wells	
1949–50	Dr G.B. Dowling	Dr R.E. Bowers
1950–51	Dr F.R. Bettley	
1951–52	Dr W.G. Tillman	
1953–54	Dr D.I. Williams	Dr D.S. Sharvill
1955–56	Dr H.T.H. Wilson	Dr R.G. Howell
1956–57	Dr R.H. Meara	Dr R.G. Howell
1957–58	Dr H. Haber	Dr R.H. Marten
1958–59	Dr M. Feiwel	Dr W. Frain-Bell
1959–60	Dr C.D. Calnan	Dr I. Sarkany
1960–61	Dr R.J. Cairns	Dr R.R.M. Harman
1961–62	Dr R.H. Marten	Dr M.A. Smith
1962–63	Dr O.L.S. Scott	Dr D.D. Munro
1963–64	Dr I. Sarkany	Dr R. Summerly
1964–65	Dr K.V. Sanderson	Dr P.W.M. Copeman
1965–66	Dr L. Forman	Dr R.B. Fountain
1966–67	Dr A. Jarrett	Dr M.L. Johnson
1967–68	Dr H.T. Calvert	Dr J.E. White
1968–69	Dr R.S. Wells	Dr J.A. Savin
1969–70	Dr E. Wilson-Jones	Dr M.M. Black
1970–71	Dr E.A. Cronin	Dr C.A. Ramsay
1971–72	Dr H. Baker	Dr R.P.R. Dawber
1972–73	Dr D.D. Munro	Dr J.J.H. Gilkes
1973–74	Dr P.W.M. Copeman	Dr R.S.H. Tan
1974–75	Dr T.W.E. Robinson	Dr D. Thompson
1975–76	Dr T.J. Ryan	Dr R.A. Marsden
1976–77	Dr M.M. Black	Dr P. Hudson
1977–78	Dr R.P.R. Dawber	Dr J.D. Wilkinson
1978–79	Dr J. Ellis	Dr M. James
1979–80	Dr F.A. Ive	Dr P. Kersey
1980–81	Dr R.R.M. Harman	Dr C.R. Lovell
1981–82	Dr J. White	Surgeon Commander R.E. Ashton, RN
1982–83	Dr W.A.D. Griffiths	Dr J. Miller
1983–84	Dr R.C.D. Staughton	Dr C.M.E. Rowland Payne
1984–85	Dr M.A. Kleber	Dr R. Meyrick Thomas
1985–86	Dr A. du Vivier	Dr S.M. Neile
1986–87	Dr J.A.A. Hunter	Dr D.J. Gawkrodger

Year	President	Secretary
1987–88	Dr F. Wojnarowska	Dr S.M. Burge
1988–89	Dr C.A. Lovell	Dr S. Jones
1989–90	Dr A. Burns	Dr J. Berth-Jones
1990–91	Dr N.P. Smith	Dr S. Whittaker

Overseas visits

Year	Place	Year	Place
1948	Paris	1949	Copenhagen
1950	Brussels, Liège	1951	Holland
1952	Munich, Frankfurt	1953	Venice, Pavia, Milan
1954	Paris	1955	Lyon
1956	Zurich, Basel	1958	Nantes
1959	Vienna, Zagreb	1960	Barcelona
1961	Warsaw, Berlin	1963	Budapest, Pécs
1964	Utrecht, Amsterdam, Nijmegen	1965	Sweden
1968	Spain	1969	South Africa
1970	Lebanon	1971	Athens, Israel
1973	Holland	1975	Iran
1976	France	1978	Spain
1979	Turkey	1980	Canada
1981	Athens, Cairo	1982	Dallas
1983	France	1984	Portugal
1985	Germany	1986	India
1988	Thailand	1989	Jordan
1990	Kenya	1991	Austria

APPENDIX III
THE DOWLING ENDOWMENT FUND

The Dowling Endowment Fund of the Royal Society of Medicine was set up in 1970 by Dr R.S. Wells and Dr W.G. Tillman with £1000 given to the Royal Society of Medicine. Subsequently, further sums of money were given to the fund by dermatologists and others after an extensive appeal, and the capital sum is now more than £20,000.

The chief purpose of the fund is to provide an endowment for the annual Dowling Oration. The first Dowling Oration was given in 1956 and has been given each year since then. Although the Orators did an enormous amount of work, they never received any financial recognition for their work. Because of this, and in recognition of Dr G.B. Dowling's many contributions to dermatology, the fund was set up to endow the Oration on a permanent basis. It was always accepted that the Oration did not have to be given in the Society's House (1 Wimpole Street) unless it was convenient to do so. It is accepted that the honorarium for the Oration is in no sense a 'payment' nor does it relate to the actual 'cost' of the talk, but is some sort of recognition to the Orator for all the work he has put into the Oration. The rules of the Society said that every Oration should have an honorarium of at least £50, but this sum has always been exceeded and the most recent Orator was given £400.

When funds allowed, it was accepted that money might be provided for other purposes that were of interest to Dr Dowling. This has generally been taken to provide funds for a young British dermatologist to visit the Annual Meeting of the American Academy of Dermatology. This is considered to be the one meeting of greatest educational value for junior dermatologists in training. These visits were set up with the full co-operation and encouragement of the authorities of the American Academy, who did not charge the usual course fees, etc. The visits have been so astonishingly successful that now funds are available from a number of other sources to enable young people to go to the American Meeting in December. There are always a good number of people who put in applications for support each year. A small subcommittee of senior dermatologists evaluates these applications.

The fund is managed and the Orator appointed by a small subcommittee, which has two permanent members, appointed by the Council of the Royal Society of Medicine, and three who change every year. One is the President of the Dermatology Section of the RSM, another the Secretary of the Section and the third the President of the Dowling Club for that year. By this mechanism many people are involved in the choice of the Orator.

When the idea of an annual Oration was first discussed, it was Dowling's wish that the speaker should be a dermatologist from a non-university hospital. His purpose was to stimulate and involve others as well as academic teachers, although this has not always been possible.

The Dowling Orators

Year	Orator	Address	Title
1956	G.C. Wells	St Thomas's Hospital, London	Esterases in cutaneous granulomata
1957	I.B. Sneddon	Royal Infirmary, Sheffield	Some unusual traumatic lesions of the skin
1958	J.M. Beare	Royal Victoria Hospital, Belfast	The pH of skin in newborn babies
1959	R.E. Bowers	Royal Hospital, Gloucester	The natural history of strawberry marks
1960	R.D. Sweet	Greenbank Hospital, Plymouth	Treatment of BCC by curettage

Year	Orator	Address	Title
1961	I.W. Whimster	St Thomas's Hospital, London	Morbid anatomy and the skin
1962	H.T. Calvert	Royal Berkshire Hospital, Reading	Atopy, old and new
1963	J.R. Simpson	Royal Devon and Exeter Hospital, Exeter	Congenital ichthyosiform erythroderma
1964	A.J. Rook	Addenbrooke's Hospital, Cambridge	Drugs, poisons and the skin
1966	S. Shuster	Royal Victoria Infirmary, Newcastle upon Tyne	Trends in dermatology
1967	K.R. Rees	University College Hospital, London	Lysosomes and skin injury
1968	I.A. Magnus	St John's Hospital for Diseases of the Skin, London	Dermatological photobiology
1969	K.V. Sanderson	St George's Hospital, London	Dynamic aspects of wartiness
1970	K.D. Crow	Princess Margaret Hospital, Swindon	Chloracne
1971	C.N.D. Cruickshank	MRC Skin Unit, University of Birmingham	O' mice and men
1972	C.F.H. Vickers	Royal Infirmary, Liverpool	Dam, reservoir or filter
1973	R. Summerly	North Staffordshire Hospital Centre, Stoke-on-Trent	In vitro quo vadis acetate?
1974	H. Rorsman	Sahlgrensa Sjukhuset, Gothenburg, Sweden	Melanocyte illuminated
1975	W.J. Cunliffe	Royal Infirmary, Leeds	The mark of diversity
1976	E. Wilson Jones	St John's Hospital for Diseases of the Skin, London	Malignant vascular tumours of the skin

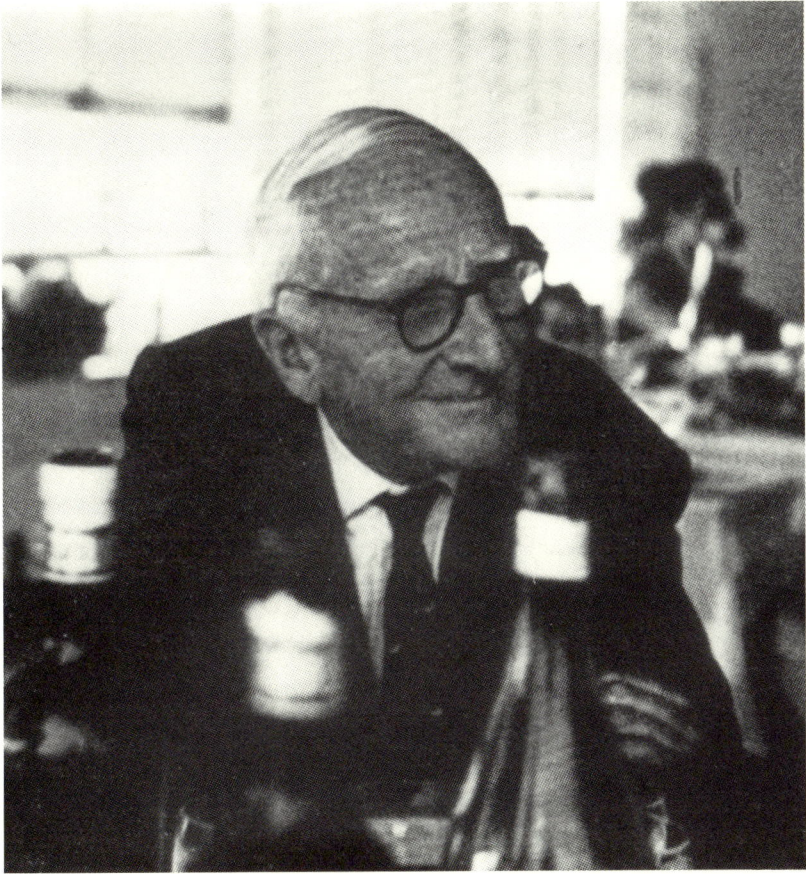

PLATE 1 Dr Geoffrey Dowling at lunch (courtesy of Dr Robert Bowers)

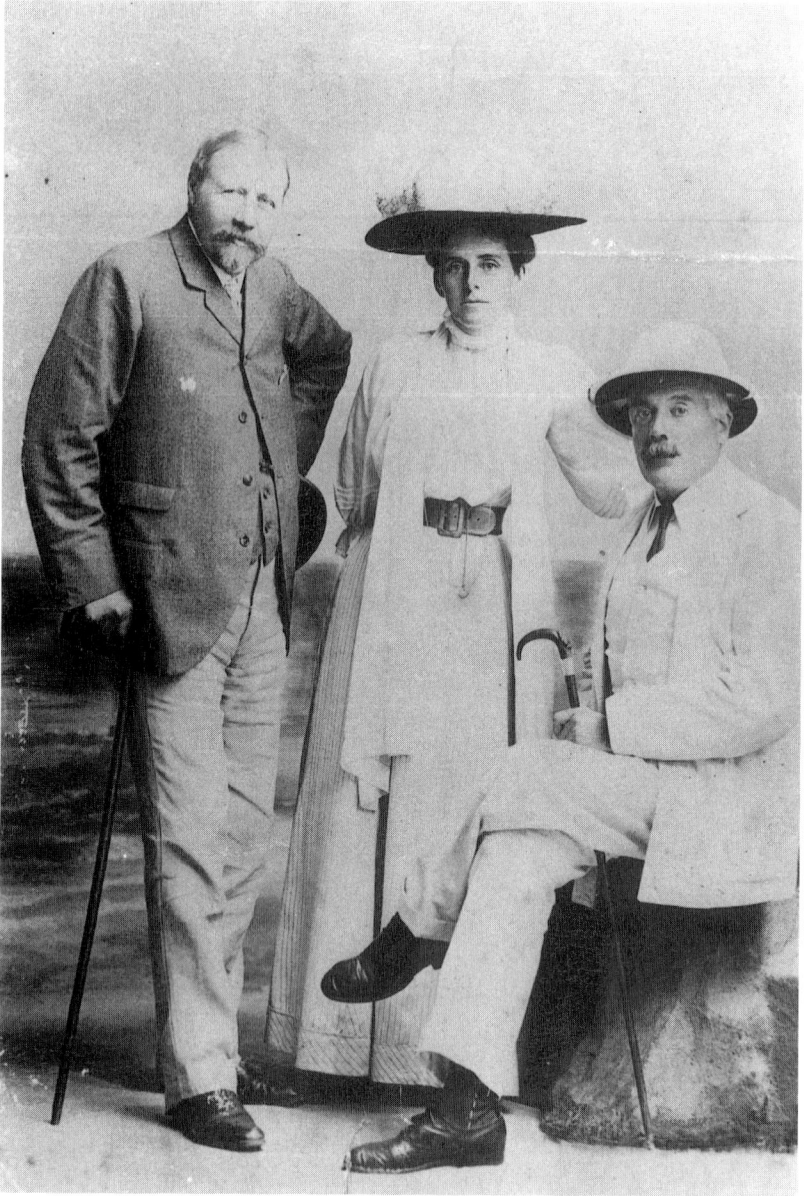

PLATE 2 Dr Thomas Barrow-Dowling (seated)
with his wife and a friend, Cape Town 1889

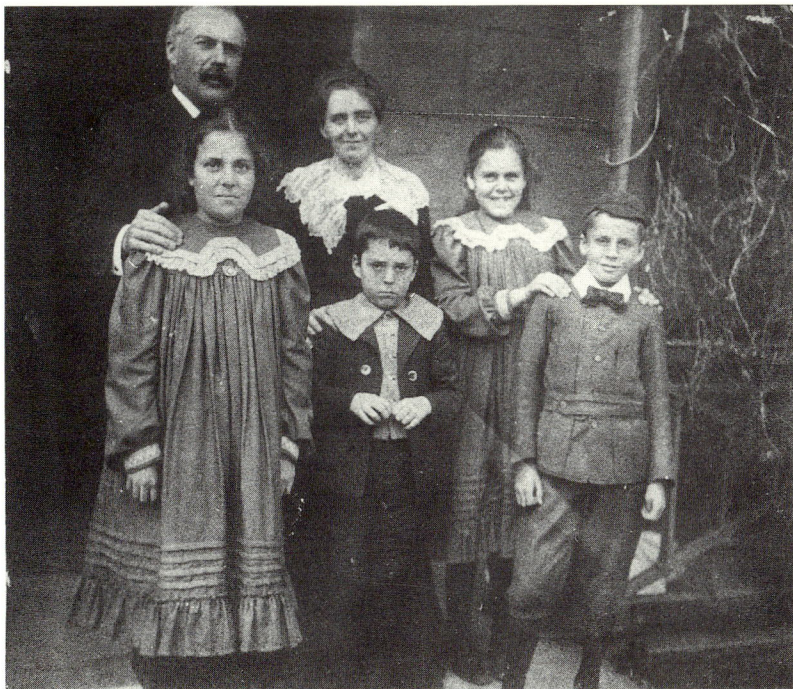

PLATE 3 The Barrow-Dowling family 1903

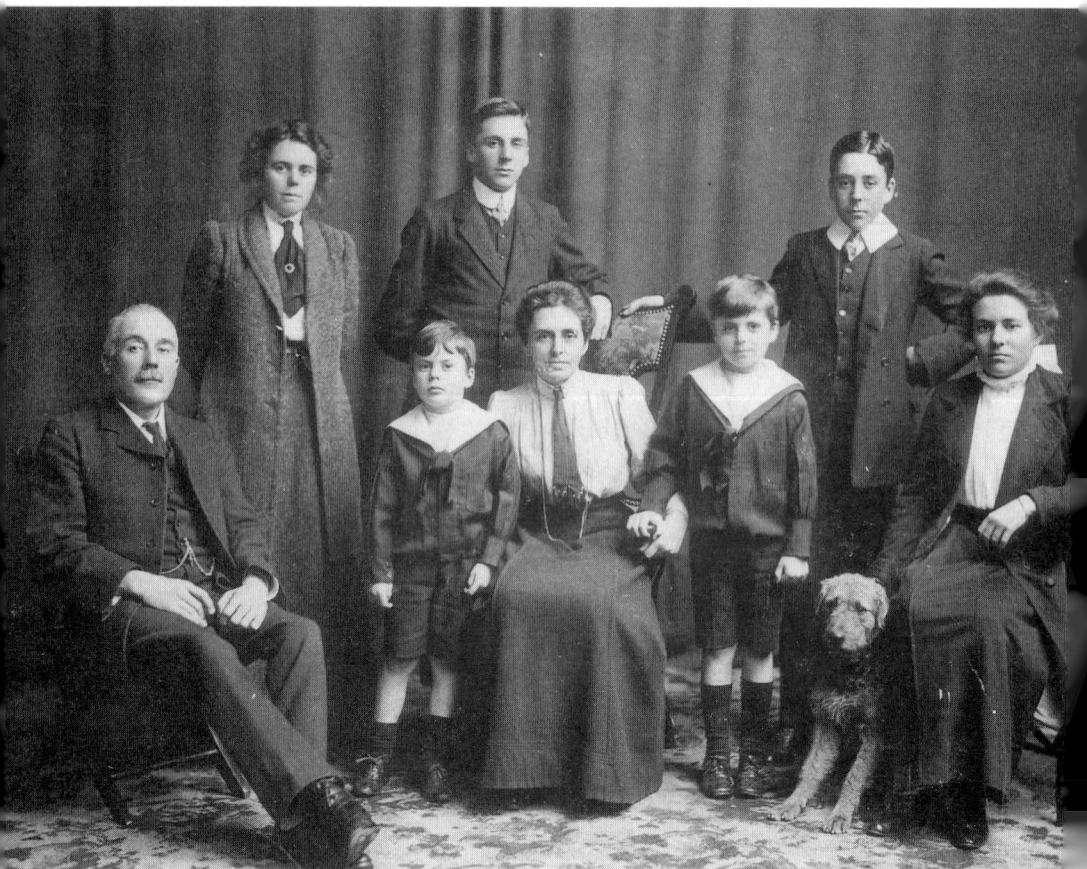

PLATE 4 The Barrow-Dowling family 1910

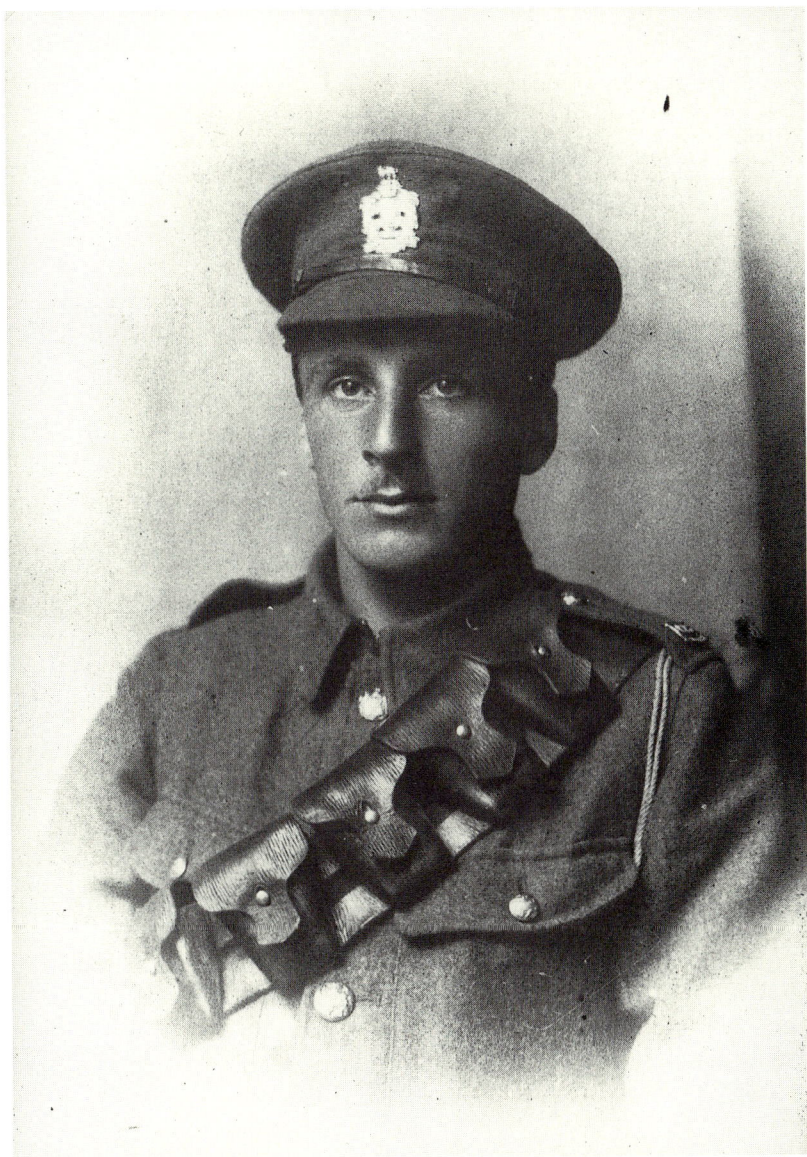

PLATE 5 Trooper Dowling 1916

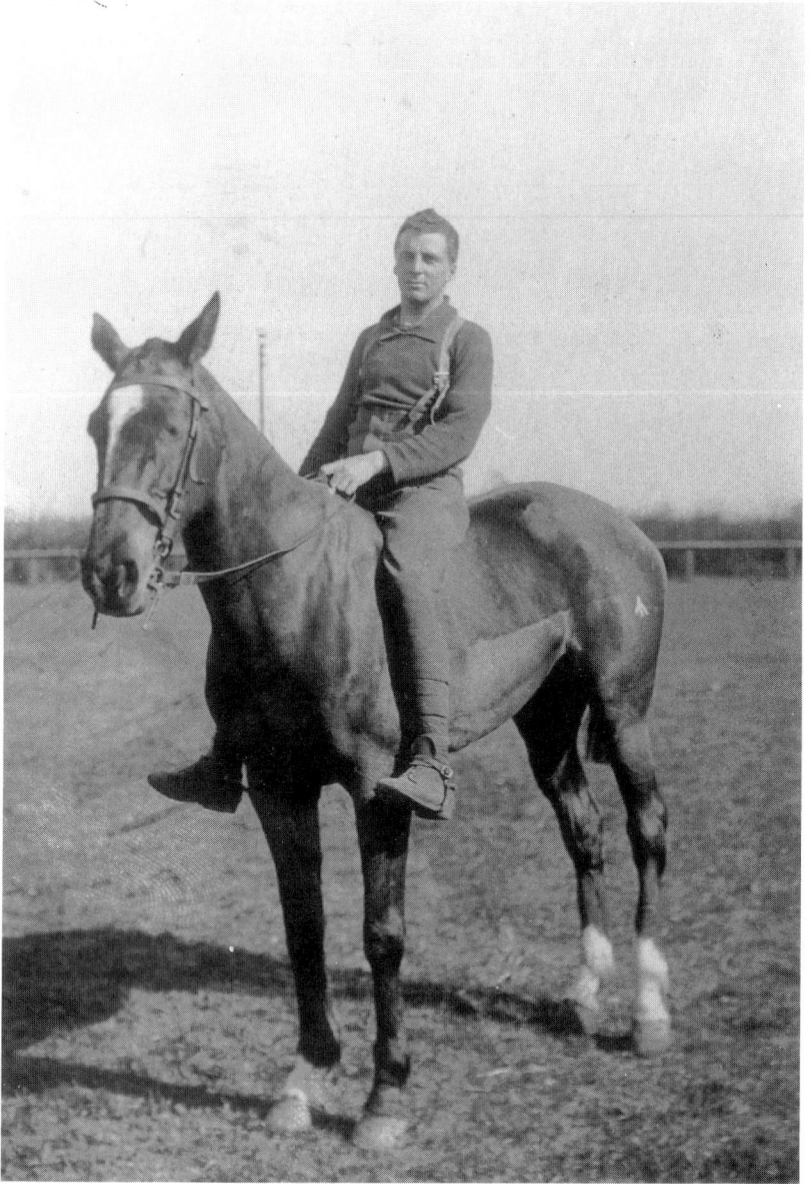

PLATE 6 'Myself on horse' 1916

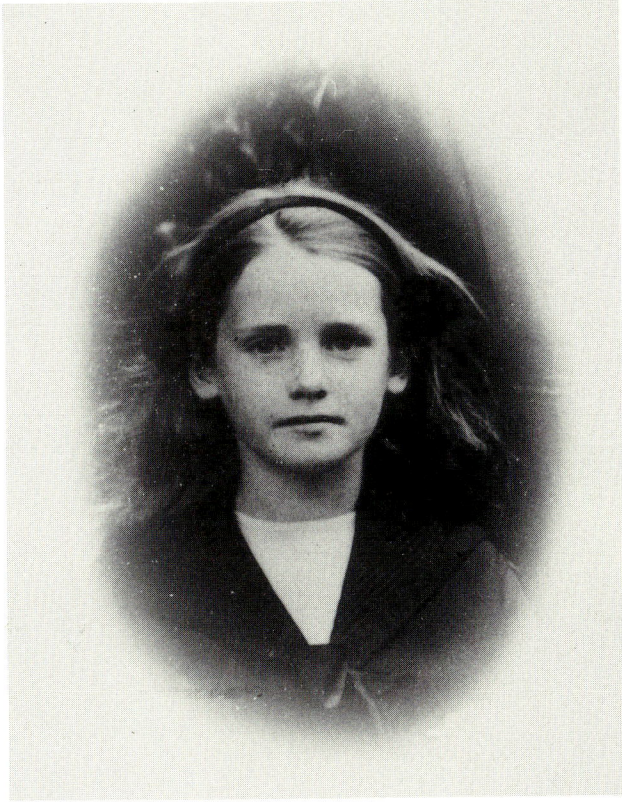

PLATE 7 Mary Elizabeth Kelly

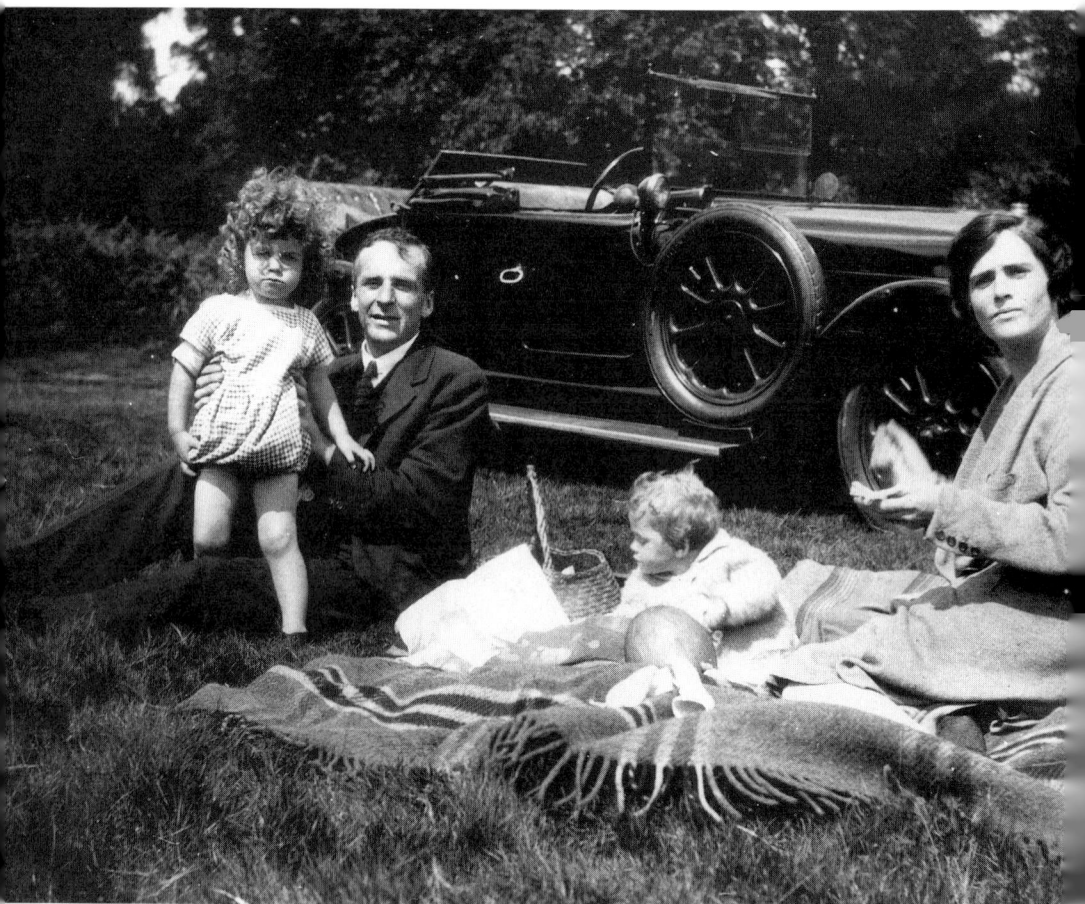

PLATE 8 A picnic by the River Thames at Wallingford

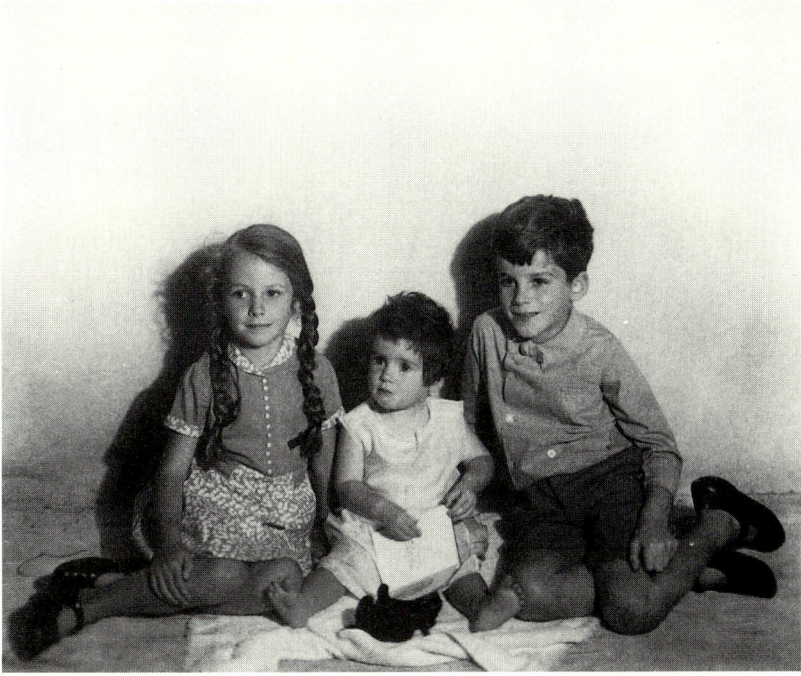

PLATE 9 Jane, La and Tom

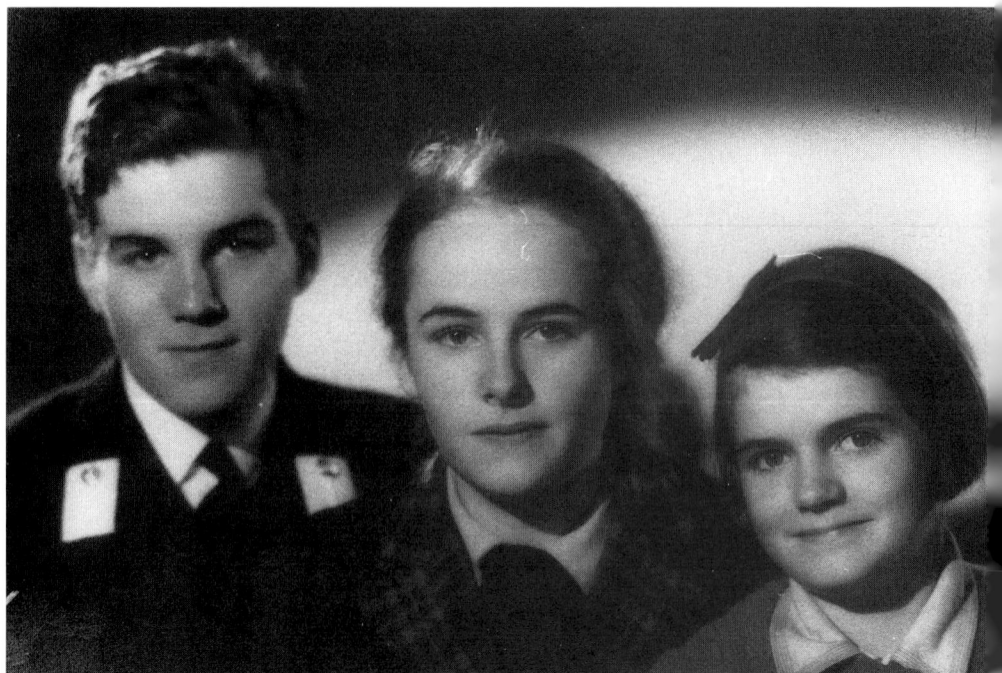

PLATE 10 Tom, Jane and La

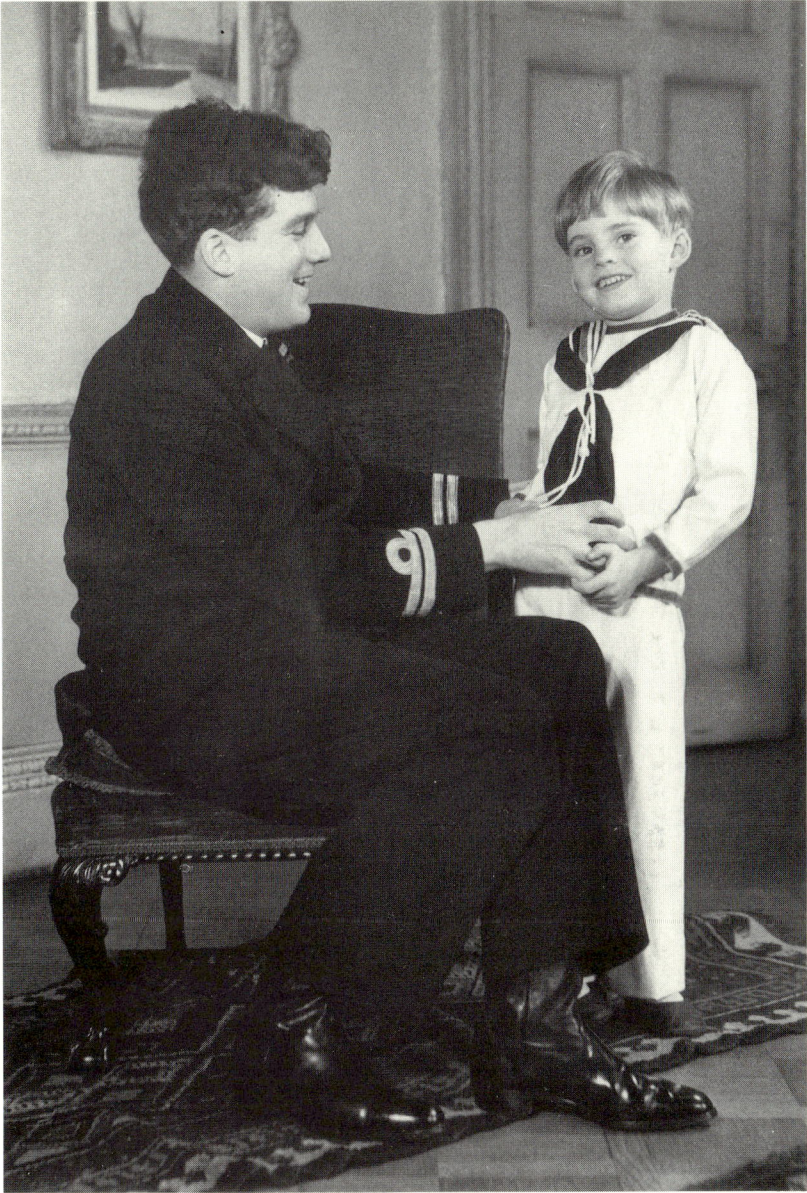

PLATE 11 Tom and Simon

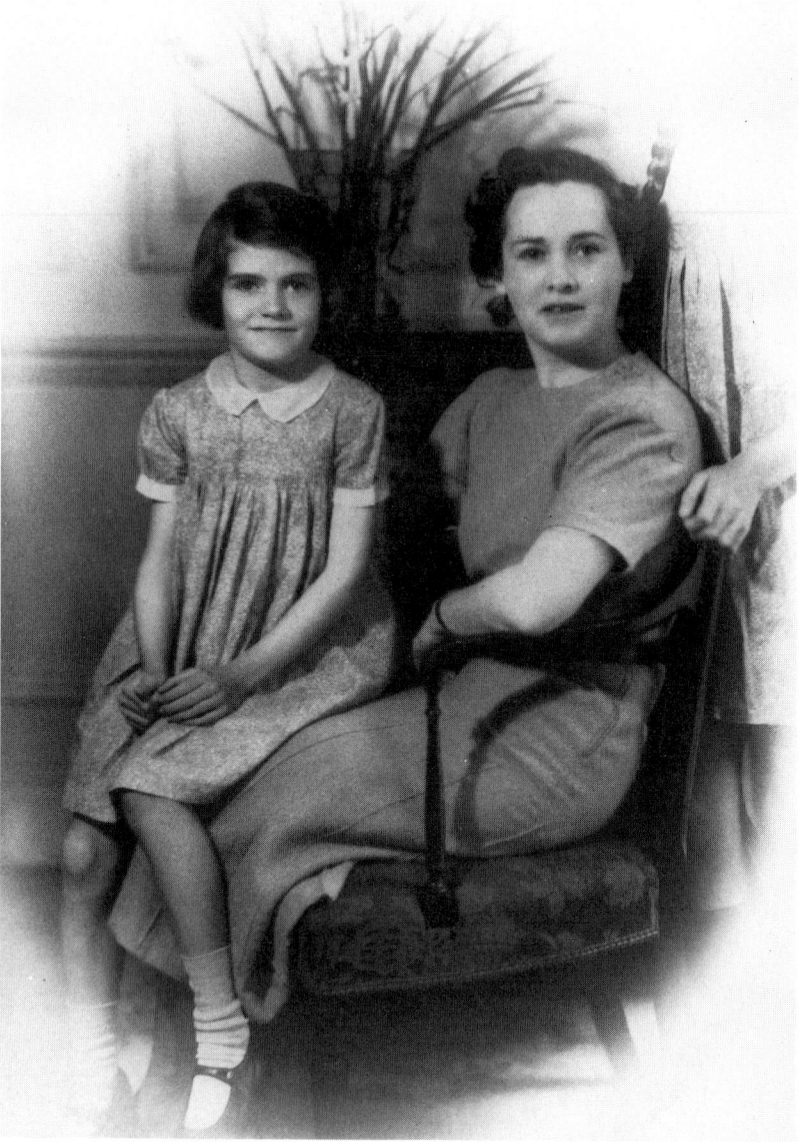

PLATE 12 May Dowling with La

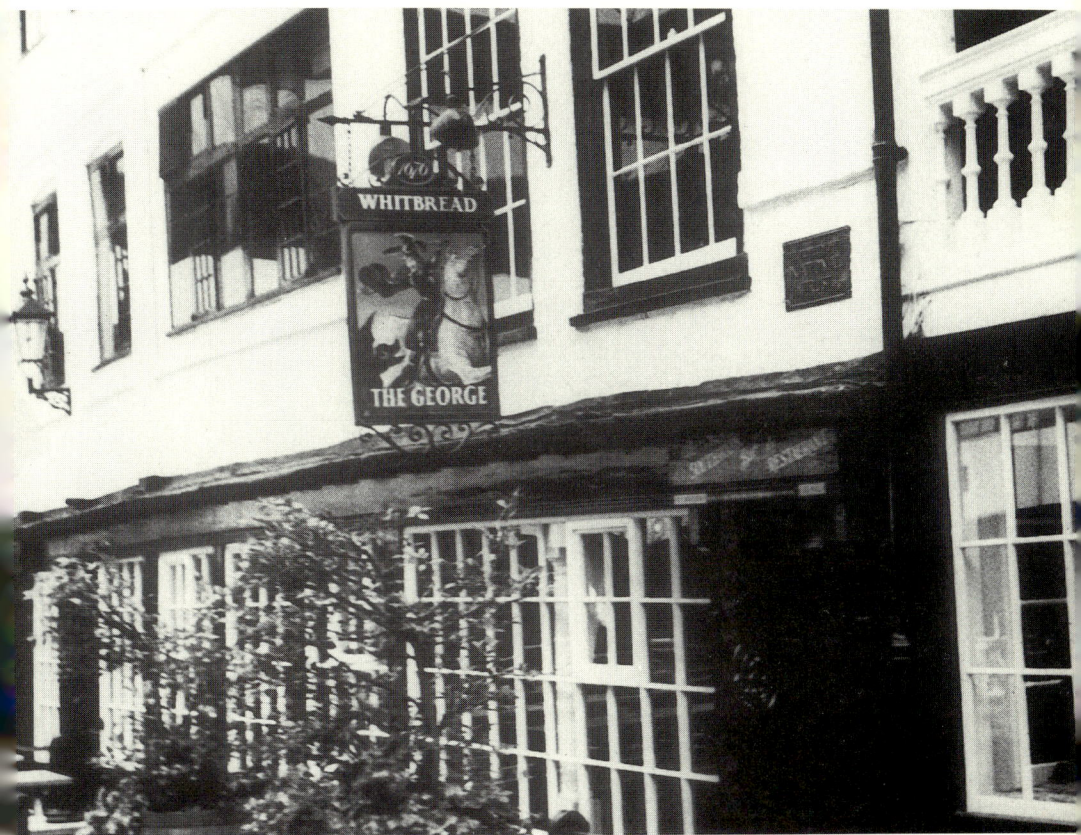

PLATE 13 The George Inn, Southwark

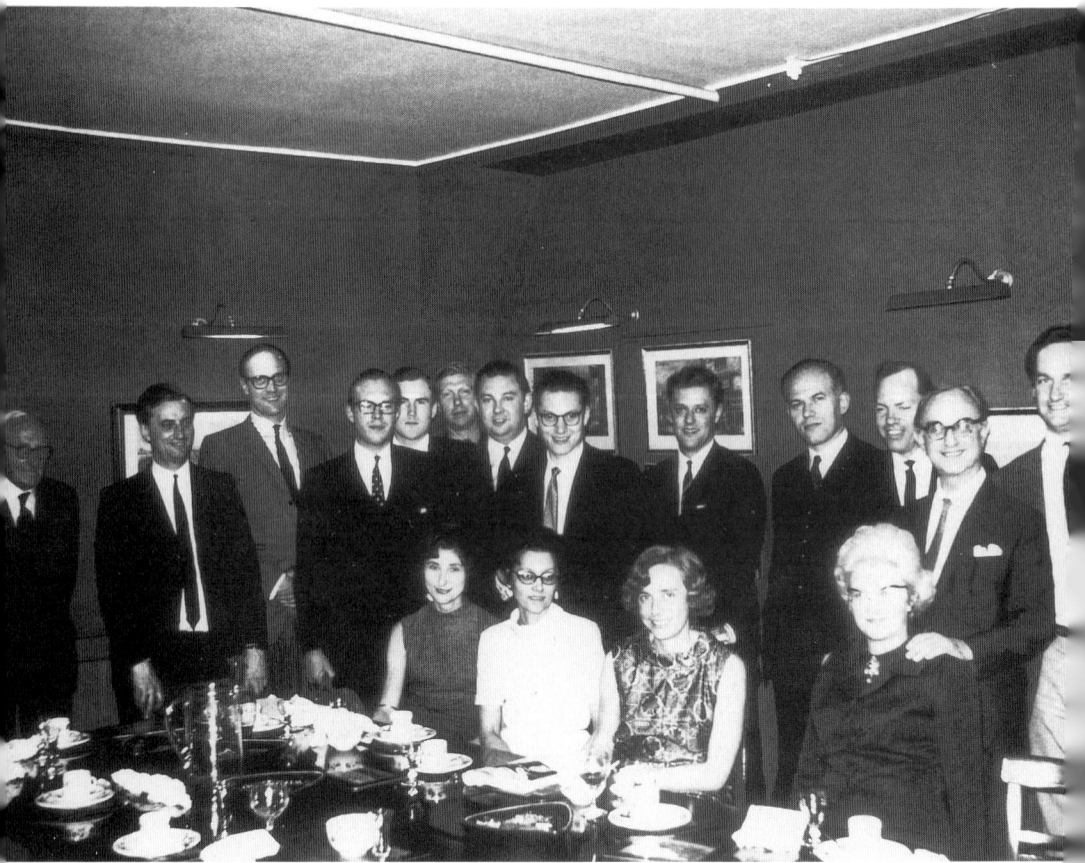

PLATE 14 Dowling Club dinner at the George Inn

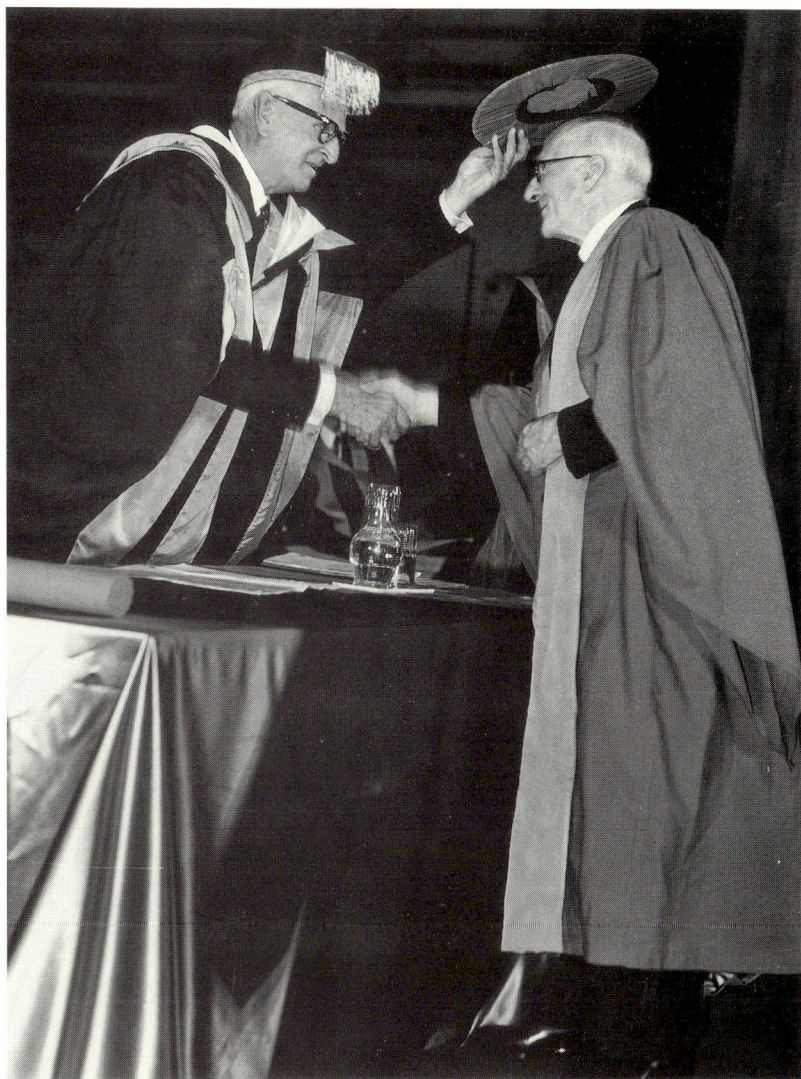

PLATE 15 Presentation of Honorary Doctorate of Medicine,
Pretoria University 1965

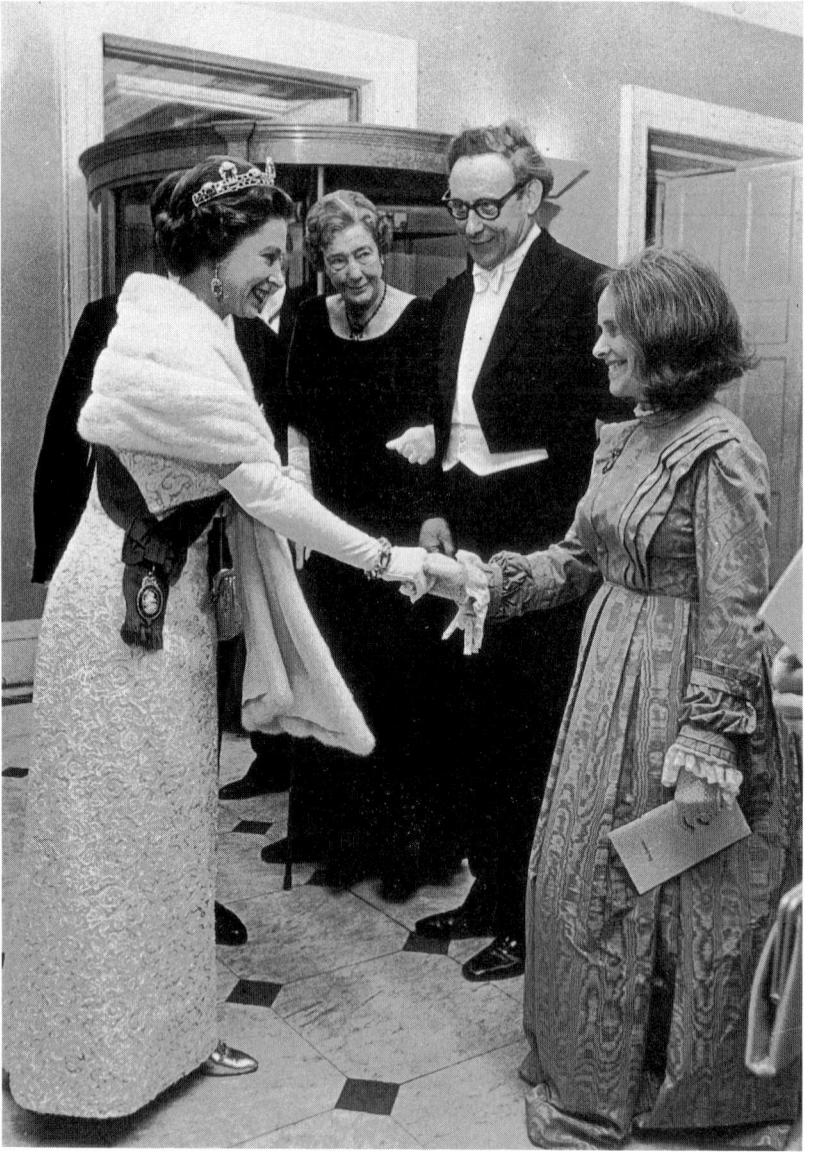

PLATE 16 Jane and Peter Greenham at the Royal Academy of Arts

Year	Orator	Address	Title
1977	Janet M. Marks	Royal Victoria Infirmary, Newcastle upon Tyne	Dogma and dermatitis herpetiformis
1978	W. Frain-Bell	Royal Infirmary, Dundee	What is this thing called light?
1979	M.W. Greaves	St John's Hospital for Diseases of the Skin, London	From molecules to medicines
1980	J.L. Burton	Royal Infirmary, Bristol	The language and logic of dermatological diagnosis — some antics with some antique semantics
1981	R.M. MacKie	University of Glasgow	The changing face of malignant melanoma
1982	J.A.A. Hunter	Royal Infirmary, Edinburgh	The Langerhans cell: from gold to glitter
1983	N. Rowell	General Infirmary, Leeds	The natural history of lupus erythematosus
1984	R. Marks	Welsh National School of Medicine, Cardiff	Device and rule
1985	T.J. Ryan	Slade Hospital, Oxford	Morphosis — occult forces and ectoplasm
1986	R.A.J. Eady	St John's Hospital, Leicester Square, London	Babes, blisters and basement membranes
1987	R.P.R. Dawber	Slade Hospital, Oxford	Cold kills
1988	J.H. Saurat	Hôpital Cantonal Universitaire de Genève, Switzerland	How do retinoids work on human skin?
1990	Prof. R.J. Hay	St John's Hospital for Diseases of the Skin, London	A thorn in the flesh: mechanisms of percutaneous infection

Chapter 12
The Writing

THERE IS an apparent paradox in the statement that Geoffrey Dowling was one of the greatest teachers of dermatology of his time, but one of its least effective lecturers. His natural diffidence and shyness inhibited his effectiveness with the formal spoken word.

This was in sharp contrast to his abilities with the written word. At Dulwich College he chose science rather than humanities, and yet his family origins in the arts coupled with his isolation from home after being sent to school in England probably meant that he spent a lot of time reading. Throughout his life he had always read voraciously, not least during his retirement years when living at Ravenscourt Gardens and never suffering any impairment of his sight.

Soon after returning to Guy's Hospital after the war he became editor of the students' *Hospital Gazette*. His special style of writing, with its simplicity, clarity and absence of waffle or speculation, was evident then. These same characteristics were to be seen in his hospital and private practice letters to general practitioners, as well as in his personal letters to friends and colleagues. This was especially true of the 'references' he sent to appointment committees in support of a registrar's application for a consultant post. Eric Waddington remembers that after he was appointed at Cardiff, one of the physicians said to him, 'We feel we know you already from Dr Dowling's testimonial!'

Although he read a great deal of dermatological literature, he was not a collector of books and had no personal medical library. In fact, he only ever bought one textbook, Darier's *Précis de Dermatologie* (presumably recommended by H.W. Barber at Guy's Hospital). He had mastered French, although he had never studied abroad like so many of his colleagues. When he was presented with a copy of *Dermatologie* by Robert Degos in 1953, he read it straight through from cover to cover. He always had a high regard for French descriptive dermatology.

In the nineteen twenties, thirties and forties he published articles regularly on a variety of subjects, and presented many cases at the Dermatology Section of the Royal Society of Medicine. Some of these were 'firsts'.

The publications before 1940 reflected the dermatology of the times — subjects such as protein sensitization and protein therapy, the role of *Pityrosporon ovale* in seborrhoeic dermatitis (the result of experimental work with J.M.H. MacLeod), the early diagnosis of tuberculosis, syphilitic nephritis and allergy. His exceptional memory enabled him to recall early observations; the 1936 case of 'pustular bacterid type of reaction', in which fungus was found in the roof of a blister; the patient shown as a case of acanthosis nigricans with Freudenthal in 1938, which he knew was something different and was later to become known as the Dowling–Degos disease.

His two main dermatological interests at that time were dermatomyositis and tuberculosis of the skin. His interest in dermatomyositis was stimulated by the fact that he himself presented the first case at a dermatological meeting in London in 1930, although the fatal case of a child aged $9\frac{1}{2}$ at the Metropolitan Hospital London had been described by F.E. Batten in 1910. Dowling described the first two patients he looked after in a paper on dermatomyositis in the *St Thomas's Hospital Reports* of 1936. Many of his sentences are so characteristic of him:

> It is not very easy to recognise dermatomyositis owing to the fact that according to the relative predominance of the muscular or cutaneous symptoms it may be regarded as muscular rheumatism, polyneuritis, acute sunburn, food poisoning, lupus erythematosus and several other conditions.
>
> We owe to Petges and Clejat the first complete description of the cutaneous and muscular changes in dermatomyositis; a description so accurate that it will always serve as a model.
>
> A band of erythema with telangiectases extended down the extensor aspect of the forearms to the dorsal aspect of the hands and fingers; here the skin was atrophic, red and slightly scaly. The appearances suggested lupus erythematosus of the face and hands and I made that diagnosis, supposing the eruption and the accompanying fibrositis to be due to a common cause.

When Walter Freudenthal, the distinguished dermatopathologist from Vienna, arrived in London as a refugee, and was provided with laboratory space by Sir Archibald Gray at University College Hospital, Dowling quickly recognized his potential. He was one of the keenest attenders at the Freudenthal tutorial sessions, and published several papers with him.

Dermatomyositis was a disease poorly recognized by dermatologists at the time. Dowling separated it from poikiloderma vasculare atrophicans and from scleroderma. His articles, but especially his out-patient and bedside teaching, in which he pointed out the clinical signs so well, have made it possible for even the most junior dermatologist to diagnose it now with relative ease. In the same way he clarified the confusion among dermatologists over various types of scleroderma, while O'Leary at the Mayo Clinic was doing the same for American specialists. Dowling pointed out that generalized morphoea was not the same disease as systemic sclerosis, even though it might cause loss of weight and atrophy of muscles and even be fatal. Furthermore, he constantly stressed that acrosclerosis was not a different disease but only a variant of systemic sclerosis. His views were assailed by others, but his confidence was not undermined and he did not change them.

His interest in and contributions on these two diseases over 20 years were recognized by the Royal College of Physicians in London, when he was invited to deliver the first Watson-Smith Lecture at the college in Pall Mall East on 11 January 1955.

It was a big occasion. These College lectures were always very formal occasions. The lecturer, in academic dress, is led into the hall by the college bedell and accompanied by the college officers and the president. When everyone was seated, the president, Sir Robert Platt, rose and said, 'I call on Dr G.B. Dowling to deliver the Watson-Smith Lecture.'

Geoffrey Dowling rose and went to the lectern. In spite of his age and position in British medicine and dermatology, he was nervous. It was a big ordeal for a shy man. But after the first few sentences he was at ease — on his own ground again. The lecture was a masterpiece. The literature of scleroderma and dermatomyositis was thoroughly researched; several decades later it still reads well. The Dowling style of writing is never better illustrated, with its simplicity, clarity and total lack of groundless speculation. All contributions and thoughts from junior colleagues were acknowledged by name. The final section was on morphoea, 'which has not been discussed partly because of lack of time, but also because at the present time there is not very much that one can usefully say about it . . . Research in this field may require new technical resources. I know of only one attempt in this direction, a piece of work performed recently by Musso at the Institute of Dermatology . . . This was a tiny step but perhaps in the right direction.'

Dowling returned to his place, and sat down to applause. There is no vote of thanks. The president stands, the bedell hands him the Cadeuceus and takes up the mace and the college officers, lecturer and president file out in silence.

Although he himself recognized the beneficial effects of vitamin D on tuberculosis of the skin after treating the first patient at St John's Hospital, almost all his publications on the subject were shared and joint-authored with his consultant colleagues and registrars, apart from some review articles and chapters in books. This applied equally to his other original contributions. These included:

'Acquired axillary and inguinal pigmentation: an epidermal naevoid abnormality not to be confused with acanthosis nigricans',* with E.L. Smith and E. Wilson Jones.

'Epidermolysis bullosa resembling juvenile dermatitis herpetiformis', with R.H. Meara.

'Atypical (annular) necrobiosis lipoidica of the face and scalp. A report of the clinical and histological features of seven cases', with E. Wilson-Jones.

Dowling was intensely interested in the history of dermatology in Britain, and particularly how it affected his own lifetime. And his analysis was as astute and accurate as one would expect.

Although he had moved to St Thomas's Hospital, it is said that he always remained a Guy's man. He relished the publication of *Mr Guy's Hospital* by H.C. Cameton in 1954. And probably this spurred him to write the excellent account of *Dermatology at Guy's Hospital (1850–1950)*. Illustrated with portraits of the leading personalities, including his revered teacher, Harold Wordsworth Barber, it is the best researched account of dermatology at any British university hospital.

He was closely associated with Sir Archibald Gray, particularly at the time of preparations for the Tenth International Congress of Dermatology in London in 1952, of which Sir Archibald was president, and Dowling was the organizer of the clinical case presentations. Sir Archibald was editor of the *British Journal of Dermatology and Syphilis* in 1915, and conceived the idea of a society similar to the Association of Physicians. Entirely due to his personal efforts and inexhaustible

---

* Now known as Dowling–Degos disease.

executive energy, the British Association of Dermatology and Syphilology (the last two words were dropped in 1950) was founded in 1920, and held its first meeting on 18 November 1921 at the Royal Society of Medicine.

Dowling wrote a detailed account of the 'British Association of Dermatology (1920–1970)', describing its birth and progress through his own medical lifetime, and it is likely that he himself attended every single meeting, whether in London or at a provincial centre. At the first meeting in London Sir Malcolm Morris was in the chair.

> The proceedings consisted of a discussion on Focal Infection in the Aetiology of Skin Diseases, and the openers were Leslie Roberts and H.W. Barber. A demonstration of cases was also held. Some 30 members were present and this was regarded as a very satisfactory attendance. The papers are now interesting only in reflecting a then current hypothesis regarding the cause of obscure disease in general. The second meeting was on a much higher plane. It was held in Edinburgh and Sir Norman Walker was the President. 'Allergy' was the main subject for discussion and Arthur Whitfield and Cranston Low were the opening speakers. Both of these were among the best minds in the world of dermatology at the time. Low (1924) on the basis of experimental observation on himself and his brother sharply distinguished the sensitivity produced by primula from anaphylaxis.* The sensitivity resided in cells and could not be passively transferred. Sensitivity to drugs and to contact with chemical substances was of the same order as that due to primula, while much of the eczema provoked by contact with various irritants was not an allergic response at all. Low was ahead of his time.
>
> A dinner was included in the annual Proceedings and after some years a President's reception was added. One of the main characteristics of the inter-war meetings was the presence from time to time of distinguished colleagues from abroad. Howard Fox was an early guest. Haxthausen first appeared at a London Meeting in 1927 and both he and Lomholt became lifelong friends of the Association. It was Sven Lomholt who, as Permanent Secretary of the International Dermatological Committee, stimulated the Association through Gray into organising the

---

* *British Journal of Dermatology* 1924, 36, 292.

International Congress of 1952 in London. Joseph Jadassohn
was the guest of honour in Oxford in 1929, and Bruno Bloch in
the following year contributed a paper on Endocrine Glands and
Skin Disease. The Association also organised the visits of the
British contingent to the two inter-war Congresses. In 1930 in
Copenhagen, a great event magnificently organised by Lomholt
and his colleagues, members met Darier, Brocq, Sabouraud,
Schamberg and numerous other prominent figures of a great
vanishing era.

The British attendance at the Congress in Budapest in 1935
was similarly organised by the Association and this event was
intensely interesting though marked by some depressing changes.
Hitler was in the saddle and many heads of famous departments
in Germany had been unseated: the same was shortly to follow
in Austria. It was possible to sense that in Hungary standards of
dermatology were very high. The production of that Congress
by Nekam of his great Atlas was, and remains, a magnificent
achievement by any standards. Stephen Rothman, a relatively
junior colleague of Nekam at that time, was to become before
very long in America, a great world figure.

As everyone knows no other International Congress of
Dermatology could be held until after the war when, in response
to strong representations from the International Dermatological
Committee, the Association agreed to hold one in London, Sir
Archibald Gray being Chairman. This Congress is generally
ranked as having been highly successful, as well as enjoyable. An
important event in the life of the Association arose out of the
Congress. At the Annual Meeting in 1934 it was suggested that a
fund should be raised to commemorate the life and work of
Robert Willan. By degrees some money accumulated for which it
was not easy to find a good use. In 1952 an unexpected windfall
fell to the Association. The Congress had paid rather hand-
somely. The Committee of Management of the Congress held a
special meeting to decide what ought to be done with this
money, and it finally decided to add it to the Willan Fund.
Gray's ideas on how at that point to use the Willan Fund are
expressed in his article (1960) as follows:

> Knowing that the Royal College of Physicians was about to
> rebuild, it was decided that it would be an excellent memorial

to Willan if the College would be prepared to name one of its rooms the 'Willan Room', which should house the works of Willan, including the original drawings of his Atlas, which the College possesses, together with other important derma- tological works. The Royal College has kindly agreed to this proposition and is planning to establish such a room in its new building. This should also encourage a closer liaison between general medicine and one of its more important specialities.

The beautiful Willan Room has in the event provided the Asso- ciation and indeed British Dermatology with a splendid home.

In Gray's clear and succinct account of the Association's history he appears to have believed that restriction of member- ship had enabled the Association to maintain a high scientific standard of achievement. In this he was perhaps putting the cart before the horse. The Association fulfilled a very valuable func- tion indeed in a number of ways but although there were out- standing contributions now and again, its scientific standard of performance in the inter-war years was not high. Scientifically in fact the Association has come to life in quite recent years, especially perhaps from the time when limitation of numbers has been removed altogether. Not only is this a beneficial change, whatever its cause, reflected in the quality of contributions at the Annual General Meeting, but the Association has organised additional Annual Meetings at which only research work may be presented. The programmes of these new Meetings have rather resembled those of the Society of Investigative Dermatology and of the American Academy but not slavishly.

Perhaps it would be out of place here to thank our friends in the United States for consistently warm and unstinted generosity to the generations of British dermatologists of the postwar years. The great debt is fully and gratefully recognised.

In later years, as one might expect, Dowling was able to use his range of knowledge and experience to review certain subjects of personal interest. The usual stimulus to do this is a guest lectureship or other form of special invitation rather than any spontaneous urge. In consequence the publication might appear in a little known journal, and not be widely read.

One of the first was a paper on 'The concept of collagen disease'.* It had been written as one of a series of 25 invited articles on 'Modern treatment in general practice' by the Editor of *The Medical Press*. Dowling used most of it for a paper presented to the West of England and Wales Dermatological Society at their meeting in Newport, Monmouth, on 22 February 1957. It was as comprehensible to general practitioners as to dermatologists. The term 'collagen disease' was first used by Paul Klemperer (a pathologist) in 1941, but was seized upon by clinicians in many branches of medicine (as they later did with the term 'vasculitis') to label and explain many disorders which had previously been regarded as of unknown origin. Most of these clinicians, unlike Dowling, did not read Klemperer's paper six years later, in which he wrote, 'This result would seem regrettable.' In spite of Klemperer's retraction, the original term has remained in common use among doctors for several decades. But there was some beneficial effect. The term did catch their imagination and undoubtedly stimulated a great deal of research into connective tissue and its diseases, which was valuable at a time when corticosteroid drugs were coming into general use.

Another such review was on Behçet's disease.† For this he read almost all of the original publications on the subject and wrote a masterly critique. If he thought that some of the published reports were inaccurate or inadequately supported by evidence, instead of stating his opinions and including the references to them, he simply omitted any mention of them. This led some readers to believe that he was not aware of and had missed the reports of these published cases. But he preferred the reader to assume that his review was deficient, rather than that he should be seen to be criticizing the authors of such reports.

In similar vein, if he was sent a book to review by an editor and he found it to be of poor quality, he preferred to return the book to the editor rather than submit an adverse review.

In 1958 Dowling was the Prosser White Orator of the St John's Hospital Dermatological Society. His Oration was entitled 'Concepts in dermatology'.‡ Having practised both before and after the scientific revolution of the 1940s, he was in a unique position to review the changes in dermatological thought during his own lifetime. It is an

* *The Medical Press* 1958, 239, 92–97.
† *Proceedings of the Royal Society of Medicine* 1961, 54, 101.
‡ *Transactions of the St John's Hospital Dermatological Society* 1958, 41, 1.

historical document, and paints a wonderfully clear picture of the ideas which were dominant in the minds of the British dermatologists during the first half of the twentieth century.

Almost every paragraph shows again the distinctive characteristics of his style. More than 30 years later it still reads well and illustrates his capacity to criticize and review opinions in a sufficiently detached way, showing respect for views other than his own and devoid of any trace of personal animosity. And in the final paragraph he ventured to predict future trends and the way forward for dermatology. It was prophetic.

The entire Oration is reproduced here.

> May I begin by saying how deeply I appreciate the honour of being invited to give the Prosser White Oration this year. I feel it all the more since I have attended the Society's meetings regularly for years, sharing with Dr Wigley the honour of being the oldest active member. I am in the habit of expressing opinions at the meetings frequently and freely, and I am duly conscious of the fact that the opinions are not always right. In spite of this hard fact, and knowing that I can have nothing fresh to add to knowledge, the Society invites me to contribute something that I may perhaps have gleaned from a relatively long experience. It occurred to me that one way of doing this might be by attempting to review the impact of the major aetiological concepts on dermatological thought and practice during the past forty years, comparing past attitudes with those that appear to prevail today. I realise that I could hardly have undertaken a more difficult task, for I cannot truthfully claim to know much more about the thoughts of the dermatologists during the period I am setting out to review, than you do. My observations must, therefore, be based mainly on contemporary literature, though I am of course better able to speak from personal knowledge on contemporary practice.
>
> 'The state in which the animal finds itself at any time' says Pickering (1950), 'is determined by two prime factors — its inherited constitution and the effects of its environment, past and present. The common causes of disease thus include:
>
> 1 Inborn and inherited abnormalities

2 Excess of a chemical agent in the environment
3 Deficiencies
4 Infection or infestation by viruses, bacteria, fungi and animal parasites
5 Physical trauma

and he envisages as an additional group, diseases which may be due to the absence or deficiency of organisms that live on the host and in some way contribute to its welfare, though of this class no established example has been isolated.

Obviously a considerable proportion of skin diseases belong to these categories, but there is a large residual pool of common and rare diseases which cannot yet be shown to do so. Their causes are unknown or at best only partly known. It is these that the major concepts of the day have attempted to explain.

When I became chief assistant in dermatology nearly forty years ago, having had no previous experience in this subject, Barber told me that the key to knowledge of the subject was the dermatological eye. With its aid it was possible to know a great deal about the state of health in one's patients. He regarded dermatological vision as a natural faculty which, if deficient, could not be acquired by any amount of diligence. Many who had the good fortune to be present must have retained a vivid recollection of Haxthausen's (1951) lecture on the subject. He took rather a different view, maintaining that the dermatological eye was acquired naturally by certain mechanisms, and these he illustrated by prehistoric cave drawings and by drawings of some of the modern artists. The essence of the argument was that in the course of practice dermatologists, like such artists, acquired the faculty of being able to pay attention only to visual essentials. I believe most of us agree that dermatologists, though by no means comparable in skill with a Matisse, do indeed recognise without conscious effort, a host of complicated looking skin disorders, while their non-dermatological colleagues have no such facility and are usually only too ready to admit it. I do not think there is any conflict in these two definitions of the dermatological eye, only a difference in emphasis. Haxthausen laid stress on the mechanism of observing differences in appearance. Barber emphasised the importance of correlating what could be seen with the expert eye with derangements which were hidden from view. Among British dermatologists of that period he, Leslie Roberts, and Whitfield were the leading exponents of the approach to obscure dermatological problems by looking inwards, that is through general concepts.

Focal sepsis

The great concept of the 1920s was that of focal sepsis. There was a vast literature on the subject and this was collected and comprehensively summarised by Leslie Roberts (1921) in two long papers. I know of no other dermatological publication in which such a complete summary has been attempted.

There is now a consensus of opinion, he wrote, that tonsillar infection and diseases of the gums and alveolar sockets may be followed by systemic disease, such as acute rheumatic fever, infective chorea, endocarditis, arthritis, and some forms of nephritis, and other symptoms such as muscular pain, recurrent headaches, anaemia, etc. Two orders of events were envisaged in the theory. In the tonsils or gums harmless bacteria could be converted into front attacking organisms having special affinities for special organs. Alternatively bacteria might not multiply in the focus; on the contrary they might be destroyed *in situ* by leucocytic enzymes with the coincident discharge into the blood stream of toxins which could evoke slowly evolving disease in some remote organs. Leslie Roberts believed that in dermatology the second order of events was the more important. Among its probable results he included lupus erythematosus, lichen planus, alopecia areata, and prurigo, as well as general changes such as increased greasiness, melanoderma and the tendency to pyoderma, adding urticaria and angioneurotic oedema as more acute manifestations of the same process. For a long and detailed study he selected lupus erythematosus, alopecia areata, lichen planus, prurigo—eczema, psoriasis and eczema of the seborrhoeic type.

In a very full and detailed account of the outcome of his work, listed under twelve separate headings, one striking fact seems to emerge, namely that the operation of tonsillectomy was frequently followed by resolution or marked improvement in lupus erythematosus, alopecia areata, lichen planus and prurigo—

eczema, a contemporary term for the eczema–asthma syndrome. Psoriasis and the 'eczema state' were not favourably influenced by the treatment.

The hypothesis of chronic intestinal stasis

Arbuthnot Lane's hypothesis of chronic intestinal stasis as a major cause of disease was contemporary with and in some respects very similar to the concept of focal infection. Controlling peritoneal bands produced kinks in some parts of the colon. These kinks, known as Lane's kinks, delayed the passage of the contents of the small into the large intestine, and the normally sterile contents of the lower reaches of the ileum became infected and the source of toxic absorption. Lane described the ill effects of this state in vigorous terms. They were loss of fat, degenerative change in the skin with the development of pigment, Raynaud's disease, apathy, stupidity or misery which may become exaggerated into a state of melancholia or even apparent imbecility. One of the most serious symptoms was loss of control of temper which made the sufferer very difficult to live with and led to much misery and crime. Chronic intestinal stasis was held to be responsible for Bright's disease, pancreatitis, gall bladder and duct disease, rheumatoid arthritis, Still's disease, cystitis, pyelitis, salpingitis, ulcerative colitis, infections of the skin of a pustular nature and a number of other maladies.

Lane was probably the most skilful surgeon of his day and he was able to put his theories to the extreme therapeutic test of removing the colon, a formidable undertaking in those days, though mostly he was content with severing the controlling bands which were responsible for Lane's kinks. In support of his views he could produce patients in whom rheumatoid arthritis and even Still's disease had cleared up after operation. I may say that Lane's theories were not at all acceptable to my medical teachers, who were convinced that the colon served some useful purpose and should not be removed without good cause. But he was a man of ideas and a great surgeon and naturally he had a considerable following.

Lane was a handsome and impressive figure. I once had occasion as a junior house officer to waylay him in the colonnade at Guy's Hospital, and this I did with a feeling of some awe.

He thrust his arm through mine and walked me along the colonnade, paying no attention, as far as I could judge, to the small matter about which I had to trouble him but, in his soft Irish voice, inviting me, whom he did not know, to visit a new surgical unit he had organised at Sidcup to deal with facial war wounds. Associated with him were Professor Tonks of the Slade School of Art, Kelsey Fry, and a young surgeon named Gillies. It was the birth in Great Britain of the new art of plastic surgery. His vision in this venture was unerring.

Whitfield (1921) emphasised the importance of intestinal toxaemia as an occasional though by no means a regular factor in skin diseases. He sought for it by testing the urine for indican, urobilin and bile salts and sometimes by examination of the faecal flora. He described in detail two cases of psoriasis and one of lupus erythematosus in whom he had found indican in the urine with creosote by mouth. He thought oral and tonsillar sepsis could be held accountable for some cases of erythema multiforme, lupus erythematosus, prurigo and eczema of the eczema–asthma class. Whitfield (1932) also described under the name 'dermatitis colonica' a new clinical picture. Unfortunately no drawings or photographs were published and unless his successors at King's College Hospital have inherited the picture it may be lost to posterity. It was described as a superficial figured eruption occupying characteristic sites, of the type which might be classed under the vague heading parapsoriasis, and it was regularly associated with a great prominence in the stool of varieties of streptococci. It could be cured by intestinal anti-biotics and suitable diet.

Barber wholeheartedly accepted the doctrine of focal infection as a major cause of disease and maintained his faith during the whole of his career. His final views were given in this lecture six years ago: urticaria, eczema and psoriasis, he said, are sometimes allergic responses to infecting organisms but very commonly are not. The closely linked erythema group of eruptions, erythema multiforme, erythema annulare centrifugum, granuloma annulare, erythema nodosum, erythema induratum and lupus erythematosus always represent primarily allergic reactions to one organism or another. Finally, pustular bacterid and pustular psoriasis are directly due to focal infection and they are exceptional in that the removal of the focus or foci is in the great majority of patients sufficient to cure without after treatment.

In modern times the pendulum has without doubt, swung away from the concept, some may think too far. In relation to such diseases as rheumatoid arthritis, peptic ulceration and ulcerative colitis, Pickering regards the hypothesis as dead and buried. Long (1956) accepts the 'post streptococcal state' as an essential causal factor in rheumatic fever basing this belief particularly on work by Rantz, Spink and Boisvert (1945). Working on military personnel these authors produced evidence to show that rheumatic fever does not occur except in patients who have had upper respiratory infection with Group A haemolytic streptococci.

To what extent the doctrine may be said to have survived in dermatology I would not venture to say. It is certainly referred to in the literature as the theoretical basis for a few chronic diseases, for example the so-called vascular allergides. More especially and perhaps with greater justification, focal infection of the upper respiratory region could be regarded as the basis for pyococcal infective disorders of the skin itself. For example, a relationship of this kind seems to be evident in a type of eczema seen sometimes in children, happily less often in these days than twenty or thirty years ago. The children are subject to chronic or recurrent upper respiratory infection of catarrhal type and at the same time to recurrent or chronic blepharitis, conjunctivitis, chronic eczema of the scalp and of the retro-auricular folds and from time to time of the large folds. During severe episodes acute pustular folliculitis may appear, most often on the legs, as well as eczema of the pompholyx distribution on the hands and feet. This malady may persist or it may remit and relapse at intervals throughout life, though it may also come to a stop almost dramatically at some time during childhood. In male adults sycosis may be added to it. This type of eczema is commonly labelled 'seborrhoeic' though seborrhoea appears to be no part of it. Though in this process susceptibility of the mucous membranes to infection is shared by the skin, this joint susceptibility cannot I feel be justly interpreted as a manifestation of the cryptic focal infection which was held to be responsible for so much illness thirty to fifty years ago. The existence of a direct relationship between focal infection and such peripheral lesions as the tuberculides, acute guttate psoriasis and erythema nodosum has never been in question and everyone must occasionally have met with other eruptive phenomena in which a relationship between manifest acute or subacute focal infection and the cutaneous event has appeared to be at least highly probable. I would judge the concept to be viable in dermatology, but by no means as flourishing at the present time as it used to be. It appears to be no longer customary to search diligently for cryptic focal infection in such diseases as lupus erythematosus, urticaria, erythema multiforme and 'endogenous' eczema, and treatment with autogenous vaccines seems to have gone out altogether. The concept of ileal stasis is, I imagine, quite dead, as well as the practice of treating refractory skin disease of one kind or another by colonic irrigation which was in vogue at one time.

The seborrhoeic state

Dermatology has one major concept of its own and perhaps many general physicians have never heard of it. Unna described the clinical features of the disease which he named seborrhoeic eczema in simple terms. 'The hairy regions are the places of its origin; the sites of predilection are behind the ears and the presternal and interscapular areas. Its lesions spread serpiginously and clear up in the centre. By degrees the active process comes to an end and the lesions become stationary.' Darier redefined the picture with great clarity enlarging it somewhat, but at the same time keeping it within certain strict confines. He did not like the term 'seborrhoeic eczema' because he did not find that seborrhoea was necessarily a part of it, and he coined the term 'eczematides' for the clinical group. Barber not only enlarged the boundaries of seborrhoeic eczema but he gave to its background the status of an important constitutional state. It is possibly for this reason that the term seborrhoeic eczema is widely used in this country while in others, especially in France, it has been largely abandoned in favour of others, such as figured eczematides, pityriasiform or psoriasiform eczematides or parakeratoses, infective parakeratoses or microbial epidermo-dermatides.

I doubt whether the concept of the seborrhoeic state, as Barber described it, is very well known to the modern generation of dermatologists, and for that reason I beg your leave to relate it in some detail . . . The importance of the seborrhoeic state, he said, is that it exemplifies how a metabolic change resulting from unnatural conditions of life may produce an environment which enables harmless saprophytes to become parasitic and produce skin disease. It enables us to study the local defence reactions of the body against these several organisms, the underlying factors which predispose to the change from saprophytic to parasitic, and the means of counteracting or preventing the change. The skin is not alone affected in the seborrhoeic state; the mucous membranes suffer too and become likewise a prey to infection. The skin organisms concerned are the spore of Malassez, the *Staphylococcus albus* and the acne bacillus. The patients are divided into two types: (1) The flushed robust and in later life plethoric type; (2) Predominately dark or mouse coloured people, pallid, thick skinned and hypotonic. In type 1, referred to as the simple type, the lips are bright red and covered with a superficial yellowish crust which he calls the 'seborrhoeic scum'. Gingivitis and chronic naso-pharyngeal catarrh, representing doubtless the associated lowered resistance to infection, are commonly present. When these mucous membrane changes date from childhood they are associated with the adenoid facies and marked hypertrophy of lymphoid tissue. On the other hand the condition may develop in middlelife particularly in those who, having been athletic, adopt the sedentary life. In the second pallid hypotonic type the lips may be pale or bluish, the tongue pale and indented, the papillae hardly visible. Caries and gingivitis are the rule particularly in the simple type.

Alimentary symptoms consist of intestinal flatulence due to carbohydrate fermentation. Increased urinary acidity is found in many patients with acute manifestations of the seborrhoeic state. Pathologically the essential change is the secretion and composition of the cutaneous fat and it is this modification which favours the parasitic modification of the saprophytes inhabiting the skin. Some similar change must modify the mucous membranes and their resistance to organisms. The causes of these changes may be inborn and hereditary, but all are potential seborrhoeics. Dietary errors, excess of sugar, starches, fats and alcohol contribute to the development of the acquired syndrome.

The toxic, type 2, have intestinal stasis, especially of the lower end of the ileum where toxic substances may be produced and absorbed. That was the background of seborrhoeic eczema and acne as Barber saw it thirty years ago. The clinical pictures evoked are very clear, but to many the concept has always appeared to lack definition and the term seems now-a-days to be used largely as a means of identifying a certain pattern or distribution of eczema whether associated with manifest seborrhoea or not. Percival (1939) tried to clarify the picture, differentiating the group delineated by Unna and Darier from the type I have mentioned while discussing focal infection, and preferring for that type such terms as infective flexural dermatitis or exudative infective dermatitis. Ingram (1938) does not agree with him, retaining the label seborrhoeic for both types with all the clinical variations including blepharitis and sycosis. Furthermore, he accepts the entire clinical syndrome as Barber described it, including alimentary features.

Much though I enjoyed hearing and subsequently reading Twiston Davies's disquisition on the scope of the term seborrhoeic eczema, which he seemed to enlarge rather than restrict, I did not think that by postulating the presence of a hypothetical circulating noxa he had provided a very promising starting point for laboratory study.

I doubt whether the majority of dermatologists accept Barber's aetiological hypothesis of thirty years ago. He tried to explain too much on little evidence other than his own clinical intuition. Indeed he said, 'Our knowledge of the metabolism of the seborrhoeic state is fragmentary and based almost entirely on clinical observations...A complete biochemical investigation of the whole problem is urgently needed and would I believe, throw light on much which is now obscure.' No such investigation has been forthcoming and the concept rests where Barber left it. All that we can say at the moment is that the broad clinical definition of the syndrome favoured by Barber, Ingram and Twiston Davies appears to be acceptable to the majority. We are faced daily with the syndrome; it is our responsibility, and any advance in understanding, however, small and from whatever angle, would be acceptable.

Psychosomatic origins of skin disease

The purely psychogenic origin of dermatitis artefacta, acarophobia and other skin phobias, of cutaneous hypochrondriasis, beautifully delineated by Gillespie (1938), compulsive excoriations and one or two other skin disturbances of a like order has never been in question. Excessive physiological skin responses to emotional stimuli, such as blushing and plantar and palmar sweating, are also accepted as reflecting personality and the mechanisms are largely understood. Those who cast the net more widely hardly ever fail to relate the rather rare cholinergic urticaria with the far more common chronic urticaria and angioneurotic oedema, though clinically the similarity is not great.

But the supporters of the concept pay very little attention to such direct effects of emotional disturbance as these. The literature on the subject shows immediately that they cast the net very widely indeed, embracing almost all common disorders which cannot otherwise be accounted for satisfactorily. Gillespie (1938) wrote:

The skin is an organ of emotional expression reacting like the viscera, to feelings of anger, shame and fear. The skin is second only to the sex organs themselves as a source of sexual excitement. According to the Freudian theory, the entire body is regarded as an erogenous area in early infancy, with special sensibility round the mouth, the anus and the genitalia. Ultimately in the normal course of events the genital area predominates, but fixations, that is, a lingering of special sensibility or interest in one or other of these areas, may occur. In later life involution or regressive processes may lead to a reanimation of interest in the anal zone with a diminution of genital eroticity. This would account for the tendency to pruritus ani and general pruritus to appear more often in later life. While accepting the major factor of congenital disposition, Gillespie notes the existence of a psychological factor in the eczema–asthma syndrome, being guided here by the observations of his colleague Rogerson who found the children suffering from this syndrome to be usually above the average intelligence and to be aggressive in temperament. Chronic urticaria also is regarded by him as a psychogenic disorder in a predisposed person.

Stokes and Beerman (1940), strong supporters of the concept, reviewed much of the important literature on psychosomatic correlations in allergic conditions in great detail. Some of the authors they quote express views which many dermatologists would find impossible to accept; Hansen, for example, supposes that allergens may work only in certain psychic constellations, the patient being sensitive at one time and not at another according to his state of mind. Dunbar relates the personality to the disease, finding in patients suffering from the eczema–asthma syndrome a marked predominance of anal and oral sadistic material, involving sexualisation of the respiratory function and great interest in the sense of smell. The patients were said to be intensely hostile and aggressive during symptom-free periods. Meara and I have failed entirely to observe these characteristics in the children at the Goldie Leigh Hospital, the majority of whom suffer from relatively severe degrees of the syndrome, nor have they appeared to be specially intelligent. Nickum is quoted as noting that hay fever occurs in the type whose abnormally large output of energy and accelerated emotional and intellectual responses tend to situations in which are produced aggressive and painful effects that jeopardise their sympathetic–autonomic balance.

Becker and Obermayer (1942) state that dermatology is unique in that only a minority of diseases can be proved to be of organic origin. They assume that all functional disease results from exaggerated cerebral impulses, and as neurodermatoses, that is, dermatoses which arise from such impulses, they list idiopathic pruritus, neurotic excoriations, dry and exudative neurodermatitis, dysidrosis, chronic urticaria, alopecia areata, lichen planus, vitiligo and rosacea, while scleroderma, recurrent erythema multiforme, aphthous stomatitis and Sutton's mucosal ulcers of the mouth are added as probable examples. The patients suffering from neurodermatoses, they say, seem to have been born with an excess of protoplasmic unrest present in every cell in their bodies. Mothers of the patients have often stated that they exhibited prenatal hyperactivity. Their psychological make up is described in simple general terms. At work they are constantly rushing, always behind and trying to catch up; they are hypersensitive, conscientious, worried. The neurodermatoses they say are not common in Europe and South America where, in comparison with North America, life is quiet.

To the views of all these writers Sulzberger and Baer (1951) are diametrically opposed. Most attempts, they say, to ascribe various skin diseases to psychic and emotional causes have fallen far short of satisfying criteria of proof which scientists would demand. Even severe and characteristically uniform psychic and emotional disturbances, found in patients suffering from some diseases, might not be the cause but quite frequently rather the result of a chronic or apparently quite hopeless skin disease, with its interminable years of maddening itching, disfigurement and many fundamental interferences with social and economic success and other ego satisfactions. After listing the conditions which manifestly are due to mental causes they dismiss from further consideration all diseases classed by Becker and Obermayer as neurodermatoses and all allergic responses in general.

Stated thus crudely it might appear that the question before dermatologists is simply whether to accept or reject the hypothesis that mental disturbance can engender skin disorders, but obviously it is a great deal more complicated than that. It is possible to agree with Sulzberger and Baer that the supporters of the concept have failed completely to produce evidence to support their claims, but we can hardly ignore the fact that the behaviour of skin diseases is often closely correlated with mental states. Sargent (1957) holds the view that, though never the cause, emotional tension strongly influences the pattern of psoriasis and the eczema—asthma syndrome especially, and there seems to be plenty of clinical evidence that this is so.

According to Pickering, the small amount of critically established fact on which the hypothesis can be based is probably accounted for by the fact that the condition of any patient suffering from a disease deteriorates when there is super-added mental disturbance. By and large I would expect that view to be acceptable to the majority of dermatologists; but we should like to know about the mechanisms all the same. Whitlock (1958), at once an experimental dermatologist with the scientific bent and a psychiatrist, is an ally to whom in England we look hopefully for enlightenment.

The concept of collagen disease

The concept of collagen disease never aimed at being an aetiological hypothesis. It sought to reduce the apparently heterogeneous morbid anatomical changes in an important group of diseases to a common denominator. The concept, based mainly on a long and detailed study of lupus erythematosus, was formulated by Klemperer and his associates (1942) in a concise and now well known paragraph: 'Until now an inordinate preoccupation with immediate causes has shut the door to an analysis of the fundamental changes within the connective tissue considered as a colloidal system. The connective tissue having been established as the seat of certain diseases it remains for the investigators to explain the system with the methods available to the biophysicist and the chemist.' Plain words, but the conclusions drawn from the new concept were evidently more sweeping than the authors expected and five years later Klemperer (1947) writes: 'The term collagen disease merely refers to the fact that the alteration of the extra-cellular portion of the connective tissue is pronounced and systemic in certain diseases. Such a designation would seem to lump together such heterogeneous maladies as disseminated lupus erythematosus, generalised scleroderma, rheumatic fever and even periarteritis nodosa. This result would seem regrettable. By calling attention to the collagen tissue as a common denominator we only wanted to indicate that this tissue may be the common anatomic site of several diseases.' Quite recently (1956) he called attention to the fact that the fibrinoid substances responsible for alterations seen in the ground substance are not the same in the different diseases, that they are not derived from collagen but are added to it, being deposited on or between the fibres and that only one of them has been identified chemically, the fibrinoid of lupus erythematosus. Thus the architect of this concept is also responsible for its partial demolition. Klemperer sees valid objections to the use of the term collagen disease as well as for connective tissue or mesenchymal disease as substitutes, but suggests that for the time being it may be acceptable as a convenient abbreviating term. The adjective 'so-called' seems nowadays a customary addition.

For Robb-Smith (1954) the immense value of the concept is that it has focused interest on the connective tissue and its diseases and has stimulated rewarding research both on the fundamental biologic aspects of connective tissue and also on the pathogenesis of the diseases themselves. With this assessment there can be no disagreement. The idea was prevalent at one time that the collagen diseases were linked in some way and merged into one another. Having no knowledge of the cause of any of them, we are unable to say whether such a link exists or not, but the facts as far as they have been clarified both on a clinical and pathological basis seems rather to emphasise the individuality of each disease and the importance of accurate differentiation. Here dermatology often comes into its own. One of the effects of the impact of the concept on dermatology is indeed the frequency with which dermatologists are called into consultation in the general wards over these cases.

The general adaptation syndrome and its diseases

No one can read the monumental work of Selye without admiration. Here at last was a concept based entirely on physiological experiments, and there could be no doubt that the physiological conclusions drawn from the experiments were correct. But when the General Adaptation Syndrome attempted to explain non-specific disease the reasoning became more difficult to follow. In any case the upshot of a long and complicated story seems now clear enough and the idea that collagen diseases and perhaps psoriasis could be attributed to deranged or derailed hypophysis–adrenal function in response to stress, seems now to have been abandoned. One aspect of the general adaptation syndrome, however, and of Hench's independent but contemporary work, must be of considerable interest to dermatologists. Hench's hypothetical anti-rheumatic agent Substance X, the ideal anti-inflammatory agent, was assumed to be provided by the body under certain conditions; these were shock treatment with triple typhoid vaccine, surgical operations of any kind, starvation, jaundice and pregnancy. That such an agent could only be produced through the defence mechanisms described by Selye can hardly be doubted, so that we have now perhaps a reasonable explanation of the disappearance of psoriasis, for example, in pregnancy and of the remarkable cures and remissions in various skin disorders which have been shown in the past to follow tonsillectomy, and other operations. Some of us may even have had occasion to be impressed by the astonishing success in the treatment of eczema achieved sometimes by nature curers by pure starvation.

I have attempted to review briefly the impact of five major general concepts on progress in dermatology in England during the span of my experience. Allergy, a term signifying various mechanisms, is not a concept and therefore it has not been discussed. If we suppose that lupus erythematosus and erythema multiforme may be allergic responses to hidden bacterial infection, the hypothesis by which we are attempting to explain these two disorders is that of focal sepsis. If it is said that the eczema– asthma syndrome is the product of hypersensitivity to allergens of the pollen type, the cart is being placed so plainly in front of the horse that no discussion is called for. There are solid reasons, in fact, for placing this syndrome in Pickering's first aetiological group. Eruptions produced by drugs and other substances belong to the second group. Whitfield's hypothesis of autosensitisation is certainly a concept which tries to explain certain events, but up to the present the allergic mechanism which the concept envisages has not been shown to exist. Throughout it has always been clear to me that the concepts have greatly influenced dermatological thought and practice. The promoters having been among the best clinicians, and at the same time men of ideas, it is natural that this should have been so. It is possible that many, perhaps the majority of us are hardly capable of practising the difficult art without thinking a good deal in terms of such hypotheses. Sometimes the idea seems almost self evident, the simplest example that comes to my mind being Whitfield's concept of autosensitisation. Without ideas it is impossible to proceed, but at the same time without facts we cannot claim to be firmly in touch with reality. If, therefore, by progress we mean advance in established knowledge of causes, the general concepts, valuable though they have been as stimuli to thought and effort, cannot claim to have contributed very much, and many dermatologists appear at the present time to wish to approach their problems from a different angle. The character of dermatological literature is changing a good deal. The subject of mechanisms, especially of hypersensitive and other immune reactions occupies more and more space in the journals, and the production in recent years of a monumental work on the *Physiology and Biochemistry of the Skin* (Rothman, 1953) also bears witness to the change in outlook.

Such a change in perspective can no doubt be attributed both to the growing influence of the Universities on medical education, and to the remarkable growth of the basic medical sciences during the past quarter of a century. Dermatologists are the same people as always, but they now have at their disposal data and means of investigation which were not available to their forerunners. Even the assembly of purely clinical facts, especially therapeutic facts, must in these days be subjected to the discipline of statistical analysis.

Barber (1953) in this lecture five years ago said that no one could appreciate more than himself the immense debt that we owed to laboratory workers or the urge to seek exact knowledge by controlled experiments and statistics that was now so apparent, but in company with others he would plead that the art of the great clinicians should not be allowed to wane. Of this danger I do not believe there need be the smallest fear in this country. Dermatologists receive in these days and no doubt they will continue to receive a far more comprehensive training in clinical dermatology than was ever before possible in the history of British dermatology, and the traditional art flourishes as it never did before. I am too old to offer advice as to how in the future to avoid sterile eclecticism in the art, by which I mean an excellent general standard of clinical ability without the power to add much to knowledge. I would, however, venture to make one observation. I do not see how stagnation can be avoided without enlisting the help of an adequate number of experimental dermatologists. Our American colleagues are well ahead of us, and indeed they appear to be ahead of the rest of the world in this respect.

REFLECTIONS

In 1969 Geoffrey Dowling was invited to take part in the celebrations
of the fiftieth anniversary of the department of dermatology at the
University of Utrecht in Holland. On 29 March 1957 the degree of
Honorary Doctor of Medicine had been conferred on him by the university for his contributions to dermatology. At the celebrations he gave
the opening address — 'Reflections' — in which he looked back on his
own half-century of dermatology. It was the only time he looked back
so personally, and it provides us with his own personal view of the
dermatological times in which he lived.

> I am deeply honoured at being invited to take part in the 50th
> Anniversary of the Department of Dermatology in the University
> of Utrecht, of which Department I am surely the proudest of
> members. I have been in dermatology for nearly fifty years,
> having joined the Department for Diseases of the Skin at Guy's
> Hospital, London, as Chief Assistant to H.W. Barber in 1920.
> Barber himself was the first physician to be appointed to Guy's
> Hospital with no other duties than the care of diseases of the
> skin and I was the first Chief Assistant.
>
> Previously the charge of diseases of the skin had been given to
> general physicians, beginning in 1850 with Thomas Addison.
>
> Perhaps the greatest figure in British Medicine of his time,
> Addison was succeeded in this department by other renowned
> teachers of the 19th century. Several years before his appoint-
> ment to the Department for Diseases of the Skin, Barber had
> been selected by his seniors at Guy's Hospital as a person of
> outstanding promise and he was awarded a travelling fellowship
> in 1913 to study dermatology.
>
> The First War followed a year of study in Paris under Darier.
>
> Though the title 'Chief Assistant' corresponds to the rather
> important 'Chef de Clinique' of the Hôpital St Louis, it was in
> my case made entirely in accordance with the law of supply and
> demand at that moment, for I knew not the first word about
> dermatology.
>
> Barber loved Darier deeply and greatly admired the French
> and their language. The great *Précis* was our bible and we also
> knew the *Entretiens*, the *Maladies du Cuir Chevelu* and other
> outstanding French works of the time.

Barber was a fine clinician, a gifted speaker and writer, and in due course he became generally accepted in England as the outstanding thinker and teacher in dermatology of his day. He had a great following who thought him quite incomparable. He was a good deal younger than the other leading figures in dermatology of that time.

Pringle was nearing the age of retirement. Adamson, a man of great and deserved repute, who is yet remembered for 'Adamson's fringe', was also among the seniors. Sequeira was the writer of a good standard textbook on *Dermatology* and he had set up a copy of the Finsen Institute at the London Hospital for the care of tuberculosis of the skin which was very prevalent in the East End of London in his days. Arthur Whitfield was the generally accepted senior leader of the time.

MacCormac among the younger group was becoming an authority on skin cancer. Later he was to describe molluscum sebaceum in the best classical style.

There were other dermatologists of repute in the twenties, but very little of what they said or did has come down to us.

But in general the generation of dermatologists of fifty years ago were the successors of those who, in the view of Professor Sam Shuster, had lived in dermatology's finest hour, those to whom we owe the first accounts of the diseases and their natural histories, the classical works of dermatology. For the dermatologists of the early decades of the century not very much had been left to describe. Their immediate outstanding predecessors were Jonathan Hutchinson, a surgeon, Radcliffe Crocker and Tilbury Fox, both professional dermatologists and, rather farther back, Erasmus Wilson, also a surgeon.

I like to include Frederick Parkes Weber among the old masters, although he died in his 100th year less than 10 years ago. I like to recall him to mind also because we shall never see his like again. His career at school and Cambridge University had lacked distinction unless a 3rd class degree in Natural Science can be counted as promising. Instead of attending to his masters in his early life be became a collector of butterflies at school, of coins and other antiquities later on. His collections of antiquities are now in the British Museum and in other museums about the world. He and his great friend and collaborator Sturge must have been among the most learned antiquarians of their time.

Parkes Weber was German by birth and he had been brought up to speak in the principal European languages. He became learned also in the antique languages because as a good collector he found it necessary to know them. Quite suddenly he gave up collecting, gave away his entire collection, and became instead a collector of rare diseases, of which a number bear his name. He was not a dermatologist but he liked dermatology better than any other part of his work; he kept many papers on dermatological subjects apart and these are now housed among other classical works on dermatology in the Royal College of Physicians of London. At dermatological meetings he spoke often and at length, invariably ignoring the red light, and even sometimes putting his hand over it.

In his 99th year he told me that he believed that it had been said of him by some that collecting might have been the moving force in his medical life, and he thought there might be some truth in this. He wrote beautifully, altogether just over 1000 papers and several books, his greatest and largest being an anthology on death, the most comprehensive ever to be written, entitled *Aspects of Death and Correlated Aspects of Life*.

Barber had no intention of attempting to copy the achievements of his predecessors. For him descriptive dermatology belonged to the past. Rather he set himself the formidable task of discovering the causes and rational treatment of the common but obscure diseases. To this end he accepted the current aetiological concepts of his age, wholeheartedly maintaining his faith during the whole of his career. Much of his writing was accordingly on lupus erythematosus, erythema multiforme, psoriasis, alopecia areata and various aspects of eczema.

Towards the end of his life he restated his beliefs in the Prosser White Oration of 1952 entitled 'What is truth?'

Discussing focal infection he said: 'Urticaria, eczema and psoriasis are sometimes allergic responses to infecting organisms but very commonly are not. The closely linked erythema group of eruptions, erythema multiforme, erythema annulare centrifugum, granuloma annulare, erythema nodosum, erythema induratum and lupus erythematosus, always represent primarily allergic reactions to one organism or another.' Finally, pustular bacterid and pustular psoriasis are directly due to focal infection and 'they are exceptional in that removal of the focus or foci is in the great majority of cases sufficient to cure without after treatment'. This had been the advanced thinking of the twenties.

Whitfield had similar beliefs. He emphasised especially the importance of intestinal toxaemia as a not uncommon factor in common skin diseases.

He will be remembered for two main achievements: first as a discoverer of fungal infection as the cause of interdigital intertrigo of the feet, together of course with his formulation of the immortal ointment. Secondly, for his hypothesis of 'autosensitzation' as the cause of the widespread eczema which so frequently follows sudden worsening of localized chronic eczema, especially of the legs. I believe that in spite of a good deal of work on it we yet remain in the dark on the mechanism of this common phenomenon. I would think that Whitfield would have been among the avant-garde had he been born a generation or two later, while Barber's innate romanticism was probably incurable. Of his 100 publications very few bear re-reading.

Archibald Gray was a very important figure in British dermatology and indeed a man of world repute in dermatology. He was appointed successor to Radcliffe Crocker at University College Hospital because he was recognised as a man of outstanding ability in general, but he had had very little experience in dermatology at the time of his appointment and he went to Breslau to get it.

His contributions to dermatology, very good of their kind, were unfortunately small in number. He did not accept the speculative hypotheses of the day and Barber regarded him as a broken reed, nothing but an externist. Gray was very soon caught up in Hospital and University administration and he was in due course knighted twice for his public work.

He made good use of his administrative ability and great influence to help to establish dermatological institutions. First he founded the British Association of Dermatology and Syphilis; a little later he was closely concerned with the foundation of the Institute of Dermatology in London. This was a post-graduate school which was intended to serve the needs especially of students from overseas. They were not well served but it was a beginning, and the Institute is in these days a flourishing school with a University Chair.

Later on he was able to establish a Readership in histo-pathology at his own Medical School for Freudenthal who left Breslau during the early phase of the Hitler regime. Hitherto little or no teaching in histopathology of the skin had been available in England. Some who sought to correct the deficiency went to Vienna where standard courses of instruction were given. The pupil, I believe, might receive some kind of certificate as a reward for his attendance, and a few inserted 'Vienna' in the Medical Directory as one of the seats of learning in which they had studied. Evidently some self-deception regarding the value of all this was prevalent at one time. Freudenthal was a first-class histopathologist who satisfied a need and set a good standard. He died not long after the war and meanwhile we had acquired Whimster. Others were soon added and this department of dermatology has been well cared for during the past twenty years.

Without any question dermatology in Great Britain was not in flourishing health during the 1920s. Shuster describes us then and even now as staggering on like a 'dropsied giant, one generation painfully following another'.

The subject was undermanned; there were hardly more than 50 or 60 professional dermatologists in the country who would attend the Annual Meeting of the Association, and much of the hospital dermatological work of the provinces was in the hands of amateurs, mainly general physicians, most of whom were poor dermatologists. Dermatology and venereology were rarely associated and the great dermato-venereological clinics of the Continent had no counterpart in Great Britain.

While unable to speak from personal knowledge, I am under the impression that even outside Great Britain dermatology was not invariably progressive and well organised. However, the clouds appeared to be lifting here and there. There was Bloch who from the outset of his career in the first decade of the century was primarily an experimental worker. Each year he produced a few or several original observations based on experiment in a wide variety of problems, for example, on the production of skin cancer with tar products, on the pathogenesis of eczema and perhaps above all on the mechanism of pigmentation. He was the first professor of dermatology in Zurich and the Swiss authorities provided him with all the space and money for equipment that he required. Bloch in the twenties became the leading dermatologist in Europe and Zurich the leading centre.

In 1930 everyone went to Copenhagen to the International Congress, the first to be held after the War. Among the old guard we were able to see and hear Sabouraud, Brocq and Darier for the last time.

Among the senior Americans Schamberg appeared to me to be specially impressive; it was rumoured at the time that he was expressing regret at having mentioned the matter of the pigmentary dermatosis. Lomholt, the Secretary of the Congress, was following in the footsteps of Finsen and led the world in organising the management of tuberculosis of the skin. Haxthausen fulfilled his promise of those days as an experimental observer, but perhaps he may be remembered best for a small work on *Cold in relation to the Skin*, surely one of the world's classics in dermatology.

The Congress in Budapest in 1935 marked two important changes in dermatological trends. Hitler was in the saddle and most of the heads of departments in Germany had been unseated; the same was about to happen shortly in Austria. The atmosphere was heavy and unpleasant. The second half of the decade in America was to be remarkable for the development of the Society for Investigative Dermatology and its journal.

This Society was officially founded in 1937 but it had been planned much earlier, especially by some of the younger dermatologists who had worked in Bloch's clinic in Zurich.

The promoters had the enthusiastic support of the progressives among the senior generation but there had been some conservative opposition. The venture was successful from the outset.

I am under the impression that America has led the world in the investigative field from those days, while according to Professor Findlay in Pretoria, who for years abstracted dermatological scientific literature for *Dermatologica*, the post-war standard of technical research in Germany has also been very high. No doubt the efforts of the pioneers in the United States were lightened by the advent from Hungary in 1938 of Stephen

Rothman, a veritable giant among dermatologists, whom we had the good fortune to meet in England during a short stay. The bounds of scientific reason may perhaps have been overstepped on one occasion in the United States when a Chair in Dermatology was awarded by 'the powers that be' to a scientist who knew not a word of dermatology and for that reason. He accepted the Chair, but preferred not to sit in it for very long.

On the subject of the scientific approach to dermatology I recall a visit which Whimster and I, with a number of British colleagues, made to Utrecht a few years after the War. Zoon had decided that his department must be manned with scientific workers. He gathered about him such a staff, including Jansen, his natural successor. We found Utrecht very impressive and enjoyable, especially as we had been warned by some Gallic colleagues that we might find the Dutch a bit stodgy.

In Great Britain dermatology has changed out of all knowledge since the War. No dermatologists have ever been trained for practice in the ordinary sense but only to have charge of hospital departments. Accordingly the number of dermatologists, less than 200, is smaller in proportion to population than in most other countries.

There are Chairs in London, Birmingham, Newcastle and Edinburgh and we look forward to the development of some more.

Training for consultant hospital posts, as a rule for a period of six or more years, includes research work, sometimes carried out in research departments not specifically attached to the department of dermatology.

During this period a number of the more able registrars and lecturers spend some time abroad, usually in America. In many cases the same work could be done at home but the experience abroad is greatly prized and enjoyed.

Those in charge of departments of dermatology are free to organise their work as they please. Having no traditional patterns to follow such as those of some of the great Continental clinics, their methods vary somewhat. Thus dermatology at Cambridge, for example, under the aegis of Arthur Rook, gathers to itself periodically for a week scientists in various fields to bring their experience and knowledge to bear on dermatological problems. Three of these meetings have taken place so far and large volumes of proceedings have emanated. Rook also has, with colleagues in both dermatology and other scientific fields, produced a large and comprehensive text book.

We think this a very valuable effort and certainly the best thing of its kind to have come out of our country.

So we hope and believe, most of us, that dermatology is developing, not rapidly but in the right direction in Great Britain. I must admit that I understand some of the language of the avant-garde in dermatology about as well as I understand Dutch, a language of which the English are known to be exceptionally ignorant, hence the term Double Dutch, meaning total incomprehensibility. None the less I have been able on the whole to observe matters in dermatology as they have passed during nearly half a century. I have enjoyed all of it.

In addition to these papers Dowling wrote many other articles on various dermatological subjects, and demonstrated numerous patients at the Dermatological Section of the Royal Society of Medicine (RSM). Showing a case at the RSM nails the problem in the memory of the presenter. Dowling remembered the first one he ever showed — an unusual case (to him) of urticaria pigmentosa. He was humbled by the total absence of comment from either the president or the audience. Another time he showed the first case there of trichostasis spinulosa, and he immediately remembered the patient he had shown with Walter Freudenthal in 1938 as benign acanthosis nigricans (which he always felt was wrong), when the same condition was shown in 1971 as 'a pigmentary anomaly of the axillae', and which is now known as Dowling–Degos disease. As one might have expected it was at a meeting of the Royal Society of Medicine that he chose to present his discovery of the calciferol treatment for tuberculosis of the skin.

His writing remained evergreen both in its quality and its style. Most of his contributions were based on close personal observation. Like Parkes Weber he had great powers of observation and visual curiosity.

In the years between the two world wars he regarded Whitfield and Cranston Low as the best minds. Whitfield said that he himself was not capable of diagnosing ringworm of the feet without a microscope. Knowing this, Dowling showed a patient at the RSM in 1938 with the clinical features of pustular bacterid on the feet, but in whom microscopy showed the roof of a pustule to be full of fungus.

It was the diseases rather than the physiology which he went for; one has to contend with the facts, plus the literature and experiments. But some dermatologists are apt to treat the literature as the raw material. He had little time for theoretical ideas and propositions not based on fact, and he was critical of studies which are interesting but shed no light on a subject. 'We don't want to know that.' Those who have done most work on a subject are the least prepared to speculate. He abhorred pomposity and pretentiousness in any form.

Many articles and even books are published under the title of 'recent advances'. But some 'recent advances' are only the latest ideas, which are not actually controlled nor have they stood the test of time. A step or two backwards could sometimes be regarded as a 'recent advance', such as the curtailment of remedies with unacceptably high risks.

Dowling was meticulous in his choice of written words, and avoided imprecise words or phrases. 'Faulty hygiene' is not capable of more than a vague definition. To regard dysidrosis as an eczema is probably the right way to look at it.

One of Dowling's most agreeable qualities was his informality, and the pleasant conversational air was preserved in his writing. He carried his ideas about with him over a long time, which is a good recipe for almost any field of work. The amateur can pick up or put down his interest. For the professional it is a commitment that overrides retirement, ignorance, mistakes — by living up the subject you live down everything else.

Dowling never let go of dermatology; he was a lifelong professional. He could afford to say what he did not know or understand, since he was committed anyway. If ever he saw dermatology being attacked in medical circles, he was ready to move in and defend it vigorously. And this happened on several occasions when he started at St Thomas's Hospital after transferring from Guy's. It helped to earn him the enormous respect he was given by the staff there in later years.

Dowling spent nearly 30 years honing his tools and incubating his skills before releasing them on to the young dermatologists in training at the end of the Second World War. Musical people know that talent lies with the young, notably in performers. Not surprisingly, he knew it too, and was rewarded in due time with seeing such talent revealed. In fact, it probably gave him as much pleasure as anything else in his life.

Chapter 13
The Family

GEOFFREY Dowling was married to Mary Elizabeth Kelly — May — in 1923. For a short time she had been a nurse at Guy's Hospital. She fell ill and was admitted to the infirmary, where the nurses were looked after by the resident medical officer; and by chance Geoffrey was doing this job. He fell in love.

May Kelly was born in Maryborough, Port Laoighse, in County Leix in Ireland. Her father, Patrick Kelly, was a leading businessman in Maryborough, manufacturing metal goods. He had three wives and 21 children and referred to Maryborough as 'Kellyville'. His parents, William and Sarah Kelly, were married on 7 February 1849. They had 10 children. Patrick, the second, was born in 1852.

Patrick Kelly married Margaret Bray on 19 November 1873, when she was 21 years old. They had nine children:

William Vincent	born	20 July 1874
Sarah Anne	born	31 October 1875 (stillborn)
Margaret Agnes	born	2 October 1877
Patrick Joseph	born	1 April 1879
Francis Joseph	born	15 January 1881
John Alexander	born	10 July 1882
Alphonsus Liquori	born	15 September 1883
Joseph Lazarianno	born	16 October 1885
Aloysius	born	12 July 1887

His wife Margaret died on 8 November 1894. Within a year he married Elizabeth Daly, on 25 July 1895. They had two children:

Sarah Mary (Sallie)	born	18 April 1896
Mary Margaret	born	17 April 1897

Just a few weeks later, after the birth of their second child his wife died, on 8 May 1897, presumably of puerperal septicaemia. The baby girl survived only for two months and died on 6 July 1897.

Patrick Kelly was married for the third time to Katherine Lowe. They had ten children:

Eileen Mary	born	27 June 1899 (died February 1900)
Kathleen Philomena	born	31 August 1990
Mary Elizabeth	born	18 September 1901
Gertrude Mary	born	15 January 1903
Thomas Augustine	born	15 May 1904
Theresa Mary	born	26 June 1905
Irene Frances	born	12 July 1906
Sheelagh Josephine	born	1 April 1908
Gerard Majella	born	15 June 1909
Anthony Noel	born	14 December 1910

May's mother's family, the Lowes, were farmers and horse-breeders in the area around Carrick-on-Shannon in the west of Ireland. Katherine Lowe was one of eight children, whose father died young, and their mother had to bring them up alone. She never remarried. The Lowes were interested in antiques, and Katherine's father encouraged the children to play games and to draw, but there was no hint of any musical talent in the family.

May spent most of her engagement at home in Ireland and, since engagements were formal and relatively long in the nineteen-twenties, Geoffrey had to do most of his courting across the Irish Sea, an activity not easy for a hard-working young doctor struggling to get on in his profession.

They married in Ireland in 1923. May was 22 and Geoffrey 32 years old. Back in London, their first family home was in Prince of Wales Drive in Battersea. It was a large corner flat and Tom remembers it as having a very cold drawing-room.

Three years later they moved to a small cottage in Nuffield village near the Huntercombe Golf Club, rented from W.R. Morris. It was one of a group of three cottages and a house, a blacksmith and a pub — the Crown Inn, a sixteenth-century coaching inn — which made up the hamlet of Huntercombe. Huntercombe had several attractions. William Morris (later Lord Nuffield, but always known as W.R.) had bought the club in 1925. There was a residential clubhouse, where a coterie of their friends stayed, linked by Guy's and a fondness for golf, who would regularly visit the cottage with their wives. W.R. was one of this circle, as were the Lazanbies and Jonah Gedge, Dowling's solicitor. John Conybeare, Robert Macintosh, Dean Johnson, William Doherty and McEvedy were frequent visitors. The fact was the club was just too far from London to pay. Clubs nearer, like Wentworth, thrived, but Huntercombe was in danger of closing, so W.R. moved in and saved it. He wanted to own a club as he did not wish to be pestered by 'motor people', so they were banned from membership! He was thought to have wanted to be a doctor when young and it was through this association that so much money was given to medicine, especially to Guy's Hospital.

The cottage was double-fronted, 'two up and two down', with an addition at the back for the kitchen below and the bathroom and spare room above. The front door was at the back facing south, where there was a brick-laid patio (called 'the bricks'), a perfect playground for the children. Beyond it was a nice-sized garden with a large yew-tree half-way down, where the vegetable garden started and where they also kept some chickens. At the end was a hedge separating their garden from the seventh fairway of the golf course.

May transformed the garden by employing tramps as day labour in return for a good lunch, and her creation is well recorded in photographs. She loved gardening, so it was surprising that they never had a garden again; but some time later she did redesign the garden at her family home in Ireland.

Geoffrey took his golf seriously and used to practise his shots on the nearby fairway, especially on light summer evenings after he had arrived back from London. On one occasion, young Tom was standing behind him, when he decided to take another viewpoint of his father's skills. Coming round his father's left leg, he was hit on his right temple by the club, which Tom later said was a mashie-niblick. Blood streamed down the boy's face. His father used his yellow tobacco-pouch to staunch the wound and carried him back into the cottage. He then drove him to the local doctor's surgery to be stitched up. More than 60 years later, the scar is still visible.

Apart from walks and car excursions, life rotated round the cottage for the next four years. Nanny Verbie came to look after the children, followed by Miss Eastwood (Essie), who came as governess and who was to stay with the family until they moved to London in 1930, returning to them for one year when La was six. Essie was a marvellous teacher. After leaving the Dowlings for a second time, she worked as housekeeper for a retired general, Leslie Jones, whom she married in

1940. They lived on a farm in Devon, where Simon had many happy holidays, always returning with 'beautiful' manners, which relapsed, according to his sisters, after 24 hours at home.

Essie taught Tom and Jane the three Rs and encouraged drawing and painting. She was so good that Jane was reading entire books by the age of four and a half. Tom was not so keen, but they were both reading by the time they went to school in London.

Their father went to Huntercombe at weekends and occasionally on a weekday in summer. He drove all the way in a large American Buick; the journey was easy in those days.

May occasionally took the children to Mass on Sunday mornings in Wallingford. In the summer they would sometimes drive there for a picnic and a swim in the River Thames. Tom vividly remembers watching sticklebacks swimming around his father's feet. He was terrified that he was going to be eaten!

Sunday lunch was always an event at Huntercombe. Geoffrey's friends from Guy's were frequent visitors, especially 'Uncle Mac' (Robert Macintosh) and 'Uncle Coney' (John Conybeare).

May and Geoffrey's third child, Alannah, was born in 1930. For this event Tom and Jane were packed off with Kiki for a holiday at Gorey in Jersey. They were told that there would be a lovely surprise when they returned home. Tom pictured a three-funnelled clockwork steamer for his bath. He already had a two-funnelled one and could think of nothing finer. On arriving home and being shown the new-born Alannah, he cried out 'Only a BABY!'

Shortly afterwards they left the Huntercombe cottage and moved back to London to start school.

Their new home was 1A Inverness Terrace, close to Kensington Gardens off the Bayswater Road. The house was very French-looking and stood out for its elegance in a terrace where most of the other houses were enormous Victorian ones, some of which had already been joined up to make hotels. It was unusual to own one's own house at that time, and the house was rented for £200 per annum, quite expensive in those days. Had May known London better, she would probably have chosen a house with a garden, but Inverness Terrace was taken because of its proximity to Kensington Gardens and also because it was reasonably near to Harley Street. The children walked across the park to school in Kensington Square, and at weekends were taken to the Round Pond, where Tom sailed his boats, or to clamber about the Albert Memorial, or to Peter Pan. Sometimes Geoffrey took La to the bandstand near the Round Pond, where there were regular performances.

In 1932 Essie left, returning in 1936 for some months when May was ill. In the intervening years the children had a series of Mesdemoiselles and Fräuleins to look after them, but when Essie left again in 1937 Delia Wood, who had worked with the family as housemaid since 1930, took over. She and her husband 'Pop' were much beloved by the whole family.

During the term-time in London Geoffrey was keen that the children should have as much exercise as possible. Jane and La went to dancing classes and swimming at the Porchester Baths, and all the children went to Queen's Ice Rink, just around the corner from Inverness Terrace.

The holidays for the most part were spent out of London, and the requirements were a sandy beach and a good golf course. In the Huntercombe years, two summers were spent in Jersey; later the family went to Herne Bay, Bude in Cornwall and Westende in Belgium, where Tom and Jane sand-sailed. When Tom was old enough to have a sailing-boat, they had a number of holidays in Budleigh Salterton near Exmouth in Devon. Spring holidays were often taken in Seaford on the south coast, where the children learnt to ride on the Downs, at Le Touquet, Paris Plage, and many times in Ireland, where they were at that time the only nephew and nieces of their many uncles and aunts. Geoffrey joined them at the weekends when he could get away.

May took the two older children in 1934 on the *Homeric*, a White Star Liner, to Madeira, the Canaries, Tangier and Gibraltar. The ship was magnificent. Tom and Jane visited the Madeira winery and duly received their little sample bottles. Not knowing anything about alcohol, they sampled them in bed that evening. May, finding her children giggling, confiscated the bottles saying they could be finished at home, where it would be 'safer'. In 1936 they spent three weeks sailing the length of the Mediterannean in the P. & O. liner *Moldavia*.

In 1937 Geoffrey and May took Tom by wagons-lits to Milan and Venice, staying at the Bauer Grunwald Hotel, and thence by a Yugoslav steamer, the *Kralj Alexander II*, to Dubrovnik, where they stayed at the Hotel Excelsior. Tom still has his Thomas Cook brochure. The holiday cost £37.10s a head. In 1939 Geoffrey planned to take Tom, with Dr McEvedy and his son Mark, via the Kiel Canal to Leningrad and thence by train to Moscow. Their visas were held up, so they booked a shorter 10-day cruise on the Canadian Pacific liner *Montcalm* to the Baltic. Geoffrey always regretted the change of plan. The next time Tom was to board the *Montcalm* was as HMS *Wolfe*. She had been converted into a very good submarine depot ship and was stationed in Trincomalee. Very little of her interior was recognizable.

Apart from the holidays, Geoffrey and May had long weekends at Huntercombe. These often took the form of reunions with the old Guy's crowd and their families. Geoffrey continued to return there until about 1958 or 1960. Tom sometimes joined them.

At Inverness Terrace Geoffrey was building up a very fine collection of gramophone records, and he used to play selected short passages of the classics to the children. He would give these movements names, like 'dancing music'. He gradually, and selectively, extended their repertoire. He was also buying paintings and encouraging the children to visit museums and art galleries.

When the war started in September 1939, the family were in Devon, where May and the children stayed until Christmas. Tom was at Dartmouth and Jane and La went to a local school for one term, before joining the Assumption Convent, which had been evacuated from Kensington Square to the Actons' house in Shropshire, Aldenham Park. Geoffrey and May bought autobikes, on which they would make laborious journeys from London to visit them.

In London heavy bombing was expected, so at the end of 1940 they moved to Stanmore in north London, first to Buckingham Cottage and then to a small flat with a garden, which was more convenient for transport. They kept on 1A Inverness Terrace, and Gerry Moy, a childhood friend of May's, moved in, after having been bombed out of her own flat. Geoffrey's letters to the children at school give a marvellous idea of what life was like at this time.

In 1943 they returned to London and moved into 55 Porchester Terrace. Supposedly, there was less general anxiety about German bombing raids but, in fact, a stick of incendiaries fell around the house, one penetrating the hall.

Simon was born, to the whole family's enormous delight, a year after the move to Porchester Terrace. Geoffrey adored the child and there are many amusing accounts of his first few months in his letters to La at school. Life revolved around him for the next few years. The family summer holidays, which had lapsed for the war years, started up again, the first being in Budleigh Salterton, then Sheringham for a few

years, Rye, Sandwich, St Ives and the Isle of Wight. In 1950, just after
Christmas, Geoffrey took Simon to Tenerife on a banana boat. It was a
great success, so a year later May joined them and they took with them
Nigel Murray, Suzanne and Ronald Murray's son, who was the same
age. Simon learnt to play the 'timpale' while out there, which led in due
course to the guitar, which he still plays.

In 1948 another move was forced on the family, when the whole
area around Porchester Terrace was being redeveloped. It was then that
they bought 24 Wimpole Street, though Geoffrey had always said he
would never live 'over the shop'. May had been keen to buy a beautiful
Regency house on the River Thames at Barnes, but the absentee owner
would not sell and 24 Wimpole Street was unfortunately chosen, probably because it was convenient. Having grown up with the Fawcetts at
66 Wimpole Street, Geoffrey must have been attracted by the chance to
buy No. 24 directly opposite. He could look across the street and see
into the shell of No. 66, then bombed, 'like a stage set'.

At first sight they both liked the house and Geoffrey bought it on
impulse for £13,000. The house next door on the north side, No. 25 —
Professor Higgins's house in Bernard Shaw's *Pygmalion* — had been
totally destroyed by a direct hit. The adjoining wall was shored up with
wooden supports and he naturally thought that the bill for any repairs
to No. 24 would be paid by the War Damage Commission. Built in
about 1790, it was a beautiful house and seemed a good investment
because two of the consulting-rooms were already let to other doctors,
each paying £300 a year in rent.

The house was bought without legal scrutiny or a surveyor's report.
Geoffrey had merely been told by a builder that the structure was
sound. Less than a year later, he arrived home one day to find a
Dangerous Structure Notice had been pinned to the front door. He was
appalled. There was a serious bulge in the façade between the first and
second floors and the whole of this west wall of the house ultimately
had to be rebuilt. The architect instructed one of the largest building
companies in London to carry out the repairs. Most of the arrangements were left with La, only 18 at the time, but she handled it as best
she could. The War Damage Commission contributed very little, on the
grounds, first, that the previous owners had already put in a claim
(unbeknown to Geoffrey), which jeopardized any future claim, and,
second, that there was dry-rot in the main wooden beam, then exposed
at the north end, across the front of the house at first-floor level, which

could not be blamed on the bombs. The final cost of the repairs was £9000, a very considerable sum in 1949. The resultant weight of a second mortgage was a crushing blow and the worry of it all, including the staffing problems, which gradually got worse, made a great difference to the rest of their lives. In 1949, Simon was only five and, in spite of his eminence, Geoffrey did not have a large private practice, as he had always preferred and concentrated on his hospital work. His future prospects were depressing.

Dowling's fees were always very modest, three guineas for a half-hour consultation, and only one or two guineas if the patient was not well-off, which led to some patients turning up in threadbare clothes.

Sometimes he saw actresses who were worried about their complexions. Geoffrey did not enjoy these consultations. He would ask them, 'Do you put muck on your face?'

When first in practice in Devonshire Place he had a secretary called Mrs Olivier. One day she ventured to mention that she had a brother-in-law on the stage.

'Who's that?'

'Laurence Olivier.'

No response.

'He's married to Vivian Leigh.'

'I haven't heard of them.'

This was after *Wuthering Heights*, *Waterloo Bridge* and *Gone with the Wind*.

Only one family from the practice became firm friends. They were the Finnegans, who owned leather goods shops in Bond Street and Wilmslow, Cheshire. They often had Christmas dinner together, usually on Boxing Day.

In the 1960s the family also joined the Wallaces for dinner on Christmas Day. The Wallaces always had a large family party. Hugh Wallace was a great raconteur and told a final story at Geoffrey's funeral. The Health Service had just been introduced and at out-patients a Cabinet Minister had appeared, asking Sister if he could be seen by Dr Dowling very quickly, as he had a Cabinet Meeting in half an hour. Sister, knowing Dowling's views on equality of treatment, kept him a few minutes and then insisted on his undressing — he complaining that it was only on his face — and gave him a gown which did not quite meet at the front. The system at St Thomas's Hospital was that patients were seen in rotation between the three of them, as they reached the top of the queue. However, he was taken directly to Dowling (by now he was going to be late for the Cabinet Meeting) and Hugh, having got wind of what was going on, sat in on the consultation. The Minister made a five-minute speech about his complaint; Dowling put on his big magnifying glasses and took a long look at the spot. Putting down his glasses, he turned to Hugh saying: 'Nasty' and asked him to deal with it. He said not one word to the Minister.

In 1958, after his research job at St Thomas's had been terminated, Dowling seemed down and called himself moribund. May invited Dr Evan Jones, one of his closest friends, to dinner. Having got through a bottle of whisky between them, Evan when leaving the house cheerfully assured May that there was nothing wrong at all, nothing that a little work would not put right. A day or two later, a tentative call from Hastings came, wondering whether he would take a locum tenens post. In his position in retirement, it was generally assumed that to go down to a general hospital would not be interesting, but he was delighted to be asked and never looked back. In no time at all, he was doing locums all over the place, particularly in Lewisham: eight sessions a week, with one afternoon a month at the Medical Protection Society. He was back to working full-time. No doubt Evan Jones engineered the whole thing.

During the 17 years at Wimpole Street, family life was loosely cohesive. The three eldest children were all grown-up and following their own careers, while the youngest, Simon, lived at home during the holidays from boarding-school.

Gradually the disadvantages of a Wimpole Street house became evident. Geoffrey had to pay a secretary and a receptionist and provide gas and electric fires. There was not then much central heating in most of the Harley Street area. The family lived at the top of the house and there were 97 stairs to climb, there being no lift. A married couple who did the cooking and cleaning lived in the basement. But after a few years, when he retired, the position was reversed, or rather the kitchen and dining-room were in the basement, but the sitting-room and bedrooms were still on the second and third floors, which did not make for easy living.

May, now in her late fifties, was depressed and disenchanted with the practical and financial problems of running the house. The mortgage was still very substantial. All of this took its toll on her health.

It was at this time that Geoffrey, who had always smoked a pipe and chain-smoked cigarettes, gave up both overnight. He developed a paunch, but lost it over a few months, and spent the rest of his life complaining about others with that 'filthy habit', flinging the windows open when anyone smoked a cigarette.

Up until 1956, when Geoffrey retired at the age of 65, a married couple cleaned the house and did the cooking, but at this time, owing to his lack of work and for expediency's sake, he decided to take on a lot of the cooking, which, though not fully appreciated by the family at the time, proved invaluable after May had died, when he lived for 10 years on his own in Ravenscourt Gardens, entertaining friends regularly with ease and enjoyment.

In November 1964 May set sail for Cape Town to visit two sisters, Tessa and Irene, whom she had not seen for 25 years. She did not feel well during the sea voyage and saw the ship's doctor, but he accepted her own diagnosis of physical exhaustion and thought that the rest would do her good. She had a wonderful holiday, but on her return in the spring she was taken into St Thomas's Hospital with pneumonia. After discharge she complained of increasing discomfort and stomach pains. In July she returned to hospital for an exploratory operation. This revealed cancer of the ovary, which had spread and was too extensive to remove. She came home from hospital and Gerry Maguire (née Moy), her childhood friend who had lived at Inverness Terrace during the war and whose husband had died the previous year, moved in to nurse her for the following six weeks. She died on 11 September. Geoffrey was devastated and consumed with remorse over his earlier reluctance to leave Wimpole Street before paying off the crippling mortgages to move into a smaller, more manageable house, which they had planned to do on her return. Had she not been away that winter, he would undoubtedly have spotted the symptoms and sought medical help earlier to make the diagnosis and have the tumour removed.

His close colleague at St Thomas's Hospital, Hugh Wallace, came to see him every day, but he was inconsolable. He never left the house. Eventually he resumed his normal life of hospital and private practice. He put the past behind him in an enormous effort of will-power. He simply said, 'One should never look back.' In a way, it was like his war experience from 1916 to 1918. When people asked about May's death, he did not answer. He never talked about it again.

Geoffrey rarely went to the theatre or cinema, though occasionally he was persuaded to join the children during the holidays, when he would usually drop off and snore, or very audibly groan. However, he very much enjoyed the Ealing comedies.

In 1948 the children gave their parents a black-and-white television set for their 25th wedding anniversary. Geoffrey seldom watched it, but at Ravenscourt Gardens he got a colour television set and he took a great liking to Cilla Black, Lulu and Goldie Horn. He made time for football's 'Match of the Day'. He appreciated the skills of soccer, as opposed to rugby, and thought it a more difficult game to play well. At one time, before the war, he was so enthusiastic he took Tom to see Arsenal when they beat Wolverhampton Wanderers 7–0, and on another occasion to see a Chelsea match.

He was also fond of rugby and would often go to Twickenham, sometimes with Frank Lockwood. Whenever there was a West of England and Wales Dermatological Society meeting in Cardiff, he stayed with Geoffrey Hodgson, who usually managed to obtain tickets for them at the international matches at the Arms Park ground.

Golf was his favourite sport and most weekends he played two rounds, usually, after the war, at the Royal Mid-Surrey Club at Richmond, a course he was introduced to by Jonah Gedge, his solicitor. May and Simon would often join him for lunch and walk round the course.

He enjoyed cricket too and loved watching at Lord's. He joined the Middlesex Cricket Club so that he could watch the Middlesex matches from the Long Room.

Dr Evan Jones, with whom he often played golf, introduced him to fishing and he nearly became addicted. He went salmon-fishing on the River Test and, with beginner's luck, Geoffrey caught a salmon with his third cast. Considerable time passed before his next success, so the owner of the beat presented him by way of consolation with a large box, apparently of smoked salmon. His initial reaction was of dismay, complaining that the rich had no idea about food. However, he was delighted to discover below a layer of smoked salmon a dozen bottles of whisky!

Geoffrey had always been interested in pictures, probably encouraged by May. He was very pleased that their nanny, Miss Eastwood, helped the children so much with painting and drawing. He started buying pictures in the 1930s, taking good advice from a dealer, although he still held strong opinions of his own. Once he wanted to buy a Christopher Wood for £70 or £80, but the dealer advised him against it — too naïve. That was a mistake, because Christopher Wood died relatively young and his works are now quite rare.

On another occasion he did not buy a Boudin for £130, at the time the price of a small car. It was just too much money for him. He regretted it many times in later years.

His collection was middle standard, all good — Cox, Collier, de Wint — but getting better, when the war broke out. After it was over, he could never again afford to return to the market.

At 24 Wimpole Street the walls were covered with pictures. One Christmas a senior registrar asked him:

'What are you hoping for this Christmas?'

'I don't mind really. As long as it is not a picture.'

'Oh, why?'

'There is nowhere to put it. The walls are full of pictures.'

The annual Private View of the Royal Academy's Summer Exhibition was always a special occasion for him. He loved the atmosphere and especially the overheard comments of artists and ignoramuses. He came to know many painters, who were often introduced by Peter Greenham, and enjoyed their company. Eileen Agar was one such.

Jane had married Peter in 1964. She had met him at the Byam Shaw School after she left Oxford. He was an RA and in 1965 was appointed Keeper of the Royal Academy. They have two children — Mary, born in 1965, and David, who is now studying medicine in Dundee, in 1969.

Music had been part of Geoffrey's life since infancy, as both his parents were professors of music in Cape Town. It was mostly church music there, which continued during his time at Exeter Cathedral Choir School. He enjoyed concerts in London and would often go to rehearsals. He used to sit in the organ loft at St Paul's Cathedral with John Dykes Bower, whose brother was at St Thomas's Hospital and ran the Hospital Choral Society. The Hospital Choir had been started and built up by Ralph Vaughan Williams during the Second World War, when most of the hospital and staff were evacuated from London to the Godalming and Guildford area. When the hospital returned to London and was working again as one unit at Lambeth, Vaughan Williams gave up his position as president of the Choral Society, and Dowling was asked to succeed him. He accepted but only as a figurehead, although he did make time to attend rehearsals and their performances.

He would sometimes take some of his children to concerts and musical events. Tom recalls one occasion when they sat through an entire rehearsal of the *St Matthew Passion*. It lasted for almost 10 hours, with a break of two or three hours in the middle. Wilcox directed at the Royal College of Music. All the great names took part — Heather Harper, Janet Baker, John Shirley Quirke. Robert Teare stood in for Peter Pears. They went to hear it all again at the Festival Hall two days later.

Church music was certainly his first love. He would always listen to the BBC programmes at Christmas and Easter.

Having built up a fairly large collection of records in the thirties, he continued collecting chamber music and long-playing records after the war. He listened to them less as the BBC service improved, and relished the introduction of the Third Programme and eventually concerts on BBC television. In later years his hearing slowly deteriorated, in spite of a hearing-aid, and he found he could not enjoy his music as much as previously. He had always had a sensitive ear.

Geoffrey had always been an avid reader but one would not call him a bibliophile. He never collected books. He probably began reading in his teens, when he must have spent many hours on his own at the Fawcetts' house in Wimpole Street. The habit stayed with him throughout his medical school years and beyond. He learnt to read and write in French. All this was an advantage when his children were growing up. He encouraged the girls to read more and wrote some of his letters to them at school in French. When Jane went to Oxford to study English, books were a common bond, which drew them closer. If Geoffrey had a favourite child, it would have been Jane.

When he met the artist Eileen Agar and her husband Joseph Bard, they spent many evenings together and Geoffrey sometimes took Jane with him. He was more interested in Joseph's discussions on literature than Eileen's views on surrealism.

After his retirement, when he lived in Ravenscourt Gardens, he spent even more time reading, especially as his hearing gradually diminished and he could not obtain as much pleasure from music as he had before. He read a great number of memoirs and books on the wartime leaders, both Allied and German, and like many people of his vintage he reread a number of books from earlier years. He especially enjoyed Marcel Proust's *Remembrance of Times Past*, which he had originally read in French.

He was fortunate in having reasonably good sight. He considered it a more precious faculty than hearing. His illnesses throughout his life were few. On a family holiday in Bude, North Devon, in 1933 he developed acute appendicitis and had to have an emergency operation. In 1964 he had a severe attack of shingles (herpes zoster) afflicting one side of his chest. He could readily diagnose it himself, but he did not expect to find how ill it made him feel, even though the fever associated with it did not last long. He was surprised by the lethargy, malaise and depression which followed it, a kind of postviral syndrome. It continued for several months, even through he returned to work, but he eventually recovered without residual pain. His final illness is described later in a letter from Dr Ian Whimster to George Findlay in Pretoria.

Chapter 14
The Children

THOMAS (Tom) was born on 23 June 1924 in Dublin, as May wished her first child to be Irish born. Jane, his sister, was born the following year from the flat at Prince of Wales Drive, Battersea, which faced the park.

At Huntercombe the children were close enough in age for everything to have to be done together, and everything had to be equal, but it seemed to Tom that a great deal was unequal, particularly regarding presents and possessions.

There was a beautiful black double-hooded pram with large wheels and old-fashioned elegant leaf springs, which gave a soft ride and a gentle rocking motion for getting a child to sleep. The two would be put into it in the afternoon for a nap, on the 'bricks'. Tom was really beyond the pram, but was put in for company.

Tom and Jane were good companions at Huntercombe. They were happy days and Tom retains vivid memories of them. He often climbed the old yew-tree in the garden.

Alice (Fawcett), Tom's godmother, visited frequently and would be put in the spare room at the back over the kitchen. Access was through Tom's room. She had a felt cloche hat. Once, during his afternoon 'nap' Tom was not sleeping, so he entered Alice's room to explore a jar of powder. To find out more about this he tipped it into the hat and back into the jar. Of course it would not all go back and the powder would not come off the hat. With powder everywhere Tom slunk back to bed and pretended to be asleep.

That was no doubt an occasion when May used the back of the brush. May relied largely on the threat, but did use it if necessary. Geoffrey, who was usually away 'making money' anyway, never seemed to be called upon to administer corporal punishment — except once when at Inverness Terrace Tom refused to eat queen's pudding. The children were allowed a few refusals of food, particularly offal and some root vegetables.

On their return to London in 1930 Tom went to the Blessed Thomas More, later St Thomas More, School in Kensington Square.

Tom and some of the boys from his school formed a gang, who played in the park. They had bicycles with small wheels which were allowed inside Kensington Gardens. One of their adventures was searching for lost dogs posted as 'missing' at the police station near the school. The 'rewards' were to be shared by the gang, who took the particulars and names of the dogs and dispersed in search around the park. Tom, like the others, would identify a dog using its name from the police description and would try to entice it away from its owners, only to be driven off angrily to mutterings, 'Well, it looks stolen to me.' They eventually forgathered, as agreed, at the Man on the House, dogless.

This, and other more unruly adventures, led in the end to a visit from a park-keeper to the house in Inverness Terrace, with a warning that Tom might be banned from the park. Thus May's wish for Tom to board at prep. school took on a new dimension. Geoffrey had not enjoyed boarding-school as a child and so kept Tom at day-school until he was 11, but the idea of sending him off to prep. school was being increasingly discussed, as St Thomas More School was only pre-preparatory. Geoffrey happened, at this time, to be called in to give advice on a ringworm outbreak at Avisford School. He was very impressed by the headmaster, Major Jennings, and his family subsequently became close family friends.

Michael, his son, met his wife Mariella through Jane, with whom she had been at art school, and Tom, Jane and La are godparents to three of their eleven children. Having such a large family precluded foreign holidays, so their practice in summer was to rent a large house in Wales or the Borders. It was from one of these, Sibden Castle in the Severn Valley, that Mariella wrote to Geoffrey for some advice about one of her boys. He wrote back that giving the advice was easy, but understanding how Mariella came to be writing on writing-paper from his mother's birthplace was a puzzle!

In January 1938 Tom entered the Royal Naval College at Dartmouth as a cadet. Geoffrey was delighted when Tom went to Dartmouth. He and May went down to see Tom on parade in 1939, but could not, as it turned out, visit him again.

In September 1941 Tom went to sea as a midshipman, boardng the P. & O. troop-ship *Strathaird* at Glasgow. Then followed a major troop convoy to Suez via the Cape, where he saw his grandfather's plaque in Cape Town cathedral.

Arriving in Alexandria, Tom served in the battleship *Queen Elizabeth*, flagship of the Mediterranean fleet. The ship was disabled by an Italian two-man submarine attack three weeks later, so Tom had an inactive battleship experience in the Mediterranean. This changed dramatically when he joined *Beaufort*, a Hunt-class destroyer, which saw a great deal of action in the eastern Mediterranean, including taking part in many convoys to Tobruk and one convoy to Malta and another attempted one.

After repairs, the *Queen Elizabeth* sailed round the Cape to be brought back to operational readiness at Norfolk, Virginia, with Tom on board. There he visited the US Naval Hospital to have recurrent warts on his fingers treated, telling the young Naval dermatologist of his previous treatment at the hands of his father. The young American knew about Dr Dowling.

After a stint in the home fleet based at Scapa Flow, Tom returned ashore for courses and then decided to join submarines. He served first in an old training submarine H32, and then the operational submarine *Vitality*. She was destined for the Mediterranean, but that theatre of operations was ending so he was appointed to *Scorcher*, destined for the Pacific. Having reached Ceylon, *en route* for the Philippines, the Pacific war ended, so Tom saw no real action in submarines.

After the war Tom served in a number of submarines at home and in the Mediterranean, *Sceptre*, *Telemachus*, *Anchorite*, *Tantivy* and *Talent*, until 1951, when he took his command course on the *Perisher*. He subsequently commanded *Selene*, working out of Portland, and *Astute* with the Canadians at Halifax, with a period of general service sandwiched between.

When Tom had command of *Selene*, Simon, by now about eight years old, came down with May to stay in Weymouth and was taken out by Tom for a day's exercise. When outside Portland harbour, Simon settled into a comfortable position and announced he was 'ready to dive'. Tom had made four rules for the day — not to use the words 'peculiar' (Simon's current favourite), 'sailor' and 'why' and not to ask questions just to keep the conversation going. And Simon stuck to the rules. When the boat did dive, he was disappointed that the angle of dive was so gentle, but he had a long and really interesting time on the sonar hydrophones, listening to the destroyers above.

On return from Halifax, *Astute* was due at HMS *Dolphin*, Gosport. May and Geoffrey were ready when the bows of the submarine appeared on time. Tom had actually allowed an extra day for crossing the Atlantic, as it seemed more important than anything else to arrive on time, as there would be so many families there who had not seen their men for nearly two years. Arriving in the Solent in good time, the morning had been partly spent painting the hull black, touching up the grey paint and polishing all the brass-work, so the submarine looked smart coming alongside. Geoffrey and May were beaming with pleasure.

After completing the staff course at the Royal Naval College, Greenwich, he was teaching submarine tactics in Malta when the rather generous early retirement terms were announced. As the Navy was contracting and Tom felt that his remaining sea-time was likely to be little or nothing (submariners did not get seagoing submarine appointments after the age of 35 in those days — it is different now) he took the plunge to retire, but it was a 50–50 decision. His father seemed disappointed.

Tom designed and built in Malta the catamaran *Bluefin*. This boat was the largest fibreglass catamaran in the world at the time and is still going strong. Built with commercial prospects in mind Tom sailed the boat home with Tom Fawcett, Robbie's son, as part crew. Serious offers to build came from France (the boat crossed via the Midi canal) but Tom wanted the boats built in England. Back home he found the English were too keen on comfort at the expense of speed and so the opportunity passed.

May intercepted *Bluefin* at St-Tropez and she stayed on the boat for some two weeks, sailing along the coast most days, but the season was running out, and Tom without crew decided to winter there as there were modifications to be made. May loved the boat and, after its return to England next year, continued to sail in the Solent and along the south coast as far as Devon for a week or two at a time. She had one fault. She would steer happily for two hours or more and then suddenly go off at right angles one way or the other. So Tom could never relax when she was at the wheel. She enjoyed living on the boat, unlike Geoffrey, who, when he first saw it at Southend, declared the bunks were like torpedo-tubes.

May shed 20 years as soon as she stepped on board. She was taken for Tom's girlfriend in St-Tropez, as she had been when she saw Tom off to Dartmouth at Exeter station. Tom remembers her skipping across the sands near where *Bluefin* was moored in the River Erme, South Devon. This was one year before she died.

Geoffrey did take a one-day sail in *Bluefin*, with a crew of Tom's art school friends, from the Medway to Bermondsey. This was nearly all downwind. He enjoyed this very much and entertained the crew at the Angel pub on the Thames before taking a bus back to Wimpole Street.

He did come once more. Joining at Lymington, he slept on board, not enjoying it, and the next day sailed with a crew of young girls, sitting in the cockpit in a folding chair very contentedly as the boat sailed downwind, again, to Hayling Island. Bob Campbell, the father of the crew, met them. He was the senior surgeon at Portsmouth and had been captain of St Mary's Hospital fifteen and also a Barbarian. Entertained at the Campbell house, Geoffrey had plenty to discuss with Bob. They found they had mutual friends as the Amersham connection revived old memories, including the surprising discovery that Paddy, Bob's wife, had been on Geoffrey's ward there as a VAD. But Geoffrey never went sailing again.

When Geoffrey was dying at St Thomas's Hospital, the children arranged that there was always one of them there during the waking hours, and Tom was with him at the end.

Jane was born on 6 December 1925 early in the morning in a nursing home in Kensington. The family was then living in Battersea. When Jane was 18 months old, they moved to a small cottage with a large garden on the edge of the links at Huntercombe in the Chilterns. Jane's earliest memory, or one of them, is of losing Tom on the links when she was two and a half. Her mother scooped her up on her back and they trotted about in much agitation searching for him, only to find he had already gone home by himself. Jane thought the fuss that was made of him on this occasion was excessive.

Early on, Jane slept in a cot beside her parents' bed. She used to climb out early in the mornings when Geoffrey was home and sit astride his chest demanding nursery rhymes. He was always very good-humoured about this and instead of turning over to go to sleep again he would go through his entire repertoire and they would intone together. This was the first step in education. The children had porridge plates with the letters of the alphabet inscribed round the edge and they learned these by heart, but this alone did not unlock for them the mysteries of reading.

When Jane was three and a half, a governess came to the house called Miss Eastwood. She had been preceded by a fairly unpopular figure called Nanny Verby. Miss Eastwood after a while was allowed to start proper lessons. Jane always remembered the day when she discovered how to read 'Sam ran to the pond'. There was an accompanying picture and the print was beautiful.

Miss Eastwood, known as Essie, introduced the children to crayons and drawing, another excitement. She taught them to make macaroons and flapjacks and led them about the links looking for sitting-rooms, i.e. little snug enclosures in the bunkers where they would plait grass and daisies. There were walks near by, Grimsdyke and ancient woodlands. There were hazelnuts in the hedgerows and once they saw a cuckoo flying low. Geoffrey had a car which took them on many expeditions further afield. The children had names for the surrounding woods, the Quiet Wood, the Pale Wood and the Green Wood. The culminating excitement was to see Wittenham Clumps on the horizon. They would twist and turn until they saw them and then call out, 'The Clumps! The Clumps!'

Geoffrey's home-coming was always a big event. When he came in, he would go through a pantomime of pretending the children were invisible and he would hunt for them everywhere. Jane found this disquieting and was always relieved to be found. When Geoffrey took her on his knee, she would remember all the injustices that had taken place while he was away and this always reduced her to tears. Then Geoffrey would pick her up and, holding her legs, would pretend to kick Tom round the room to make up for it all. He was always benign, always a supporter; each child felt this.

Many Guy's doctors came to Huntercombe at that time. Jane remembers her third or fourth birthday party with Dr Mackintosh and Dr Conybeare standing round her high chair. They seemed to be tall, laughing, invulnerable figures.

Jane and Tom were sent off to Jersey the summer La was born. They were taken by their aunts. When they got home, they found a Fräulein nursing a baby with narrow feet, about whom they had not been warned. In the autumn of that year, all three children developed whooping cough and Jane and Tom were sent to Ireland for five months to recover. They were never to go back to Huntercombe.

This was not their first visit to Ireland. They always felt at home in Maryborough and were made much of by their grandmother and the rows of uncles and aunts. They had a great deal of freedom and were allowed to go about alone. Cars were few. Jane had her fifth birthday there and wore a favourite dress, her apple frock. Geoffrey sent them two fat books at this time, one red, one green, Hans Andersen's and Grimm's *Fairy-Tales* with curious Germanic illustrations. Their youngest aunt, then about 16, spent many hours reading with them. She used to take them to the old library in the town, where in a little room up two steps was a hoard of ancient fairy-tales. She also told them the gospel stories. Geoffrey came over at Christmas, and the following Easter Tom and Jane were woken up early one morning by their mother, who had just arrived to take them home.

When they got back to London, Essie was there to welcome them, La had grown into a person, the house smelt of new paint, and Kensington Gardens in late spring flowering were just across the road. They were taken straight out to see Peter Pan.

That summer they developed a new routine, lessons in the nursery followed by walks in the park, a more formal life than either Ireland or Huntercombe. Tom was sent to a day-school in the autumn and Jane, after her sixth birthday, followed him. The schools adjoined one another in Kensington Square. Jane was eager to start school. It never occurred to her it would mean losing Essie. But so it was, and Essie was replaced by a series of Mesdemoiselles. She was to come back, however, for some months in 1936.

One of May Dowling's sisters, Kiki, lived in London and worked for a long time as Geoffrey's secretary. She was often at home and had almost as large a hand in bringing up the children as their parents. She was extraordinarily good-natured and devised endless outings. Jane missed her severely when a few years later she went to Africa to get married.

In the early days at Inverness Terrace, Geoffrey used to come into the nursery at the end of the day and get down on all fours and play with the children. He was always welcomed with excitement. Alice Fawcett was a frequent visitor too. She would take Tom and Jane to the zoo and then back to the large tall house in Wimpole Street, and later on to the Fawcetts' house in Chester Terrace, where they would slide down the banisters from top to bottom. Once they scratched them and Alice got into trouble. There were always 'Playbox' biscuits for tea. Two maids would stand to attention throughout the meal. Mrs Fawcett was quite an alarming figure. She wore long dark clothes and a velvet band round her neck and she had a stick. After tea the children would play on the old rocking-horse and with the immensely complicated Victorian dolls' house that was kept in the basement.

Life was not all London, however. The family went to Ireland and, three summers running, to Bude in Cornwall. It was a favourite place among Guy's doctors. One year Geoffrey developed acute appendicitis there and was operated on in the cottage hospital nearby by Mr Sinclair. A week later he was playing golf. The following year Jane had her appendix removed in the same hospital and caught pneumonia. She had a happy convalescence doing a large jigsaw of Cape Town, which Geoffrey had bought for her, and reading. After Bude the family went for several years to Seaford in Sussex. The air was bracing and they went at Christmas and Easter as well as for eight weeks in the summer. Geoffrey and May both insisted on fresh air. There were long walks into Newhaven with heavy spray pouring over the sea-front. The children's appetite became sharp and at six o'clock in the evening May would preside over a table groaning with high tea.

Sometimes they went to fairs. When Geoffrey had supplied them with money to have their rides, Jane would see him unobtrusively slipping coins into the hands of deprived urchins who were watching the merry-go-round with longing. Geoffrey was not an overprotective father. He had bought Tom a Folboat canoe with a small sail in Bude and Tom also had this in Seaford. He used to go across to Newhaven in it and no one seemed to think this was dangerous. Life-jackets for sailing and hard hats for riding seemed to be unknown. Once Geoffrey, with too much confidence in his ability, took all three children out in a sailing dinghy. About half a mile out to sea they capsized. Jane, who was about nine at the time, caught La, who could not swim, and handed her as they surfaced in the water to her father. Geoffrey thought this showed presence of mind. Tom climbed on the upturned hull and signalled for help. When they were brought ashore, a little crowd had gathered, including some reporters. Geoffrey was rude to them. He wished to keep the story a secret from May, who was in London at the time packing to go to a medical conference in Budapest.

About this time Geoffrey's mother came on a winter visit from Cape Town to Inverness Terrace. Jane took to her enormously and danced for her indefatigably in the drawing-room to the music of Mozart. The music was never the right music for the steps and it was a question of dancing under difficulties. The grandmother was appreciative and told

Jane how she had met Pavlova when she came on a tour of South Africa. Later on Jane was sent a beautiful photograph of Pavlova with a small Christmas tree in her arms and a message 'To Minna' inscribed on the bottom. Unfortunately this was to get lost in wartime removals. Jane danced quite seriously for six years, going to Miss Mclaren's Dancing School in Scarsdale Villas. She danced in various London theatres in inter-ballet school competitions and twice in the Albert Hall in *Hiawatha*. Her great ambition was to go and learn to dance in Russia.

By the time the war came the family had taken to going to Budleigh Salterton in Devon for the long summer holidays. Here Tom sailed properly with Jane for his crew. Alice Fawcett would sometimes share these holidays. May was always at her happiest by the sea. She took Jane over to Torbay for the National Dinghy Championships in September 1939. Tom sailed *Joanna* round from Exmouth and there followed three days sailing in bad weather. Then, as war seemed imminent, the championships were cancelled and everyone went home, much to Jane's relief.

For the first autumn of the war, May and the girls stayed on in Budleigh Salterton. Geoffrey returned to London and Tom to Dartmouth. Riding was suspended for the moment. They had all ridden in Sussex and in Devon. May herself used to ride in Rotten Row when they first moved to London. Afterwards she would ask Jane to pull off her boots. In Budleigh she hunted with the East Devon Hunt until one day she was rolled on by her horse. She also bicycled long distances with the girls. She looked very young at that time. In the autumn evenings she would teach her daughter *gros point* and *petit point* beside a frugal fire of pine-cones.

Jane and La went to school in Budleigh Salterton for one term. After Christmas they went as boarders to their convent school, which had been evacuated from Kensington Square to Aldenham Park in Shropshire, the seat of Lord and Lady Acton. In the summer of 1940 May came to stay for several months at the Acton Arms near by in Morville. Geoffrey paid short visits and Tom spent the summer holidays from Dartmouth there. The whole family helped with work on the land, cutting down thistles, making hay, getting in the harvest, picking plums. Geoffrey gave the children a family tree showing how, through his mother's cousins, the Fleming Baxters of Sibdon, he could trace his descent from the first Sir Edward Acton in the seventeenth century when there was a double marriage between the two families; an Acton son married a Fleming daughter and a Fleming son married an Acton daughter, Elizabeth Acton, of whom they had a portrait at Sibdon.

Geoffrey was a natural educator. In the war years he wrote weekly letters to Jane and La at school which show what a detailed interest he took in everything they did. Whatever he was reading he would try to make Jane read too as she was growing up. Thus they read a lot of history and, when quite early on in the war Geoffrey took up French rather seriously, Jane too was sent French novels to read, mainly nineteenth-century ones with many of the words pencilled in in English above the print. Geoffrey always had a terrible French accent but he learnt to understand the language well, listening throughout the war to 'Ici Londres' on the BBC. He also sent Jane a collection of history of art books for her to study at Aldenham on the National Gallery and the Tate Gallery, and a case of records of some of his favourite music. Although he never said, 'You must do this' or even 'I want you to do that', such was the force of his personality that he had only to indicate what he would like for it to happen. This was to make it all the more difficult for Jane to go totally against his wishes later on by entering an Order of enclosed Dominican nuns on the Isle of Wight. Jane left school at 16. The plan had been to go straight to the Slade School of Art, but instead, following Geoffrey's wish, she spent a year at a crammer's (tutor's) in Baker Street and went up to Oxford to read English when she was 17.

Geoffrey had a great friend at Oxford, Dr Alice Carleton. She was a demonstrator in anatomy as well as a dermatologist. He greatly admired her wit and Jane was to get to know her well during her undergraduate years. Alice would give celebrated parties for medical students at her house in Banbury Road. Charades were enacted in an uproarious manner. Once Alice took Jane with her to the President's Lodging in Trinity College. Again Alice got the charades going. They did the Rape of the Sabines and then the Foundation of Rome. Alice as the wolf got down on all fours to nourish Dr Frank Sherwood Taylor and Professor Zulueta, who were Romulus and Remus. Alice had a brilliant talk which she gave periodically on how to reconcile the book of Genesis with evolution. Geoffrey was more than surprised to hear about this. He had not realized she was a devout Catholic. She once told Jane she always thought of Geoffrey's marriage to May as of an eagle married to a humming-bird.

During the three years Jane was up at Oxford, she went part-time to the Slade and Ruskin, then housed together as one art school in the Ashmolean Museum. Albert Rutherston, the Ruskin Master, was an old friend and patient of Geoffrey's. When she had got her degree at Oxford, she went on the Byam Shaw School of Art in Notting Hill Gate, where she was to spend three happy years. The family by this time were living in Porchester Terrace near by. Simon had been born at the end of Jane's second term at Oxford. He spent many hours in his early childhood trailing round the National Gallery with Jane, lured on with promises of ice-cream.

When Jane was 23, she went to St Dominic's Priory at Carisbrooke on the Isle of Wight. Geoffrey was profoundly upset by this decision and refused to visit her for two years. Jane took solemn vows and stayed eight or nine years, eventually coming out because of ill health. Dr Evan Jones and Dr Shorvin of St Thomas's Hospital saw her through this difficult period. She stayed five months in hospital and went to recuperate for a further five months with the Jennings family at Avisford.

Finally in 1958 she returned to the Byam Shaw Art School for a further three years' training, supporting herself meanwhile by doing part-time teaching jobs. She attended the Central School of Arts and Crafts to learn print-making and began to exhibit in various London shows. Geoffrey would break off from his work to visit her in the National Gallery, where she was copying a Rubens. Geoffrey now became a tireless exhibition-goer.

In August 1964 Jane married Peter Greenham, who had taught her at the Byam Shaw School. She had known him since Ruskin days. He had recently become Keeper of the Royal Academy Schools. Geoffrey and May walked on air at the time of the wedding. Their first child, Mary, was born on 7 August 1965, but May only lived five weeks after the birth of this eagerly awaited first grandchild.

The Greenhams lived in a studio flat in Blenheim Crescent for the next three years. Geoffrey came every Saturday afternoon and pushed Mary out in the pram. Jane paid several visits to Old Bosham in Sussex and sometimes Geoffrey came too. He remarked that it was just the sort of place May would have chosen — a house whose garden wall was lapped by the tidal waters of the estuary.

In 1966 the Greenhams rented a large wooden summer house in the mountains near the Austrian border of Italy. Geoffrey flew by night to

Milan, took a train to Verona and was met early in the morning by Jane
and Harold Strub, the cellist, who was staying with them. As they drove
alongside Lake Garda and up the valley towards Rovereto, surrounded
by high mountains, Geoffrey said he had never seen a place that re-
minded him so much of South Africa, the highest compliment he could
pay. He was delighted with the large house, its heavy Austrian furniture, the surrounding woods, filled with cyclamens and mushrooms, and
the mountainous aspect, and perhaps more than anything by the Italian
people who looked after the family: Gemma, the housekeeper, who
became devoted to Mary, and the postman, who used to arrive during
breakfast on the balcony. He would throw aside his postman's bag and
spend the next quarter of an hour wooing Mary, who refused to be won
over. Passing people whom they met on their walks remarked that
Mary was well made and had pretty white teeth, all of which delighted
the proud grandfather. He thought highly of Italians in general because
of their reverence for family life. This was a happy holiday for Geoffrey,
the first he had taken for many years. He stayed three weeks and grew
more and more energetic, taking longer and longer walks each day.
Once, on an impulse, he decided to scramble down the mountain in a
direct line to Rovereto at the bottom of the valley, avoiding all roads
and zigzags. He was away several hours and, just as the family were
becoming anxious, he reappeared rather triumphantly in a taxi, having
been too exhausted to walk home. He particularly enjoyed the long
evenings on the balcony with Harold Strub, who was a gifted raconteur
and made Geoffrey feel he was in touch again with the world of
professional musicians.

The Greenhams moved from London to Charlton-on-Otmoor in
1968. Geoffrey became a regular visitor. He had friends to see in
Oxford, Dr Renwick Vickers and Dr Terence Ryan, and he liked to visit
the Otmoor pubs. He particularly liked to come at Easter, when he
would sit in the garden as much as possible, enjoying the spring air.
On one occasion Jane heard him talking to Mary outside the kitchen
window.

'Why have you got only one tooth, grandpa?' said Mary.

'Because I'm O L D,' said Geoffrey.

He first saw David (his second grandchild) when he was one week old.
He leaned over the cradle and said almost reverently:

'Perhaps he'll be an artist.'

Jane said, 'Perhaps he'll be a doctor.'

'There are plenty of doctors,' said Geoffrey, 'Let him be an artist.'

He acted as general practitioner to the children, prescribing whatever Jane demanded and undertaking to have tests done when she became an over-anxious mother. He was particularly supportive when Mary swallowed a sixpence when she was two. He would ring up frequently for the bulletins. Mary was swept into St Thomas's Hospital, an operation threatened, but finally she passed the sixpence and all was well.

He twice visited Brancaster in Norfolk, where the Greenhams rented a rectory for the summer holidays. He was fond of Norfolk and found it surprisingly unchanged since his boyhood. The rectory, a pleasant white Georgian house with roses rambling over the porch, stood back a quarter of a mile from the sea. To reach the beach you walked across the marsh. There were splendid sands, a bird sanctuary and, on good days, truly Mediterranean colour.

Geoffrey would sit in a canvas chair on the shore for hours developing a deep tan. He usually brought some work. On Sundays, the quiet beach would be invaded by swarms of families from London. They would arrive with transistors, picnics, babies, grandmothers, uncles and aunts and take over the place for the day. The adults would fling themselves on their backs and shut their eyes. The children were ignored. One such child made for Geoffrey's lap and sat there like a cat among his papers. They stayed together contentedly for about twenty minutes looking out to sea. Then the child clambered down and Geoffrey resumed his work. He was very fond of children and often used to say after a day at the hospital, 'I saw a delightful little girl today. Such a pity she has to grow up like her mother.'

The little girl, on further questioning, would turn out to have been about eight weeks old. Similarly, when Simon was a small child, Geoffrey would refer to Jane and La as the Ugly Sisters. He would take Simon aside and say, 'Aren't your sisters awful?'

The last time Geoffrey came to stay at Charlton-on-Otmoor, he was brought over by Terence Ryan, with whom he had been staying. He was quite unwell, and did not talk very much. As he was leaving, he pressed some money into David's hand. David, then six years old, looked at the coins with an experienced eye and broke out into a big smile.

'That's something he understands, anyway,' said grandfather with satisfaction.

He was particularly pleased with the plans for David's education,

first the Dragon School and then Magdalen College School in Oxford.
But he died a year before David started at the Dragon. He was glad,
too, to see Mary having an athletic childhood, riding, skating and
swimming. Once, years before, when he had been pushing the infant
Mary out in her pram in Notting Hill Gate, he had met Dr Wallace.

'This is a remarkable young lady,' he said, 'who will go far.'

Communication between Geoffrey and Peter was sometimes difficult
as Geoffrey became increasingly deaf and Peter refused to shout.
However, they had a healthy respect for one another and Peter always
signed his letters to him as 'Your affectionate son-in-law.'

Geoffrey rather disliked clergymen but, although he was an ag-
nostic, he never entirely outgrew earlier influences and sacred music
remained his first love. He ranked Bach's *St Matthew Passion* highest of
all the music he knew and often took the family to hear it. Once he and
Jane listened to a performance of this in the organ loft in St Paul's
Cathedral. Dykes Bower, the organist, had a brother at St Thomas's
Hospital and both were friends. Geoffrey was himself an unbeliever but
he had the aspirations of Christianity and used to say to his patients
with intractable diseases, 'This is your cross, you must bear it.'

Along with his beloved friend, Dr Evan Jones, he respected the faith
and dedication of the Nursing Sisters at St Thomas's and, without being
able to subscribe to the dogmas of religion, they both thought there was
nothing to touch a genuine Christian life.

In politics Geoffrey was a mixture of radical instincts that went
along with deep respect for tradition. He used to claim to be a liberal
and lamented the loss of the party. He was in fact quite left-wing,
deeply interested in Communism and thirsty for social justice. He
believed passionately in the National Health Service, which latterly
became his whole life. He was delighted one day when a black shop
assistant in Woolworth's said to him:

'You're a hospital doctor, aren't you?'

'Yes,' he said, 'how did you know?'

'Because you look like one,' she replied.

He told this story many times with tremendous pride.

He continued to behave characteristically in his last illness.

'You're doing very well,' Jane said to him after his operation.

'Doing well, my foot,' he said, 'I'm very ill indeed.'

Alannah (La), initially self-named Lala, was born in London in 1930.
Being pushed in a large black pram across Hyde Park hurrying to get

Tom and Jane to school in time, dawdling back via the Flower Walk, the Orangerie or the Round Pond are among La's earliest London memories. Then came school, or rather the Montessori class, which seemed to be constant play. Not having had Essie to push and encourage her, but Tom as an amusing, kind and considerate playmate and Jane to read to her constantly, she happily 'played' until Essie was brought back to get her going on the three Rs.

Soon the round of dancing classes and from 1938 skating at Queen's Ice Rink occupied the weekends, and she would often drag her father to listen to the bandstand near the Round Pond on Sunday, not so much for the love of music at the time, but to get him to herself. The interest in music was encouraged by the present of a lovely five-octave piano, which, as neither Tom nor Jane played, was solely for her; and in the evenings before bed Mozart was interspersed with nursery rhymes on the gramophone, until the music became so familiar that the two intermingled. When at boarding-school a few years later, she was seen with tears pouring down her cheeks as she listened to a crackly rendering of *Don Giovanni*; this was mistakenly interpreted by the nuns as outstanding musical appreciation, rather than acute homesickness. On one memorable occasion during the war, their father took the children to hear Myra Hess play at the National Gallery and, years later, they walked over Hyde Park from Porchester Terrace to concerts at the Royal Albert Hall.

As a child, La rejected vegetables on a regular basis, but a penny bribe worked wonders and on one occasion, when alone with her father lunching with the Fawcetts (possibly the others were away on a cruise), spinach, the most detested vegetable of all, was served. She caught his sympathetically conspiratorial eye and was later well rewarded.

Holidays were a source of great excitement, particularly the build-up, as the family always left with trunkloads and great canvas sacks of lilos, all-covering bathrobes, roller skates, riding clothes, bicycles, Tom's collapsible canoe, games, painting books, jigsaws, even tapestry canvases, which May constantly worked on during the long summer evenings. As a child, May's own family had always spent the summer in Waterford, so the memories of packing up for a family of nine children must have made the Dowling family departure appear a trivial problem. May was particularly keen on exercise and thought nothing of walking miles over the Downs from Budleigh Salterton to Sidmouth, and regularly cycling round the Devon lanes or riding on Woodbury Common.

Two magical holidays, which stood out above all others, were an Easter holiday at Le Touquet and a summer at Westende in Belgium. The beaches appeared to stretch for ever and Tom and Jane sand-sailed. Geoffrey crossed over on the ferry to Le Touquet at weekends, bringing on one occasion the newest Babar book in French, *Babar en famille*. He was very keen that they should all learn to speak French.

The war came as a shock. The girls' evacuation to a large, stone-faced, freezing cold, seventeenth-century mansion in Shropshire in January 1940, which proved to be one of the coldest winters on record, reduced La to a state of unimagined misery and homesickness. As the spoilt youngest both at home and at school, she pined away, spending half the first term in bed vomiting, rather to Jane's embarrassment and great general concern, but, under the awesome eye of a wholly unsympathetic Parisian Mademoiselle, whose concerns were understandably elsewhere, she finished up considerably underweight and being stuffed with Radio Malt. The summer, fortunately, was a memorably beautiful one and a large number of the children stayed at school for the holidays, owing to the London Blitz, when the house came to life as a lovely family home. They swam in the lake, played croquet and tennis and roamed the beautiful countryside. Her mother moved for some weeks to the Acton Arms, the local pub, where a number of the parents stayed. Tom joined her from Dartmouth for the holidays and Geoffrey visited them on his autobike whenever possible. His bike problems were well described in his letters, a lifeline for La, who fortunately kept a large number of them. Her misery must have deeply disturbed him; he always reckoned that the place for children was at home, but there was no choice and gradually school life became acceptable. From Christmas 1941 they were able to return home for the holidays.

In December 1943 La was put under the care of Dr Evan Jones and the resident assistant physician at St Thomas's Hospital with tuberculous glands. London was still under the constant threat of air attack every night, but Geoffrey wanted her close at hand. They had just moved from Stanmore back to London and May was six months pregnant. After three weeks of observation the doctors fortunately decided not to operate, reckoning that the glands would calcify, which they eventually did, and she was sent to stay with Robbie and Anne Fawcett and their three young children to convalesce. Robbie's own parents had shortly before stayed at Porchester Terrace with the Dowlings, while waiting for their flat to be completed.

Simon's arrival in the spring was a source of total delight to all the family. During the first summer holidays, when he was four or five months old, the house in Egham where they were staying resounded with coos and gurgles. Geoffrey took every opportunity he could to take him for walks, or car rides if he would not go to sleep. It was a warm and very happy summer and during the ensuing holidays Simon was the main-spring of the family's lives. Very soon the holidays resumed the pre-war pattern of sand, sea, golf and high tea.

Back at school La was now allowed to have a friend's pony. Geoffrey was keen for her to have as much fresh air and exercise as possible and her early childhood riding on the Downs and Exmoor stood her in good stead.

Outdoor holidays were encouraged and in the summer of 1945 she camped in Scotland and the Outer Hebrides with Jane and her friends from Oxford. Immediately after the war, in 1946, the three of them cycled through France with their parents' blessing, rapidly withdrawn on their return as La was accidentally left behind in Paris. There were few trains at the time, so Tom and Jane stayed overnight in Calais waiting for La to arrive with all the bicycles, luggage and money for the next day. It was a short-lived but major drama, when parental wrath was poured on their heads. La, to this day, claims total lack of culpability in the affair.

The blue of the Mediterranean and the warm sea were already well known to Tom and Jane, but to La it was unbelievable. Her blue serge school bathing-costume appalled Tom, as he eyed the local beauties, imaginatively wearing two scarves as bikinis. This journey was soon followed by a visit to Italy. La drove out there with Tom in his new Morris Minor coupé. He was on his way to Malta and then La joined Jane and some art student friends in Tuscany and went on to Rome. She loved Rome and arranged to return to study the piano and learn Italian in return for English conversation, later going on to stay with a Florentine family, where she developed a lifelong interest in architecture and wine.

Tom and Jane's lives had followed a clear pattern since childhood. La felt outstripped, both academically and art-wise, from the nursery, so concentrated on music, but was fairly relieved when on her return to London from Italy she failed to get into the Royal Academy, knowing that she had really neither the talent nor the single-mindedness necessary to make a successful pianist. She took a secretarial course at

Queen's instead, and continued to play for her own amusement. She also sang in the St Thomas's Hospital Choir, when her father was the president of the Choral Society.

Her first assignment on completion of the secretarial course was at the Family Planning Association. She was blissfully unaware of the nature of 'the planning' — to her father's immense amusement — and stayed for one day. Soon afterwards, she started to work as his secretary and took charge of every aspect of the medical household. There were several other doctors consulting in the house at the time, and May was often away with Simon for long holidays. Geoffrey had no love of his private practice, but no patient would have guessed this as he approached them with outstretched hand and a welcoming beam. In hospital, five to ten minutes per patient normally sufficed, but in the consulting-room the statutory twenty to thirty minutes had to be given to each. The really loquacious ones got a row of crosses across the tops of their notes.

Geoffrey's X-ray machine had been a gift from May's father when he started in private practice. By the mid-1950s it had become an antiquity approached with great caution, when used occasionally by a colleague standing in for him for some reason. In 1965, when 24 Wimpole Street was sold, La disposed of it at Geoffrey's request but to Hugh Wallace's great sorrow. He had planned for it a resting-place of honour.

After four years of working at 24 Wimpole Street, La felt the need for a change and mentioned the possibility of going around the world to her father.

'People who go around the world are a bore' was his response.

Soon afterwards an extended trip to Turkey and Greece was mooted and agreed to with enthusiasm. The journey through Turkey with a friend was unusual in those days. Rose Macaulay's book *The Towers of Trebizond* had inspired it and, unknown to them at the time, their own fairly eventful journey was followed up daily as a feature in the national press. Tom, serving in Malta at the time, was later given a résumé of the trip by a Turkish naval officer.

At one point, having strayed into a military area, La and her friend were taken into custody in Erzerum. Their questioning in Turkish proved uninformative, so an interpreter was produced, a local doctor. Looking later in the day through the bookshelves in his house, La noticed a volume with her father's name on it; it was Conybeare's

Textbook of Medicine, which he was then editing. At last, their identity was established and thereafter they sensed that they were *persona grata* with the police.

Their next stop was Konya, where they arrived by train at midnight. The few beds in the town were full, so the taxi-driver, on being asked by La in her fractured Turkish to take them 'somewhere, anywhere', took them to the local brothel! Happily, as ever, they were being trailed by the police, so a fate worse than death was averted. The following day the then vice-president of Turkey, who was paying an official visit to the area, scooped them up in Ugup and entertained them. Subsequently they followed in the wake of his entourage, before heading for the south.

On her return form Turkey and Greece, La decided, with her mother's encouragement, to apply for an interior design job at Asprey's. She found from the outset that she loved it. Laurence Olivier was her first client; Victor Borg had her falling about with laughter the next day and on it went. Their clients were mostly the British establishment or from the Middle East. Her lunch-hours were well spent studying the furniture catalogues in Sotheby's sale-rooms opposite, as a comprehensive knowledge of antiques had been a requisite for the job, but had been wholly lacking.

After 18 months she started a company, Mansion and Mews, with a rather more experienced colleague. Interior design and decorating were becoming fashionable, but there were not many companies in the business, so they were instantly in demand and had to expand. After four years, as La reckoned 'small was beautiful', the partnership was disbanded and she started her own company, Alannah Dowling Interior Design, which has grown over the years. It took her to Norway and Japan to work on hotels and a shipping line, to India where she worked and witnessed the demise of the Raj, to Los Angeles and very often to Turkey, which she loves.

One of her first clients was her Uncle Tom (one of her mother's brothers), who had bought Westfield House in County Leix in Ireland. Her success gave her father great pleasure. He had been extremely dubious at the outset, when she first went to Asprey's, asking if she might ever earn as much as £12 a week.

Her experience was most useful when, after her mother died in 1965, it was decided to sell 24 Wimpole Street. La managed all the arrangements and helped her father to find a smaller house. After endless searching, she advertised in despair in Roy Brooks, then a very popular newspaper column, for a two-storey Georgian house with a garden. The result was remarkable; they were spoilt for choice. She only showed Geoffrey two, and the first time they walked up to 52 Ravenscourt Gardens he said, grinning, 'This is it.'

The house was bought for £12,000. Geoffrey said that she could spend £2000 to £3000 more on renovations and in a few weeks' time he moved in. A new kitchen was built on, the house was rewired and centrally heated, bookcases etc. were installed and the house was re-decorated. Geoffrey's only request had been that it should look like Wimpole Street, so the same colours and curtains were used throughout and he loved it.

Geoffrey's last 10 years there were very happy. Simon lived there initially, moving later into his own house. La saw that everything was kept in good order, a simple task after Wimpole Street. Geoffrey appreciated this, but took nothing for granted and never failed to express his thanks for errands performed, or even for visits from any of his children or friends.

Towards the end he ate nothing and was clearly in pain, but would not admit it, wishing to see no one, so that nature could just take its course. On reaching St Thomas's after an unfortunate, but logistically unavoidable, twenty-four hours in Charing Cross Hospital, he beamed on the sister in casualty, murmuring, 'Now I am home.'

Simon was born in hospital in Woking on 17 March 1944 when the family were living in Porchester Terrace. His early years are well documented in Geoffrey's letters to La at boarding-school (Chapter 15).

Geoffrey Dowling's weekends were passed largely in Simon's company and Simon's earliest memories revolve around golf courses, art galleries and Kensington Gardens. He had a particular interest in boats and 'engines' (the Science Museum). One of many games they used to play involved travelling at the front of the top deck of a bus. Simon could choose red or green and, if the bus went through a green light, that would be a 'point' to Simon. Simon was quick to realize that green nearly always won in the end, and so invariably chose green, resulting in happiness all round.

Tom recalls an amusing anecdote about this time. He had been away in the Mediterranean for a couple of years and on his return suggested that he and Simon should have a punting holiday on the

Thames. The venture was to be a secret, so he suggested the boat trip to Simon, saying that there was no need to ask, they would just leave a note. But Simon said the parents would have to give their permission, and the best way to get it would be for Tom to ask Mummy, and he would ask Daddy 'as Daddy always gave him everything he wanted'!

When Simon was seven, his Christmas presents included a surprise, in the form of a trip shortly after Christmas with an unspecified destination. Geoffrey and Simon took the train to Dover, and then transferred to a small boat which set off into the harbour. There was great excitement. The boat drew up to a ship anchored just inside the harbour entrance, and they clambered aboard. It was a Norwegian banana boat, 4000 tons, with space for twelve passengers in luxurious mahogany-panelled quarters shared with the ship's officers, bound for Tenerife. The trip out took four and a half days, during which Simon had the run of the ship, from the bridge to the engine-room, and the benign tolerance of the entire ship's crew. The holiday in Tenerife was characterized by Geoffrey sitting in a deckchair on the beach, wholly unaffected by the sun, reading endless medical textbooks, with Simon constructing shingle causeways in the rock pools, interspersed with walks into the banana groves, a drive up the mountain through cloud up to the volcano, and so on, all with a very real sense of adventure, as tourists were practically unknown.

Two years later a return trip to Tenerife was made with both his parents and with Nigel Murray (Ronald and Suzanne Murray's son, and a chum of Simon's). But Tenerife had by then been 'discovered' and changed beyond belief, and the magic of the first trip could not be recaptured.

Geoffrey did the minimum to discourage harmless misbehaviour. He was highly amused by exploits such as that when Simon and Nigel made the clock at Rye church, while exploring its mechanism, strike one, firing starting pistol shots to add to the confusion while making their getaway on their bicycles. He was nevertheless expected by Simon to give the final 'say' on all matters, which he was generally reluctant to do.

Geoffrey fostered Simon's natural interest in music in various ways. In particular, they often went to concerts together. Neither paid uniformly wrapt attention on such occasions, with Simon finding much of the music new and unfamiliar (it extended across a very broad spectrum from baroque to modern) while Geoffrey would invariably cough, shuffle about, rustle the programme and groan very audibly, particularly during pieces they had not specifically come to hear, to the consternation of all around. He was visibly pleased by Simon's singing and piano-playing performances, both at Avisford School, where he had followed in Tom's footsteps, and later at Ampleforth. He then bought him a Challen baby grand to encourage practice when Alice Fawcett temporarily retrieved the Bechstein. Geoffrey's appreciation of music was by no means catholic; he disliked pop, loathed the jazz 'big band' sound, and was very resistant to Spanish guitar music (perhaps this was because Simon also played the Spanish guitar, to the detriment, Geoffrey thought, of the piano).

In his first year at Ampleforth, Simon developed an acute Asian influenza illness and lapsed into a coma for three days. He was taken to Leeds General Infirmary and his mother went up to stay by his side. He gradually recovered. He had possibly had an added herpes simplex virus infection which was complicated by encephalitis. His father was desperately worried and consulted his neurologist colleague at St Thomas's Hospital, the late Dr R.E. ('Nervous') Kelly, who assured him that the prognosis was good and that Simon would make a complete recovery; which he did. Simon was very intrigued by his regular examinations by the neurologists. They would usually scratch the soles of his feet, which made his toes turn up. The doctors looked grim; so one day, at his father's suggestion, he turned his toes down; they were delighted!

Simon was studying engineering at Edinburgh University when May died in 1965, and he moved with Geoffrey from Wimpole Street to Ravenscourt Gardens the following year. Subsequently he bought a house with a friend in Balham but, like all the family, he was a constant visitor to Ravenscourt Gardens, where he usually played the piano for his own but certainly for Geoffrey's pleasure too. It was Simon who found on a visit to his father that his condition had seriously deteriorated, and with his agreement called an ambulance and escorted him to the hospital, where his condition was at last officially diagnosed.

Simon married Shaan in 1980 and in 1990 they had a baby girl, Eleanor, almost a century after her grandfather's birth.

Chapter 15
Letters to the Children

WHILE JANE and La were away at boarding-school during the Second World War, Geoffrey gave them wonderful support, not only by weekend visits whenever it was possible, but also by letters. He well knew the enormous pleasure that children in those days derived from letters from home.

Fortunately, La has kept more than 50 of them. They show great charm but also his parental skills as an educator. He wrote to children as he spoke to them. He treated them as adults. He would tell them what was happening in his life as well as asking about theirs, and sometimes he wrote in French.

In June 1940 Jane was 14 years old and La was 10. When Jane left school, Geoffrey continued to write regularly to La, latterly giving her regular news about her new brother, baby Simon.

June 1940

Dear little Pets,

There is a great hullabaloo going on overhead but last night was as quiet as anyone could wish for; the train was only forty minutes late, a record for quite a time I was told.

I don't think I brought home any letters for Delia,* anyway I looked in my pockets this morning and could not find any. Delia was in very good form, having had a good night's rest; but she turns up at the same time in the morning whether she has had any sleep or not. I hope both of you will never depart from your present admirable habit (made necessary by the system of rigid discipline under which you are being brought up), and develop the demoralising habit of going to bed and getting up late, both late. Anyway a Brownie always pays attention to anything her daddy happens to say.

---

* Delia worked as the cook and general factotum for the family from 1930. When they moved north of London to Stanmore at the beginning of the war to avoid the raids, she worked at Lyons' and visited them often at the weekends, invariably bringing them useful additions to the larder from work.

After this advice I don't really know what to say next. Tom wrote today explaining how my engine works, I told him when I wrote how I imagined it managed to go, but I don't think I was quite right; Tom's diagram is quite professional.

I am sorry I had to rush away yesterday, I was just feeling my way with the fish game, anyway the brownies had their meeting so that was over in any case.

I don't think I have anything more to say, so I think I will turn in.

I enclose £1 for pocket money, I hope it will be enough, if not you will have to say later on.

Good night Pets,
Lots of love and kisses,
and good wishes for
future birthdays
and Xmas's
from Daddy

October 1940

Ici Londres!*

Voici d'abors un message personel: Le père de Jeanne D. et La D. déclare que ces deux enfants sont de très gentilles petites filles.

Je repète, Le père de ces deux jeunes filles affirme catégorique-ment qu'elles sont tres sages et tres gentilles; et quiconque dit qu'elles ne le sont pas, est fort ignorant.

Et voici maintenant les nouvelles: Mummy est restée depuis quelques jours chez son amie Marie T. Elle espère que M. ait pu mis en réserve assez de pétrole pour qu'elle puisse aller voir ses filles bien aimées (darling daughters).

Tom vient d'écrire une lettre, sans auto et sans timbre, dans laquelle il dit qu'il y a un foule de voyageurs dans son bateau, mais que Clover et lui se sont installés dans un cabin, qui est assez confortable, et pourvu d'un sabord.

---

* Geoffrey listened to 'Ici Londres', the French Resistance programme, throughout the war. He was keen for the children to speak French and bought the 'Babar' books in French (*Babar en famille*, etc.) as soon as they were printed.
  Before the war the children had two holidays in France and Belgium, at Le Touquet and Ostend, from where they were taken to visit the trenches from the First World War.

D'ailleurs il dit qu'on peut manger ce qu'on veut.

La lettre fut ouvert par le censeur, mais rien n'y etait coupé.

Ceci termine les nouvelles.

I found a parcel yesterday containing some lovely potatoes,* which I am going to have for my breakfast. Thank you very much Pet.

Heaps of love and kisses,
Daddy

Have just received your letters, thank you.

Yesterday I went to fetch the motor bike† that has been annoying me so much and for so long. Its original object was to enable me to see the pets at Aldenham, that was in June, and it has never gone a foot without being pushed. The worst of it is, it really looks quite good, it is not old or knocked about, it has been overhauled from top to bottom, but it will not go. I have written to the works to ask what to do next, having explained the symptoms carefully. I am not optimistic, but if eventually it does go, it would get me to Bridgnorth in about four and a quarter hours, as quickly as a car, and considerably quicker than the train.

I enclose Tom's letter, send it on to mummy when you have read it, envelope enclosed, and don't forget.

Piles of love and kisses,
Daddy

26 October

My dear Pets,

Mummy is still rather seedy, and was really very poorly during the week; but, she now seems to be getting on all right, although not as fast as one would expect in a flu, she still has a cough and a little tempy.

I hope the cubs are going on all right and being kept in order, do they have uniforms?‡

---

* Some of the children at the school had their own gardens, so La sent samples of her labours home for approval.

† Geoffrey and May had bought autobikes in order to stretch their petrol ration.

‡ Jane started a pack of Wolfcubs in the village of Morville, near the school.

The potatoes were delicious, like new ones, but I suppose they were really small old potatoes, or is that wrong.

There is no news at all, I have done nothing the whole week except go to London, Amersham, Chertsey etc. and come home to see to Mummy, listen to ICI LONDRES, go to bed, get up, have breakfast, go for a bicycle ride etc.

The Brains Trust are getting more and more above themselves; I expect they realise that it is a popular broadcast. Joad said today that he was glad a certain question had come up, because it was one which philosophers from the time of Pythagoras or someone had tried to answer; what he was about to say would answer it for all time: much applause. A week or two ago, he remarked over some question, I hold certain quite definite views on this subject, views which however I do not intend to discuss now. That's big of you, said the question master.

Mr Rutherston writes to ask me a nasty difficult question about himself, I'll bet the Brains Trust could not answer my letters, I mean the letters I get. I must say he seems to be more interested in his own very minor troubles than in the future artistic careers of my daughters, which are certainly more interesting. However he did as a matter of fact ask after them and their progress.

I must now struggle with that letter, and then I think I can go to bed.

> Night night pets, tons of love
> and kisses from
> Daddy

29 November 1940

My dear little offsprings,

This is just to send you a little money. Five bob is for the old girl, poor old thing, only fivepence left, the rest is for Jane, ten bob for birthday and five bob for pocket money.

I shall try and remember to put some stamps in to-morrow.

I am very sorry to hear that Spitfire* is nearing the day when he will be considered more fit for eating than for rearing. I am

---

* The children's school was evacuated to Aldenham Park in Shropshire. Jane helped to feed the pigs on the home farm. 'Spitfire' was her favourite.

afraid he has become something of a pet. I wonder whether Lady Acton feels any pangs when she has to say farewell to her more attractive specimens.

No news, so night night little lumps,
tons of love and kisses,
Daddy

22 December 1940

My dear Pets,

I have changed the tape in your honour to this beautiful purple, and I really feel quite pleased with the look of it, that is Tom did most of the changing, each of us trying to push the other's fingers out of the way. Tom is making an aeroplane, and as we are all in one room, and all of us like to be as close to the fire as possible, there is a bit of a muddle.

I went to Basingstoke today on Mummy's bike, and at the beginning of the return journey, everything possible went wrong; the clutch would not answer, the carburettor flooded and to get the thing to fire, you had to get up a lot of speed; this was impossible because of the clutch, and I had to get along by asking for pushes. Finally I got a really good mechanic to fix the clutch at Staines and felt I should get home all right; however shortly after dark the light failed, and I had to do about eight miles with no lights. Anyway I got the thing home, 55 miles, and now I think I can face the worst for the future.

I expect Mummy has told you about her job, she has done it for a fortnight, and is a terrific success. She has to get up at 7.30 in the morning, and start out in pitch darkness. Mummy went to Whiteleys a day or two ago, and addressed the girl at the counter, 'Good morning, Madam'.

I don't know what to give you both for Christmas; I got some blocks from the remnants of the shop from which I got the paints; a land mine hit a block of flats just behind the shop and knocked most of its insides out. The blocks were among the things rescued. I haven't collected them but will go there tomorrow. I hope the shop has held on to them for me. This land mine pitched right on Gerry Moy's flats, destroyed three quarters of them including half of Gerry's flat itself, they happened to be in the other half, and escaped with a bad shaking. They are now going to live at 1a, Inverness Terrace, so all your belongings can be left there and will be looked after.

I am very sorry there can't be a stocking this year, and hope the bit of money will make up for it. It is also very sad that we can't be together, but anyway I would rather you were at Aldenham than here; it really is difficult to find anything interesting to do here, and Tom will find it rather dull; he is left to himself all day with Mummy and me at work.

Tom has a comic picture in the Britannia Magazine, it's very good.

I think that is all the news, so now I shall set about trying to get Tom to bed, which is about as difficult as ever, and say,

> Good night Pets? [*sic*]
> tons of love and kisses,
> and a Happy Xmas,
> from Daddy

Sorry about the question mark after Pets, it ought to have been a comma, but I made a mistake with the typewriter.

7 February 1941

Dear little spring lambs,

I was hesitating between lambs and onions, but thought onions rather undignified. Well I arrived home to-night to find that the vegetable stew that we had last night and the night before, and of which I, having been concerned in making it, was rather proud, was giving off bubbles of gas, and smelling like a marsh. I am sorry Spitfire can't have it, I am sure it would be all right for him.

I have the Cezannne book and am sending it on immediately; when I read it I marked some of the words, but I can't read my writing, so perhaps you will fill in these words for me.

I am starting on the garden very soon and would like to know how to go about it, so any information, based on experience will be welcome.

Delia came down here last week-end, and had the kitchen clean and tidy in no time; certain deposits of dust here and there were attributed to me. It was assumed that someone must be responsible, and who could that be but me? So there you are, there is scarcely any justice anywhere. At any rate both Mummy and Delia admitted that my porridge is as good as possible. And now I must stop boasting.

Well now I will say goodnight, and lots of love and heaps of kisses and good wishes.

Bye bye, little ones,
from Daddy

April 1941

Dear little April showers,

I have not written to you for weeks and weeks, the reason being that I have to write my business letters, and I am never finished with them. I am very pleased to hear about all the interesting events; somehow I doubt whether my garden is really properly prepared, there are heaps of stones, and the ground was not manured. Mummy says that the garden must not be watered at night because the frost might kill the plants, and then I must not water in the morning because it is not good for them to have the sun on them after watering, or some reason like that; so what time am I to water the garden? Anyway it has been so cold that no plants could be expected to do their best. However there are a lot of little tiny leaves appearing, all the same whatever the vegetable. I think I shall have to pick up the stones very carefully, but it will be an awful job.

I am delighted to hear about the picture; was it a drawing or was it painted? If you will keep your best pictures, I will send them to Mr Rutherston, he asked me to show them to him, and I am sure he would be genuine about anything he said.

I have just been reading Le petit Chose, by Daudet; it is very charming though unsophisticated, like a story by Dickens, David Copperfield for example, but of course quite short. It has an enormous number of words in it, like all Daudet's books: I suppose that is why he is considered so suitable for school work. Anyway I have marked the words I had to look up, written their meanings over them. So I shall send it to you to read: my efforts will save you a lot of labour. Never let a word go by without settling its meaning, or an idiomatic phrase. Anyway I suppose you ask Mademoiselle. I shall send it shortly, and I hope you will manage to read it during the term.

I enclose some stamps, I don't think mummy sent any.

Tons of love and kisses,

Daddy

2 November 1941

Ici Londres!

Voici deux messages personels.

1. Bons baisers à Jeanne D.
2. Bons baisers à La D.

Et voici la suite de nos informations. Madame Whitfield dit dans sa lettre a maman, qu'elle espère que son enfant sera, quand elle grandira, une bonne petite fille comme La D. Elle dit qu'elle n'a jamais vu un enfant aussi bonne que celle-ci.* Ceci termine nos informations.

Clover's father wrote to mummy to say that he thought the boys must be now be in their ships, they were due on the 19th. They have been posted in the gazette.

I think Mummy has the things you asked for, shoe trees etc, and she will be sending the photos.

Do you want to come home for Xmas, or stay at Aldenham; of course if there is any sign of approaching bombing here, we should leave you where you are, no disturbed nights for growing children.

Is there any drawing activity this term, are Mr Simmon's classes still going on?† Nobody has said anything about the artistic tendencies of the children this term; I hope the Brains Trust did not discourage you.

This week they were asked a question nobody could answer, by Jefferson Fargeon, why did a horse get up from the ground feet first, and a cow hind legs first. The answer came from Sweden from someone who listens evidently, but whether it was right or not I do not know. One of the questions was, why did you take to writing. Joad said that he wrote to provide himself

---

* Madame Whitfield (née Miss Curry) owned the house the family had taken for many years in Budleigh Salterton.
† Jane went to art classes in Bridgenorth.

with books to read in his old age; the others were more modest, Campbell said that his wife nagged him to have a shot, because after the last war he was out of work, he was extremely surprised when his first story was accepted immediately, and he was asked for more. Gunter said that it was his way of earning a living, and Huxley that he also began to write it to supplement his income, and anyhow he was not really a writer, except in a subsidised sense. He is going to America I am sorry to hear.

I hope you will both write to Miss Curry. She said that Rumbles is in fine form, and has a beautiful coat.* I don't suppose he is the least bit grateful for all the attention that has been lavished on him. . . .

I hope there won't be any disturbance about Xmas time; the gramophone is back, so you can play Don Giovanni, and learn some others too, and as for pictures, the days are so short, and the weather so gloomy that I shan't mind your spending the afternoon at them sometimes, in fact I might go myself on a Saturday afternoon.

Night night Pets

Daddy

9 November 1941

Dear little bits of things,

Tom has written and though I don't know where his letter is at the moment, I shall try and find it before posting this; I hope he is well away from submarines by now; I expect the escort took the letters when the convoy was left to go on on its own.

I am ashamed to say that I only posted on your letters to Delia yesterday, however I shall do so immediately in future; I have been a bit rushed and muddled with having a few extra jobs to do like cooking breakfast while Mummy has not been well, and it leaves me feeling unpunctual when I finally do leave the domestic scene.

. . .

To-day's quip in the questions: Joad: 'I often realise that I have bored someone.' Question master: 'Impossible.'

---

* Rumbles, the family's cat was taken from Inverness Terrace to Budleigh Salterton for the summer holidays in July 1939 and stayed there.

I hope all the potatoes are pulled, it must be getting a bit too cold for it; anyway it is no doubt very good for you.

I told you I think that we have a pretty good daily girl, and Missus as well, so the place looks quite tidy most of the time except for my papers all over the place.

I suppose poor old Pet is being good as usual at school; but what a handful at home; how can one explain how such a good girl can be so difficult to get to bed, and how she could want to spend so much of her time at the pictures, instead of listening to Ici Londres.

Night night pets,

Tons of love and kisses from,

Daddy

December 1941

Dear Little ones,

I am being pretty successful in the kitchen, and Mummy admits that the meals are delicious. We have a girl now who cleans up every day, and she is good; she is broad Irish and comes from Galway. Missus still comes on Mondays and Thursdays.

. . .

ICI LONDRES

Le bulletin d'informations que vous allez entendre sera diffusé par Papa a l'intention de ses charmantes petites filles, Jeanne D. et La D.

Nous voudrons savoir ce que c'est que J.D. desire qu'on lui donne a l'occasion de son anniversaire, à part des amitiés; il est bien neccessaire de le savoir aussitôt que possible, parce que le jour s'approche. Et qu'est que c'est que L.D. voudrait comme prix de consolation?

Voici un message personel. Bien arrivés les lettres de J. et La, nos remerciements, continuez.

Nous n'avons pas de nouvelles, de Tom. Ceci termine nos informations.

Tons of love and kisses

Daddy

February 1942

Dear Pets,

It was very nice seeing you, and finding you both flourishing. I hope Mummy has managed to get a lift to Morville or was able to pass that way on her way to Hampton-in-Arden; I expect she managed it somehow.

I was charmed with your respective drawings; I thought Pet minor had made great strides, and as for Pet major, I hope Mummy has got the big drawing; I could not have carried it on the bicycle.

I shall be sending the other book by Daudet, though I like to read a bit of it now and again; it is very funny. I would like to make a photograph of the big picture, I have to write and thank Kiki for some tea she sent, very thoughtful of her, and I thought I might send some of the better late snaps, and that picture. I imagine however that with a brood of her own, a little of the excitement of having photos of nieces and nephews would be diminished; however she will like them all the same.

I am only judging by the comparative lack of excitement with which pictures of my nieces etc are received by me; but then I don't know them, and they are not at all interesting to look at.

I have not got a stronger bike yet, they seem hard to get, however, if I do it will be quite easy to ride to Morville in four hours, much less than it can be done by train, even to Wolverhampton, and naturally much cheaper; so I have not given up hope.

I must go to bed now, so good night my pets,

lots of love and kisses from,

Daddy

P.S. Mummy rang up this morning, and told me that she can't see you, question of petrol. I have been pondering over this architect business, not a bad idea at all, since for long after the war there will be a lot to do. But I would rather have it the other way round, about two years of art school, if that is any use, followed by the professional training. It seems to me that what you do between 17 and 20, in the way of art is likely to stick to you like glue, just as Tom will never lose his touch at sailing.

There now follow some extracts from letters sent to the children between October 1942 and February 1944.

October 1942

. . .

Yesterday, no the night before, Tom turned up with one of his friends; they hitch hiked all the way from Portsmouth and took about 4 hours to get to London. The friend was Eddie. Yesterday we went to the Albert Hall to a concert, all Grieg, as it was his centenary and it was conducted by Sargent. Myra Hess played the concerto and King Haaken was there. Then we went to the Academy for half-an-hour, and then they caught a train back.

. . .

Jane took her cubs bathing yesterday in an open air swimming bath, only four came, the parents not allowing their offspring to do anything so dangerous, except for the four. They boasted all the way to the bath about how long they stayed in etc, but when they got there it was very difficult to persuade them to put a toe in the water.

We have had strawberries several times, and cherries, and the last few days we have had green peas and lots of asparagus, so we are doing pretty well.

Tom still keeps on about the barge and is engaged in drawing them. He gave a picture of a Thames barge to this Wren servant. Fancy they have a Wren per two boys, and at breakfast, a newspaper is put in front of them with the toast etc.

. . .

February 1943

. . .

Tom came home with two boys last weekend and what do you think? He bought a dear little puppy and wanted to hitch him to one of the chairs in the drawing room while they went out, but we would not have it and put him in the kitchen, there he was alright for a while but when we got to bed he very soon began to set up a more or less continuous wail. Meanwhile Tom and his friends stayed out until about 3 in the morning and I had to nurse this ridiculous puppy to keep him quiet, so when Tom arrived I was quite annoyed . . . Next day Tom and I went to

Oxford to see Jane, we had a good time walking around with her, but we were tired, at least I was. The boys came to supper that evening and helped Mummy with the washing up, after that they all went off by the 11.15 train taking the puppy with them and some more gramaphone records. One of them wrote today saying that the puppy was very well and enjoying himself, and not making much noise.

. . .

December 1943

. . .

We had a letter from Tom during the week. He went sightseeing to Edinburgh last weekend with Hank and Charles Poynder and the puppy. He says the puppy is a great favourite and is thoroughly spoilt, the Wrens look after him while the Subs are working.

Mummy is a terribly good cook these days, and she has learned how to make good marmalade, the best I ever tasted.

. . .

Dinner is nearly ready. Delia is doing it as usual on Sunday and in a short time Mummy will begin to coo.

. . .

February 1944

. . .

Delia was in tonight so I was able to give her your letter.

I spent a long while this morning in the Times Book Club looking for books for you, and really you wouldn't believe it there just aren't any, only deadly looking books about Hitler and Russia and so on in the way of new books, and all the old ones have gone, anyway there are such heaps in the bookshelf that none of us have read except possibly Jane who seems to have read nearly everything. There wasn't any point really in getting any more.

Delia wasn't so gloomy about the news as usual, but was sure that at the earliest possible moment Hitler will send some more raids over London, that is, when he is less busy.

I am now reading *Sense and Sensibility*, and am at the stage

where no one can make out where Willoughby has gone to or
Colonel Brandon, it's all very mysterious.

. . .

REFERENCES TO SIMON

May 1944

. . .

Well Simon is a very sweet baby; he weighs $11\frac{1}{2}$ lbs now and
makes pleasant noises and kicks, but I regret to say that he
sometimes makes noises indicating that he isn't happy, and to
persuade him to stop you have to pick him up and walk him
about. He likes this and very often drops off to sleep while you
are carrying him. Alana, the Hungarian cook fortunately likes
him a lot so she is very pleased to walk him around on all the
occasions that offer. He gives Mummy lots of smiles and he
smiled at me once or twice, anyway there is no doubt that he is a
very sweet fellow. Mummy uses all the expressions that she used
to apply to his brother and sisters when they were infants.

. . .

May 1944

. . .

As a couple of patients have not turned up this afternoon I am
improving the occasion by writing to you. I can't think of any
interesting news, although I could tell you quite a lot about
Simon's misdemeanours. He has developed the habit again of
waking up fairly early and yelling his poor little heart out as if he
were in acute pain, but I don't think he is, he only wants a bit of
a carry round and to sleep in his Mummy's bed, which he does
regularly. He is now going out for walks and has got his appetite
back.

. . .

1 October 1944

Dear Sweetie Pie,

Jane tells me that you are behaving very well and taking egg
and various other things, but you must not forget that you have
to have your oil as well. Will you tell your Mummy that I have

had a conversation with Dr. Wallace about teats, and he says he will bring some of the good ones, the ones about twice the size of any others, to London this week, I hope on Tuesday. Would you also tell Mummy that Mrs. Finnigan says you can have Barney's cot and she is going to get it out of store. I don't know what it is like, but I expect it will be alright, anyway you will have to be sure to appreciate it and never to raise objections to being put in it and ask to be pushed around. Jane says you stayed quite quiet with her and made comfortable noises but when Mummy appeared you demanded to be picked up and Mummy gave in.

. . .

Tell Mummy that Delia has been round to-day and yesterday and looked after Jane and me; she cooked us a beautiful apple pudding. Tell Mummy also that on Friday I went to the best sock shop I know and asked for socks but they only had feet and ankles and said it was all I would get, so I did not get any but would like some of the old ones Mummy has of mine if she would not mind; to-day I washed a pair and I have two others so that will be alright until they get holes in them,

Tons of love and kisses
from Jane and me
Daddy

7 October

Dear Sweetie Pie,

Thank you for your nice letter. I had a conversation with Dr. Wallace the other day and he said he had sent you ten big teats and if you chewed those up he would get you some more. So wasn't it lucky we went to tea, not that going to teas is usually a good idea, it isn't generally because mothers always think their sweetie pies are something extraordinary and visitors or people you go to tea with think they are quite ordinary. But in this case it was very lucky because Mummy forgot your bottle and that was how these special teats got to be known to her.

Jane and I are getting on alright only Jane had one of her slight tempys and I got breakfast the other day, and what do you think, when I came in with the tray what do you think I saw, you would not believe it, well, there was a pair of stockings on the floor tangled together, and there was a pair of stockings also arranged anyhow on another chair and a lot of other things in a sort of incoherent condition on another chair so I looked very sad at all this and I expect the next time I go in her room everything will be all beautifully arranged.

Delia came in and said we were going to have raids all the winter, and asked Jane would I want her to come in at the weekends because she was sure I would much prefer to have Luis. She made us a nice potato pie and a steamed pudding and brought us two eggs and some bacon because Pop gets some at weekends where he works.

. . .

Will you ask Mummy to get grey socks if she can and the very best sort of material because it isn't worth getting ones that wear out quickly and you have to mend them rather often if you get bad ones, also if she could get some toe caps made at the same time it saves them getting holes in the toes.

Dr Freudenthal is coming to tea to-day he asked after you when I saw him a few days ago and said what a lovely boy but you have to be careful with those sort of remarks because lots of people say things like that to children's mothers and fathers because they couldn't very well say what a homely boy and hope to remain on speaking terms with the mothers and fathers at the same time.

Lots of love and kisses
from Jane and me
to you and Mummy
from Daddy

The photos will take about a month to enlarge, but it can't be helped.

14 October 1944

. . .

Aunty Alice has come back and is full of enthusiasm about Simon, whom she considers to be exactly what a baby ought to be. I got Dr. Wallace to send him some teats, the big ones, and he wrote back a nice thank you letter, saying that he had a tooth and would henceforth be able to enjoy his meals, anyway Dr. Wallace was very pleased with the letter.

. . .

October 1944

. . .

Mummy says Simon puts his toes up in the air in the morning then looks at them for a time, then tries hard to sit up and just manages to have a look round to see if Mummy is awake and if she is she says she can't resist getting up and taking him into her bed where he gives her beams and chuckles. It seems to me that after all her experience Mummy ought to realise that she is certainly going the right way towards spoiling Simon. Poor little fellow he will have to be unspoiled again mainly by his brother and sisters I am afraid, and of course his daddy who had the same job with the others.

You will be pleased to hear that the Ici Londres, les francais parlent aux francais broadcasts came to an end tonight, but another one called something else is to take its place, but I probably won't want to listen to these new people; the old ones are going back to France.

I expect I shall be going to fetch Mummy and Sweetie Pie back next week end; I can't see Mummy managing all the luggage by herself, but it won't be so bad as going there with the long queue and all the business of getting a seat for certain and then in the wrong part of the train. I expect I shall find him changed a bit, probably smiling a bit more and also yelling more heartily when he feels like it. When you come home for the holidays he will be beginning to crawl and we shall have to have fireguards and all those sort of things to keep him out of danger.

. . .

6 December 1944

. . .

Tom was with us all last week and went barge hunting on two days, but without finding one, except one which leaked and would have to have any amount of money spent on it. Some of his friends have been coming along and one, Dutton, is staying with us at the moment. He and another called Mangel something, took charge of Simon yesterday evening and I must say they did it very well so that he didn't rush at me as if I were his last hope. And he had to have several drinks of orange stuff out of a cocktail glass.

. . .

April 1945

. . .

I am glad to know that dear old Simon is finding his new surroundings pleasant [they were in Ireland] I suppose there is a fair amount of room for him to move about in, and nice out of doors . . .

Kensington Gardens is now closed to the public on account of the coming Victory Parade, and is a huge camp or will be in due course, so poor Simon could not go there.

. . .

May 1945

. . .

Simon is very difficult just now as he can climb up stairs and can open any cupboards. He opened the drink cupboard and threw some glasses about breaking them, and he also found some stuff for cleaning paint off the floor and spilt it on himself thereby causing some alarm, but nothing much happened. He has only been a puppy once since he got back.

. . .

May 1945

. . .

Simon is getting more and more of a handful. The other day he pulled all my papers out of the desk onto the floor and then made a pool on them, and just as I was leaving in the morning and only had time to salvage some of the things that were still dry. He still won't bother to say anything except NO and then he seems to mean what he says.

. . .

June 1945

. . .

Mummy and I did not see any of the celebrations: it would not have been possible for both of us to see them as we could not have taken Simon; so we went to Amersham and had lunch at the Crown. As a matter of fact it poured with rain the whole afternoon and it would have been very trying in the streets.

However the parade seems to have gone off very well. Mummy will probably go and see it at the pictures today.

Dear Simon now orders me to go away and generally speaking it is only really peaceful here when he's asleep.

. . .

October 1945

. . .

Uncle Tom is expecting the family for Xmas and wants Mummy to go a bit early in order to avoid the crush.

I don't know where Tom is now, but I think he must be pretty well on the way home, perhaps Egypt, then next week Malta. I expect someone wrote to tell you that he put up a picture in chalk of the Depot ship and sold it for over £12, and then made another one and presented it to the flotilla captain. I am glad he keeps on doing it.

Simon keeps well but is not any easier to manage; he got hold of a pot of ink the other day took the top off and emptied it all over himself. However he is eating fairly well, at least he has about two good meals a day, and his pint of milk. He is walking pretty steadily now and seems pretty safe taking himself up stairs.

. . .

November 1945

. . .

Dear Simon is quite a handful, still unable to find words to express his feelings and his numerous wants, he does say Lala gone away, and no bed or no bath, or whatever it is he doesn't want.

. . .

February 1946

. . .

Margaret Lockwood's wedding rather occupied our spare time one way and another. I had to give her away and the reception was at 55. I don't know how many guests were there, but a pretty good lot, enough to fill the room up pretty tightly. Simon liked it and was very annoyed at being banished now and again to the kitchen. Everyone drifted off at about quarter past five; we took Mrs Pattersen home, had a drink with her, the best man, and a few others, then Mummy and I went with Mrs P. to the English Speaking Union and had dinner. So it all went off very well, but Mummy and I felt a bit jaded.

Simon is being good but very demanding as usual. I am glad to see that he is very careful about going downstairs and when going up, which he likes doing, he likes to have someone with him. Dr Wallace looked in last week and showed him how to play bears. This was not a very good idea as he pulled me down on the ground next day and made me play. However I think he may have forgotten as he hasn't asked me for the last few days. It is very hard on my knees.

. . .

February 1946

. . .

Simon I regret to say is generally speaking rather naughty. Jane and I took him to the National Gallery today hoping for the best, but we had no luck. He started barking and would not stop; then he played around the big radiator, playing hide and seek with the attendant, that was alright but when we went to another room the attendant was old and crusty and frowned heavily, so we thought we had better hold his hands, so then he played that awful game of sitting on the floor. We gave up and came home. At present he and the puppy are chasing each other round the chairs etc and I am finding it a bit difficult.

. . .

March 1946

. . .

Simon is very sweet these days but not particularly good: I expect Jane told you about the startling incident at the Crown Hotel, Amersham. Aunty Gertie said 'Would you like the fish lovey' to which the gentleman replied in a loud and emphatic voice NO FISH, so that the entire room looked around in a startled manner.

. . .

May 1946

. . .

Yesterday we went to Harrow to call on Colin McEvedy. We found him in, a rather large boy with a pink face and a good mat of pale hair on the top of his head, and a Harrow straw hat the rim of which was mostly adrift. I regret to say that he has outgrown his clothes so that there is a bit of a gap between his waistcoat and trousers and these are a bit tight round the middle as well. Anyway he was very nice and took us to the school restaurant where we had tea, then he took us to a small picture gallery belonging to the school, certainly a lot of extremely good water colours. We looked at them and let Simon wander around. He saw something however which took his fancy, a small bust, this he seized and it toppled, while Mummy watched in agony too far away to do anything, but it righted itself and all was well.

. . .

October 1946

. . .

Simon spent the afternoon mainly with me as Mummy had to go to a christening, so Jane and I first went to the Academy with Simon and he had quite a good time climbing on top of the benches, then I took him for a walk in the Park which was alright except that he would not let me hold his hand crossing the road on the way back, then we had tea during which he was most polite, holding the last piece of bread and honey and asking me and Jane if we would like it, and when I said no thank you and Jane said the same and I said, would Simon like it, he said no thank you and put it down again. Then I took Jane and Simon to South Kensington to some friends of hers and having to consult the map of London on the way to find the address, he was most helpful, showing me where London Bridge and various other places were or where he supposed them to be.

Then I took him to see the French Tapestries at the Victoria and Albert Museum and when we got in he said, 'I want to see the engines'; so I told him that they were shut, but he said they were not and he wanted to see them now. He went on and on about this and so I had to be taken out of that Museum across

the road to the other one where the engines were going beautifully when you pressed the button. Having arrived home he
informed Mummy who came home just about the same time
from her christening that a baby had wet the drawing room floor
and proceeded to get his sponge and wipe the polish off the
perfectly dry floor. Mummy was relaxing after her christening so
she did not stop him doing it physically, but tried the effect of
telling him it would spoil his sponge and she would not be able
to get another, and the floor would have to be polished all over
again, but he did not mind all this insisting that a baby had done
it and he must put it right. So at last Mummy decided that he
must have his bath and he yelled the whole time and when I
asked Jane if she thought anything might be wrong, she said the
cries signified anger and astonishment. Mummy said she did not
want a naughty boy in her bed, so he put himself in mine and
there he is now fast asleep.

Mummy and I went yesterday to a football tournament at
Twickenham and during a rather long interval between the
semifinals and the final a lot of little boys and girls ran on the
ground and played with little balls etc. When it was nearly time
for the last match the megaphone said would the children please
move off the ground back to their seats because the final was
about to begin, so they all did except one little boy of about six
or seven, who either didn't hear or was dreaming, so then he
was all by himself when the megaphone said again very loudly,
would the young gentleman at present occupying the centre of
the ground kindly return to his seat, so he woke up and ran like
a hare and everyone cheered and clapped.

My Biro pen has run out in one week, so I must have been
writing like anything, or done about a thousand crossword
puzzles. [He did *The Times* crossword puzzle every day.]
. . .

December 1946

. . .

Well it will be only a fortnight before you come home to see
your family again and particularly your dear little brother who
grows sweeter and sweeter. He tells long stories quite seriously
about how he went up to the sky in an aeroplane and took us

with him. Anyway he is a dear little boy who would very much like to see his big sister again.

. . .

March 1947

. . .

Tom is at home and spends most of his time looking after his little brother, takes him to the zoo or for walks by the river or fishing at Amersham or for a ride on the Thames. I must say that brother takes it all as a matter of course and doesn't seem a bit grateful for all the attention he gets, but he expects to get it all the same.

. . .

March 1947

. . .

Mummy wasn't very well last week and had a week's rest. Simon was looked after by Jane and behaved very nicely. One day she took him to the art school and he sat down quietly in a corner painting or making sausages out of clay. One of the students spent the day painting him in different attitudes and we have the picture; we are very pleased with it.

. . .

June 1947

. . .

I am sure you will want to hear about dear Simon's progress. He is still very good and Mummy thinks he is very clever in various ways, especially in finding his way about, he told Mummy in a taxi that the taximan was not going the right way when it turned down Queensborough Terrace. He certainly holds wonderful conversations with his telephone, with suitable pauses, 'No, she is out tonight' . . . no . . . yes. Then he will wait a bit and ring someone else.

. . .

July 1947

. . .

Jane and I are going to St Pauls on Tuesday to hear St Matthew Passion. I think we are going to have a pass to sit on

some seats just outside the organ loft, we should hear there very
well. We heard it at the Albert Hall last weekend and went on to
the platform to look at the harpsichord, having been invited to
do so. You can imagine that your sister was pleased when we got
there to find her favourite tenor, Peter Pears rehearsing something for the afternoon with a cello and the harpsichord. Tom
and I sat comfortably below in the morning and Jane and June
took our seats in the afternoon when we went to the gallery. I
took a stool and a cushion.

. . .

November 1947

. . .

I am glad you had a good Solomon concert, he is a wonderful
player and a pleasure to listen to always. Just now we are
concentrating on the St Matthew Passion for which I have two
seats at the Albert Hall on March 14th. There is a new set of
records in German which I have bought, 31 sides, and they are
quite easy to follow with the score. By the time the concert
comes we shall know it pretty well.

Poor old Simon has a cold that has been going around for
weeks and he looks a bit pallid, Mummy has it too so I think
they are giving it to each other. He loves going to school.

. . .

Chapter 16
The Golden Years

THE INTRODUCTION of the Welfare State, the extensive nationaliza-
tion programmes and other social changes after the Second World War
have affected the British working population in a variety of ways. Many
more people, including doctors, became civil servants, with a retirement
age of 65 and a pension. For some it was a godsend, a happy release,
but for others it spelled apprehension and anxiety. What were they
going to do after the age of 65? It was no different for large numbers of
other employed persons, but hospital doctors were not used to the
decision being made for them. They expected to resign or retire when
they wished to give up.

When Geoffrey Dowling was approaching retirement age in August
1956, he had other anxieties. He still had a 12-year-old son (Simon) at
boarding-school, not a very large private practice and no pension from
the National Health Service. To be eligible for a pension one had to
have been in the service for a minimum of 10 years — from July 1948.
Others in his position requested a special extension of their employment
for a year or more to complete 10 years and thus obtain a pension.
Geoffrey needed only another 16 months, and it would certainly have
been granted. But he made no such request.

His colleagues at St Thomas's Hospital were naturally concerned,
and at the same time they wanted him to continue on the active
dermatological stage where his reputation was at its height. They
arranged for him to work at St Thomas's supported by a research grant
from the Hospital Endowment Fund. Paul Naylor was then a senior
lecturer in the department of dermatology, with his own full-time
research laboratory in the department of medicine. Dowling expressed a
desire to work with him there, and Paul accepted.

At the time of his retirement, he was at the peak of his most
distinguished career but he himself never seemed to attach much importance to this. Paul remembers tentatively asking him if he had
considered writing a book summarizing his views on various dermatological topics, which would be based on a lifetime of experience. He
replied somewhat tartly that people no longer wanted views based on

experience but they wanted facts! He went on to express a very strong
wish to become involved in research. It quickly became clear, however,
that 'research' to Dowling did not mean clinical research — the collection, classification, and correlation of data collected from patients and
clinical records, which he regarded as very much second-best; nor did it
mean histological work, which he regarded as an important special
investigation for helping to solve clinical problems; but it did mean
learning established techniques, evolving new ones, using apparatus
and actually making measurements. The professor of medicine at St
Thomas's Hospital at the time, E.P. Sharpey-Schafer, was always
agreeable to providing space for anyone who wished to follow their
own ideas in experimental work, but insisted that they act as their own
technicians, and indeed regarded this as an essential part of training.
This discipline was usually sufficient to discourage all but the most
genuine and enthusiastic of workers. It was interesting that Dowling
quickly realized the importance of 'thinking with his hands' and took to
manipulating apparatus, washing glassware, weighing chemicals and
arguing about technical matters with his new colleagues in the department of medicine. They were an extremely aggressive and intellectually
formidable crowd, as may be judged by the fact that, during the 15
years or so of Sharpey-Schafer's reign, no fewer than 10 of the group
who worked in his department progressed to Chairs. This new-found
consuming interest of Dowling's continued to be leavened by his
customary modesty and ability to mix on equal terms with junior staff,
while referring to people of even moderate seniority as 'those important
people'.

He usually managed to plan his experiments in such a way that at
coffee break and tea-time he could slip away to the canteen with the
juniors, explaining that the extraction procedure, or whatever it was,
would take another 20 minutes or so. He loved to talk about the
results of his experiments, which he did constantly. When clinical
colleagues could not understand the points he was making because they
had no idea of the techniques in which he was involved, and few had
ever worked in a laboratory, he would look at them pityingly and
explain afterwards to Paul that it was high time that clinicians became
more involved in measuring things themselves so that they would
talk less hot air about matters which they didn't understand! He was
particularly censorious about information acquired by reading rather
than doing.

His ability to transfer his interest from patients to the laboratory was most remarkable, particularly as he was so distinguished in the first sphere and such a newcomer to the second. This change involved not only the acquisition of new facts and skills but also the ability to develop a completely new outlook — something which so many of a later generation and half his age have found impossible.

Towards the end of the second year in Paul Naylor's laboratory it became evident that the research grant would not continue. Geoffrey's anxieties rose to the surface again. He became quiet and morose at home. The family noted it with some alarm — so much so that they invited Dr Evan Jones, his best friend from St Thomas's, to come and see him in 24 Wimpole Street, fearing some major illness. After the consultation his diagnosis was short and clear:

'Nothing the matter with him. Nothing that a good spell of work won't cure.'

Shortly afterwards requests for consultant dermatologist locum tenens work appeared — in Brighton, Lewisham, Farnham and so on — and he never looked back.

It was in the early nineteen eighties that legislators in the United States decided that compulsory retirement at the age of 60 or 65 was a restriction on the liberty of the individual and should not be permitted. The proposal naturally met with the approval of President Ronald Reagan. And so the over-65s were given a free rein to pursue any business, professional or other remunerated activity they wished. They were to be known as the Golden Years.

And surprisingly, against all the odds, they did become the golden years for Geoffrey. He began working half the week at Lewisham Hospital in 1964, and the following year at Farnham Hospital. About this time his wife became ill with cancer, and she died in September 1965. With La's help, he was trying to sell the house at 24 Wimpole Street, but the sale was not completed until after May died.

Eventually he moved to the delightful little house at 52 Ravenscourt Gardens in Hammersmith. In November 1970 it was declared a 'Listed Building of special architectural or historic interest' by the London Borough of Hammersmith.

His daughter La had organized the purchase and, with her special abilities as an interior designer, built on an extension and made a new kitchen and dining-room, as well as redecorating the whole house. With her constant support, and being fully occupied in clinical dermatology,

Geoffrey gradually found great happiness again. He did his own shopping and very often Ken Sanderson took him to the local supermarket on a Saturday morning. Fortunately, he had learnt to enjoy cooking, particularly for friends. He especially admired Katie Stewart and practised many of the recipes from her book and articles in the *London Evening Standard*. Like most amateur chefs, his efforts were not always crowned with success and accidents do happen. He was especially fond of cold vichyssoise soup, which he made in a Kenwood electric mixer. On one occasion the machine was not correctly closed and the vichyssoise ended up on the kitchen table, the walls and his suit! Fortunately, he had a Mrs MacKenzie, who came in three days a week to clean up and do whatever was necessary.

He loved entertaining, going to parties and giving parties. He seemed to have a constant stream of visitors, and would always want to have a party for those from overseas, like Joy Shultz and George Findlay, who would bring him news from South Africa. For such events, his daughter La was constantly available to help. She would arrange the menu, doing much of the preparatory work in the kitchen and usually disappearing out of the back door as soon as the first guest arrived at the front.

His sons Tom and Simon frequently stayed there, but did not always know who else had been invited. One evening George Findlay arrived back late from the theatre and let himself in. Not wanting to disturb the house he did not switch on the light. In the drawing-room he found a stranger in the dark on the sofa, whom he thought must be a burglar. A brief fight ensued before he found it was Tom!

At about this time, mice appeared at Ravenscourt Gardens. The children blocked up every single hole they could find, but to no avail. A mouse would calmly walk across the front of the curtains as Geoffrey watched television. Something had to be done. La bought him a kitten, Puss Puss: the mice left. Geoffrey and Puss Puss became firm friends, though it was often referred to as 'you miserable beast' or 'you horrible animal', but with affection. The owners of the adjoining house took Puss Puss in when Geoffrey was taken to hospital, and it was still alive years later.

Until 1968 Jane would visit him every Saturday with Mary. Peter would arrive later to bring them home. When the Greenhams moved to the country in Oxfordshire, Geoffrey would visit them frequently.

Surprisingly he enjoyed the train ride from Marylebone to Bicester, saying it was his favourite journey.

Like most Londoners, Dowling experienced the local disease of being burgled. On a sunny summer afternoon he was dozing in a deckchair in the garden, but had left the front door open. When he woke up he found that his hi-fi record-player (a leaving present from the staff of St Thomas's) and other articles has disappeared.

He had his extensive record collection there and enjoyed many hours of his favourite music. But inevitably as time passed his hearing deteriorated. He gave up going to concerts — the sound was too distorted. But his sight, albeit with spectacles, remained relatively unimpaired. And he had always been a voracious reader.

The house had a nice little garden, with a lawn surrounded by trees and shrubs. He had the usual implements and an old-fashioned lawn-mower, with which he would cut the grass himself. And he would often snooze after lunch in a deckchair. It was happiness again for him. Bliss.

FARNHAM HOSPITAL

During the years of the Second World War, Hugh Wallace lived at Woking and did the dermatology clinics at Farnham Hospital in Surrey. In 1947 he began to spend more time in London and the skin clinic was first run by Robert Bowers and then by some of the other registrars from St Thomas's Hospital. The clinics were very busy and it was a long and tiring day's work, travelling down from London. In those post-war years there was a lot of scalp ringworm in children, and the dermatologist had to include a visit to a convent orphanage to cope with a small epidemic of it, armed with a Wood's lamp, epilation forceps and microscope slides. But they enjoyed the work, partly because of the help from the medical and nursing staff there, as well as from a very attractive and efficient medical secretary.

Eventually, after the introduction of the National Health Service in April 1948, Dr John Morgan was appointed as consultant dermatologist to the area in 1949. He built up the department with the help of two general practitioners, Dr Bardsley and Dr Donald Turnbull.

In September 1965 John Morgan resigned on health grounds and Geoffrey Dowling (now aged 74) was asked to carry on the clinic as a locum consultant. It was now a very busy clinic indeed and lasted all day on a Wednesday each week. It catered for the population of Farnham, Aldershot, Farnborough, Camberley and Cove, about 150,000–180,000 inhabitants.

If the registrars from St Thomas's Hospital found it hard work, how did Geoffrey cope? He was living in Hammersmith at the time, he had to get up at 5.00 am and take the Underground to Richmond, from where he travelled by train to Farnham. He took a bus from the station to the hospital in time to do a ward round at 8.00 am, before starting his clinic at 9.00 am. He inherited a very long waiting-list, which was cleared within a month as he always maintained that anyone with a skin problem could not be kept waiting. He worked in the clinic until 1.00 pm and then, after a quick lunch, wrote letters to the general practitioners and returned to Ravenscourt Gardens by the same route, usually arriving home at about 7.00 pm, totally exhausted. In later years, he sometimes travelled down on a Tuesday evening and spent the night with the senior physician, Dr J.W. Todd. Until 1970 he had the help of Dr Turnbull and then Dr E.L. Smith, who had been a senior registrar at St John's Hospital, Leicester Square.

In spite of the difficulties, Geoffrey enjoyed the work and the very pleasant atmosphere of the clinic which John Morgan had built up over six years. There was an old people's home attached to the hospital, as well as an infectious disease hospital and Trimmers Cottage Hospital, where he would sometimes be asked to see patients.

One suspects that the Department of Health administrators were not really aware of his advanced age. There were certainly no complaints from patients or staff on the grounds of efficiency or punctuality. But eventually Dr Robin Felix was appointed as consultant dermatologist to the whole area and he replaced Geoffrey (now 83) on 24 March 1975.

LEWISHAM HOSPITAL

Dr John L. Lyndon was the consultant dermatologist to Lewisham Hospital until he resigned on 30 September 1964 to go to work abroad for health reasons. The Ministry of Health did not want to appoint a permanent replacement immediately and Geoffrey Dowling was asked to do the work as a locum tenens consultant. He started on 1 October 1964 at the age of 73, and worked there for five or six half-days per week until 31 October 1972, when Dr Dorothy Vollum was appointed to the permanent consultant post. But he continued to do the sessions whenever she was away over the next two years.

So he was associated with the hospital for eight years, and there is no doubt that he enjoyed working there. The area was densely populated and he conducted a skin clinic almost every day (except Wednesdays, when he went to Farnham), with a special clinic for leg ulcer patients on a Friday morning. He did a minor surgery session on another day, when he carried out all the usual tasks of a registrar, removing warts, taking biopsies and so on. He responded whenever asked to take part in teaching for general practitioners and postgraduate students. He made a special impression on one of the clinic's nurses (Staff Nurse Sroka):

> What I remember most about him was his kindness and caring for both patients and staff, his sense of humour, and great stamina for his age.
>
> He was always punctual for his clinics, even though he travelled by public transport. He had a great memory for patient's names. He loved to go to see a good rugby match in Cardiff when his favourite team was playing. The only thing I ever heard him say really annoyed him was having to listen to a patient who couldn't give a good history of their illness. He was loved by everyone in the Skin Unit and greatly missed when he retired.

At Lewisham Geoffrey was very pleased to find two physician friends on the staff, one from Guy's and the other from St Thomas's Hospital. Dr T.M.L. Price had never met him before but certainly knew of his reputation as a dermatologist.

> I must admit I wondered how this world-renowned figure would fit in to the life of a district general hospital. I need not have worried; he came for one or two years and stayed for seven or eight, I forget which. We loved having him and he was happy to stay.
>
> I have memories of him coming into lunch, quietly, looking like Mr Punch. He would remain a while in silence, apparently not listening. We would even forget he was there; the conversation would carry on around him. Then quietly during a pause he would join in. Whatever he said was perceptive, always worth listening to, often witty and funny, and never malicious.

His teaching, of course, was a delight. He had the capacity that many very intelligent people share, of making what they say clear and apparently simple when it is really nothing of the sort. As a professional colleague he was invaluable. He particularly appreciated the Skin Unit at Lewisham because the out-patients, the wards and the daily dressing clinic were all in the same area, and the nursing staff was the same for each.

I was twice his guest at the United Hospitals Club, a dining club composed of London general practitioners and consultants from St Thomas's and Guy's Hospitals; he made an exemplary host, by enjoying the evening so much himself. I remember on one of these occasions walking past St Paul's Cathedral with him in the full moonlight on the way to his train back to Hammersmith, and the overwhelming recollection is of geniality and amusement. On this occasion neither of us would have been wise to drive a car but, in fact, he did not own one.

He was a familiar sight waiting for, or getting off, buses outside the hospital in Lewisham High Street, a long way from Hammersmith and in all kinds of weather.

We were very fortunate that he came to Lewisham in the first place and that having done so he stayed for so long.

Dr J.S. (Sam) Staffurth knew him in five different lights throughout his medical career.

Firstly, as a student during the war, I think I went to only two or three of his out-patient sessions, and I cannot remember much about them except that he had his famous binocular magnifying glasses at that time. He was difficult to hear and he did not make much impact on us.

Secondly as a patient, when I was doing my first house job I got chronic impetigo on my chin which he quickly got right with a short course of superficial X-rays, and I recall that he prescribed the dosage himself.

Thirdly, I got to know him fairly well in the immediate post-war period at St Thomas's Hospital, the time when he trained so many young dermatologists, many of whom were my contemporaries and friends. I am sure you know with what high regard he was looked upon by all of these. I do not remember an unkind word about him, and his every dermatological utterance was treated as gospel. They certainly all held him in very high regard.

At this time we had an informal golfing society that used to meet once every six weeks or so at Hankley Common. It was composed mainly of senior registrars of the medical disciplines, and it was nearly always attended by Dr Evan Jones and Geoffrey, and occasionally by other members of the staff. At this time he was a moderately good club golfer whereas the rest of us were pretty hopeless. I know he got a great deal of amusement from watching our wild shots, listening to our comments and our general behaviour. He recalled these times to me vividly on the last occasion that I met him properly, which I will mention later. He was an unusual character because he was so friendly to everyone, so encouraging, quiet and humble, lacking any pomposity, and yet it was evident to us all that he was a great man. Dr Evan Jones was, of course, a great man too but in a quite different mould, being a cheerful extrovert. He and Geoffrey were great friends and it was their combined presence that added so much to these meetings. Both of them were friendly to us all without any suspicion of standoffishness, and yet both were so much respected. At this distance, these informal golf meetings were one of the happiest times that I recall from that period.

Fourthly, I knew him as a colleague at Lewisham Hospital when he came to do a long-term locum in the mid 1960s and he stayed for five or six years. I was instrumental in getting him there through Hugh Wallace, but I cannot recall any of the details. However, from the moment he arrived, he fitted into our hospital and behaved as though this was the most natural place in the world for him to be. In no time at all he had large out-patient clinics, and I remember him complaining like everyone else at the large number of patients that 'they' required him to see, but I do not think he ever did much about stopping it. At this time he lived in Hammersmith and he had to get right across London to Lewisham. I think he often left home before seven in the morning. At the same time he also went to Farnham once a week, which necessitated getting up even earlier. At that time he was certainly attending the Dermatology Section Meetings of the Royal Society of Medicine regularly (I once showed a patient

there with him), and I believe he went to St John's Hospital
nearly every week. I understood from Hugh Wallace that he got
rejuvenated by coming back into clinical work and he certainly
seemed quite content. The rest of us were good but otherwise
ordinary consultants, who did not match up to his intellectual
capacity, but he treated us absolutely like equals. He often came
to our weekly meetings and it was always stimulating to have
him around. It was at lunch time during this period that we
realised what a quiet wit he had, for he was very amusing and
penetrating in his comments, and when critical it was either
about his peers or the administrators.

My fifth period of knowing him was briefly when he was
my patient. On one of the mornings he was due to come to
Lewisham Hospital he had a paper he had been asked to submit
to the *Guy's Hospital Reports*, and the morning in question was
the deadline for the paper. He must have finished it the previous
night for he got up even earlier and took the train to Guy's,
where he handed in the paper personally before coming to
Lewisham to do his routine out-patient clinic. It was during the
middle of the clinic that he began to feel unwell, Sister laid him
down on the couch, and sent for me. I recall that he did not have
any pain or shortness of breath or any particular symptom; he
was not particularly shocked or hypotensive, but there seemed to
be something amiss and an electrocardiogram showed that
he had a silent coronary thrombosis. It was with the utmost
difficulty that we persuaded him to come into hospital at all, but
he finally consented to stay for one night. The next day when he
was clinically stable I was quite happy for him to go home, and
so his daughter La kindly came and took him back to his house,
and looked after him for the next few weeks. I think he did not
come back to Lewisham after this episode for, in fact, he was
beginning to feel his age beforehand and had talked about
leaving us. It was my utmost regret that I lived so far away from
him that I was not able to see him very often, but I did manage
to look after him during the rest of this illness, for in a way it
was quite a minor affair.

The last time I saw him properly was when he asked me to
luncheon at home one day, which we had alone and which he
cooked to perfection. Unhappily, I cannot remember the reason

for this but I think there was quite likely no particular reason; it was merely that he wished to see me and share my company, which of course he did with countless other friends. He did not consult me during his last illness and I did not manage to see him then as I did not learn about it until he was rather ill. I gather that he did not report his symptoms till it was too late to do much about them. I am sure this is likely to be true and indeed I think it was possibly wise, for at our luncheon he had intimated that he had lived long enough, he had had a marvellous life and he did not wish to go on living too much longer.

Finally, I only saw his portrait in the Willan Room at the Royal College of Physicians the other day and I must say it is one of the best portraits of anyone I have ever seen. It is a very fitting memorial to him.

Chapter 17
In Dowling's Own Words

THE CORRESPONDENCE between Geoffrey Dowling and Dr George Findlay contains over 60 letters written by Dowling between 1958 and 1975. While George was at St John's Hospital in 1957, Dr Hugh Wallace hinted that it would be good if 'Uncle Geoffrey' could somehow be invited to visit the country of his birth, which he had not seen for nearly 50 years. Fortunately the British Council was willing to offer him a travel grant and the University of Pretoria an honorary doctorate. In this way, Wallace's suggestion bore fruit. This started an exchange of letters, both before and after his visit to South Africa in 1959.

Some of the genuine Dowling flavour can perhaps be conveyed in extracts from this correspondence. He did not seem to mind what he said or wrote. It varied from extravagant praise to what he called 'fair comment' — a euphemism for something highly unflattering. For the rest it dealt with mutual interests in dermatology, music and other subjects, as well as mutual friends.

11 June 1958 — To Dr John Cowley (Johannesburg)
... truthfully I have not much to give, being now content to pay respectful attention to the youngers and betters.

... George Findlay has his roots in the South African aristocracy, but he also has a low-class root in a sumptuous ironmonger's establishment which I admired in my childhood, situated in Parliament Street, Cape Town.

3 October 1958 — H.J. Wallace to G.H. Findlay regarding a visit to South Africa
It is very kind of you to take all this trouble but you would, I know, be rewarded if you could have seen the reception that the idea alone got from Geoffrey Dowling.

27 November 1958 — Dowling, on being invited on the visit
I am overwhelmed and thrilled and hardly know what to say. I am afraid 'thank you' is about all I can think of at the moment. I never

thought that I would see the small part of South Africa that I know again and certainly not under such circumstances. It is about the greatest compliment and kindness that I have ever received and certainly I have never had much to grumble about in that respect.

3 February 1959
I have a mother (about 90) who will be staying with friends during the time I shall be in those parts [Johannesburg] . . . I have also an elder sister (71) . . . She and the Dutch farmers at Paarl where she worked for a long while as a school-mistress were buddies; but she married a Scot named Anderson — recently died.

30 April 1959
. . . James Marshall has not changed. He is very alert and quick on the diagnostic mark . . .

1 July 1959 — From report of a dermatology lecture tour
in South Africa
The Department at Pretoria . . . is the most effective in the Union. Loewenthal . . . comparatively little use has been made of his remarkable gifts. In Natal . . . the Department is atrociously housed and grossly understaffed. The Groote Schuur Skin Department is more amply equipped with staff than any other similar clinic in the Union.

The specialty is undermanned and overworked . . . among them is a handful of the highest calibre by any standard.

It occurs to me that a system of reciprocal exchange whereby a registrar from South Africa might be exchanged for a year or perhaps longer for one from London would be valuable experience for both. The South African would gain . . . to say nothing of the liberal philosophy with which our young dermatologists are at the present time richly endowed.

9 August 1959
You are most wise to set up a laboratory and consolidate your Department's status.

Kogoj is a very good dermatologist . . . he and his boys are intelligent, as honest as the day and totally devoid of arrogance, to say nothing of being most warm hearted and friendly.

Degos . . . may be getting faintly portentous, but he quite truly is very hard worked indeed.

21 August 1959
Focal infection depends so much on the patient's personal ideas on his naso-pharynx.

Seborrhoeic eczema — what seems to be an unnecessary division into small compartments is made . . . mainly because I want to see if petaloid and other members of the Darier eczematide group are mixed at all frequently with various other features . . .

26 August 1959
With focal infection the answer must be an unequivocal yes or no, and I am not at all sure that it is an easy question to answer.

If we thought diet mattered we should have to eliminate variations in excess or deficiency and would probably never get the right answers.

18 December 1959
. . . I have just had a Symposium sent to me to review. I think there is some good stuff in it, but I wouldn't like to meet these speakers much and certainly would not choose to live among them.

. . . dermatology of the 30s: the alleged slump period of English Dermatology.

7 January 1960
In Johannesburg, the title of first assistant, equivalent to a senior registrar, for a person of Alphonse's [Loewenthal] calibre and renown is on the face of it ridiculous.

Lang 'of Africa' asked me to write to the Dean about his set-up and say whether or not I thought it fit to train post-graduates for a Master's degree in dermatology. I honestly did not know whether he wanted the answer to be yes or no.

The saying among dermatologists that dermatology is a branch of general medicine is a platitude, like the one about treating the whole patient and not just his skin . . . Some of them must find an underlying general cause for everything; e.g. alopecia areata must be an endocrine disturbance, nummular eczema is psychosomatic, etc.

17 October 1960
. . . Music . . . I like it all if it is all right of its kind, except ultra-modern which I don't understand and find disagreeable. I always thought my mother really good on music, her playing being bang on musically

though she could not do everything owing to technical limitations. My younger son (16) . . . compares himself favourably with Backhaus while admitting that Backhaus has the edge on him technically.

. . . I don't think Ian's [Whimster] intolerance means necessarily that he is any more musical than we are, could even be less . . . I shall go and see him in his little ivory tower in the West Wing [of St Thomas's Hospital] . . . The absence of output is very disappointing; very rarely he is persuaded to speak to the dermatologists and when he does he more or less shakes the foundations of the building, and then is quite happy about it all for a little while. I don't understand the reticence and anyway it doesn't pay. I like Ian and admire his talents very much . . .

. . . Regarding your cross-over observations [influence of lesions on one half of the body upon the other]. I have thought for years that this happens regularly whatever the treatment and I would never have anything to do with paired treatments for that reason. I suppose if we knew the mechanism of the cross-over we should be making quite an advance.

12 January 1961

. . . the house physician, from Cape Town, asked me what his duties were to be, my reply being to see patients and ask for help if he thought he needed it. He said he did not know anything; I said neither did I.

. . . the difficulty is to find anyone to do research, who has the necessary liking and talent for the type of work.

. . . eczema limited to the hands. Our people have the greatest difficulty over these cases, and quite a few reject an external factor altogether.

. . . I know nothing about Wolf [Dr Tillman] having had for a short time only the loan of some records sung by Elena Gerhart. I could not understand them at all. Newman said you have to know German poetry to follow these songs.

29 June 1961

. . . The George Club has just been to Poland . . . I am sure it is the relative juniority of a number of them that makes them always acceptable abroad.

24 October 1961

. . . I saw Ian Whimster on Saturday last when he was doing the annual talk of the George Club and very well he did it. He talked away on some theme that seemed well on the way to solve the major problems in principle leaving only the details to be filled in by people like us, the whole theory being based on observations he makes on lizards which he keeps more or less as pets.

... George Wells sent me a rough draft of his Parkes Weber lecture to look at and I have read it through once with considerable enjoyment, the pleasure being due to the fact that it is written in good English and without graphs or charts or tables and I found to my surprise that I can understand what he has to say ... George will have a medal presented to him for this performance which looks like a bar of milk chocolate. I believe it develops patina in time but at present it looks unpleasant.

12 November 1961

I am afraid I don't understand what is in the minds of the physician-dermatologists of the North [of England] ... They go on plugging their clichés as though preaching a new doctrine while Sneddon doesn't, and Sneddon is the best of the lot I think and very good indeed at that.

...We know that good clinical dermatologists make the best histologists.

...Wallace was forced to begin his next sentence with 'with respect', his way of saying don't talk rot.

4 March 1962

...it is disgraceful in these days to appoint a hack dermatologist to a university top appointment. Of course it is also wrong to allow the retiring man to take any part in the appointment of his successor.

25 July 1962

I have had a couple of tasks recently which have taken up a lot of time, mainly I am sure because I am slow. I have had to write obituary notices on Parkes Weber and Henry [Haber]. I did not mind doing Parkes Weber and found it interesting but it meant a lot of work going through his bibliography, writing to his School and to Cambridge and so forth. Haber's death on the other hand was quite shattering. He had about as much guile in him as a small boy of the kind that you see at cricket matches and a lot of people were very fond of him. I have never seen such concentrated grief at a funeral.

11 January 1963

... the advanced thinking of some of our men, which is that whatever the skin does we must look for something wrong somewhere else and that is why it is essential that we should learn all about the liver, etc. and not bother too much about superficialities and skin sections.

... Homecomers say that our rather absurd little gimmick with the *Telstar** [at the Washington International Congress] was the most entertaining part of the programme. Degos wrote me a note at Christmas saying it was 'émovante'. But Grupper when he has occasion to write begins Cher Monsieur et tres honoré maitre, so you don't know where you are with these people.

17 April 1963

... I think of the coast from Muizenberg to Simonstown as unique and incomparable. I was reading Bligh's diary about the Bounty recently and I was rather surprised that he could stay in Simonstown for quite a long while and enjoy the break without remarking on the beauty of the Peninsula, but he seems to have been not very good at enjoying anything.

... I did not know that I had said that I thought biochemists useless to us; I always hope they may be quite otherwise but the quality is obviously very variable. Robert Thompson is the kind that could be most helpful to us but some others have had a shot and failed utterly ...

... Our piano tuner is not cantankerous but depressing, but I suppose he goes round hoping to find something worth tuning and very rarely being rewarded, most of his jobs corresponding to our warts.

... My present interest in natural science ... is Gilbert White on the Natural History of Selborne, a place I know ... I was interested to find that the language is the same as Parkes Weber's with no wasted or obscure words. I find it very entertaining in spite of my not knowing a house martin, woodlark, redstart, etc. and never likely to know them.

... George [Wells] and Edward [Wilson Jones] do the job together [histopathology] and if the truth be told, better than Henry [Haber], but that is just as it should be, and old Henry would be happy to know it.

... I do a lot of holiday [locum tenens] hospital work for various

---

* At the Dermatology Congress in Washington DC in 1962 there was a television discussion of patients in London shown via the *Telstar* communications satellite. Dowling was in charge of demonstrating the selected patients.

people . . . there is hardly any way of tying up loose ends left at the end of the job. The incumbents say they will keep one informed, but they never do . . .

. . . I asked the head of the concern [Ciba Ltd.], Miescher,* not Guido, his brother, how it was possible to get hold of so many high class research workers, and he said they were not high class at all, and someone else had to think as well as understand the apparatus. One thing is certain, that it is difficult to do research work and diagnose and treat a lot of patients at the same time.

. . . We are finding it difficult to explain the great prevalence of atopic disease in West Indian immigrant children or rather children of immigrant parents, while the statement that it hardly occurs there may be wrong . . .

12 August 1963
. . . Thank you for the talk given to the Americans. It was first class, but I thought perhaps too clear. I imagine that what they would like would be something of which not a word could be understood.

. . . David Williams . . . likes big music and does not fancy very much the very simple stuff that we share a liking for. Anyway, he is a kindred spirit as far as we are concerned, i.e. you, Magnus, me etc.

26 August 1963 (David Williams and George Findlay had sent a Pretoria tie to GBD)
Messrs. Findlay and Williams
Gents' Outfitters

Dear Sirs,
   I am very much obliged to you for the neckwear which is indeed of remarkably fine quality and elegant design.
   You may rely on my future custom and you may use this letter as a testimonial.

---

* Prof. Guido Miescher was the head of the department of dermatology in Zurich, Switzerland. His brother was head of the international chemical company Ciba Ltd. before it merged with Geigy Ltd. and became Ciba-Geigy Ltd.
   After the George Club overseas visit to Zurich in 1956 Charles Calnan and his wife returned to Zurich to study a particular laboratory technique. They took Dr Dowling with them (in an old Ford Prefect car) and drove non-stop from Calais to Zurich. They stayed for two weeks with Dr Theo Inderbitzen, who had spent a year in London working

8 May 1964

...I remember now that 1914 was the starting year of the Cape Town Orchestra. We used to go down to the jetty on Saturday evenings to hear it...I have always thought that Cape Town must provide more music than most other places of its size, here or anywhere else, and the buildup began about 1912 with the College, then the Orchestra, both to some extent I imagine among other things aimed at offsetting my father's seeming monopoly for such a long time. It was a pleasant place for a musical life except that there was so little monetary reward to be got out of it.

...Shuster is going to Newcastle...I think it is probably the most satisfactory appointment yet since he has tried, and not without success, to learn clinical dermatology.

22 June 1964

...I got the Bartok quartets and have played a couple of them without any discomfort though I doubt whether I will get much comfort either out of these.

...My daughter Jane...is teaching English to students of art most of whom are more or less illiterate...they don't come to grips with English at all readily. The examiners ask them to explain 'fall on your feet' or 'deterrent'...One of the bright students said that 'deterrent' meant encouragement.

7 August 1964

We [George Club] went to Hungary...Clinically we seemed rather ahead and I suppose we ought to be as we are so much less isolated than they are and so much in the habit of holding numerous clinical meetings. Their science aspect seems to be attended to mainly by the Party men who I suppose are looked on as a cut above the old fashioned clinicians, professors or no.... They are very addicted to Gipsy music...During a visit to a cellar, I am sorry to say that the girl colleagues broke into song, the sound they produced being a disgrace to

---

with Dr George Wells at St John's Hospital. Ruth Inderbitzen was the daughter of the Miescher brother who was the head of Ciba Ltd. Dowling enjoyed the whole trip enormously and uncomplainingly put up with the rigours of the journey in his registrar's car. One day Ruth announced that there was little in the house for lunch.

RUTH: Would you prefer to go out to lunch or have omelettes and salad here?
DOWLING: We should prefer omelettes and salad here.
They were delicious.

any place but terrible in a musical country...Our Prime Tory... spotted his enemy, the Party man, whose duty it is to select medical students for training. He was a good looking chap and friendly, who as a member [of the Party] would put your thumbs in the rack and feel it more than you, owing to his dedication etc....Asked by one of the tactless British colleagues how much of a problem in Hungary was the homosexual spread of V.D. The answer was that this did not exist in Hungary.

17 January 1965
...in Cape Town, the surrounding country and coast being the most beautiful in the world would seem tempting to me.

   ...I would think South Africa is really a good training ground for dermatology and I doubt whether such a variety both of clinical experience and environment exists anywhere else.

7 June 1965
I have just been in Holland...Nijmegen seems to be the most advanced of the Dutch places...and I imagined Mali to be about the most impressive of the Dutch professors. There is a lot of very expensive machinery in the department, and to run it, science experts from other departments are brought in...after three sessions the English dermatologists had had about as much as they could take...

   I trust you did not with rough colonial downrightness tell Sargent that in your view Boult handles English music better than he could.

18 July 1965
Our grandchild is expected in 3 weeks, my daughter Jane looking more blooming than I have seen her look in many a year. Meanwhile another part of my news is terrible. Poor May is slowly dying of ovarian malignancy. She knows exactly what is going on and while sad at having to leave us is by no means dismayed at the thought of dying...I would expect her to see her grandchild but it is so difficult to know what will happen. It is extremely distressing and I find it something of a relief that I have quite a lot of dermatological hackwork to get on with...

13 September 1965 (Death of Mrs Dowling)
...This is only to let you know that poor May died in the weekend [11 September]. She was extraordinarily stoical throughout. Knowing

exactly what was going on because she had been constantly with two of her women friends who gradually went in the same way, she none the less kept up her interest in her friends and their doings until about the last week when she became desperately tired. She never wandered for an instant. I know that we will be in your thoughts which is a comfort but I would prefer not to be written to.

16 January 1966
... George Wells is very good indeed ... I never seem to hear him say a slipshod thing.

24 February 1966
Mrs Ryle viewed me with some distaste, I fancy, until John Ryle [later Regius Professor of Physics at Cambridge] asked me to help over their youngest child, a small girl. We had a consultation over this child, Ryle, his wife and myself, during which she informed us both that while we obviously both thought we knew a lot we were in fact utterly ignorant. We bowed, and I did my best with the child ...

28 May 1966
I am leaving this house [24 Wimpole St] very shortly. I am dreading it, because it is about twice as difficult to get to it [Ravenscourt Gardens] as it is now. On the other hand it is far more like a home than this set-up.

12 November 1966
The Times Book Shop ... it has occurred to me that this solid looking business may be running down by degrees in spite of the thick carpeting and air of refinement which clients like myself like so much.

25 November 1966
... the Committee on Dermatology ... did decide that the avant grade type of contributor should be asked always.
    ... I am regarded as suitable, because I make no comments.

30 August 1967
... I can't understand why you should not be properly paid, i.e. spared the labour of having to extract money from patients to pay for your own service to the Medical School.

... Thank you for the diploma ['The Basutoland Dermatological Society'] which I propose to have framed. I am attributing the splendid and dignified design to Fred Scot [dermatologist at Bloemfontein], he being an artist of impeccable taste and erudition, and the elegant wording to yourself. I propose to send it to Wallace, and perhaps to Whimster and Magnus. I will explain to all that criticism is not asked for and if proffered will be ignored.

4 September 1967
I would send notices to Wallace, D.I. Williams ... to Sagher [Felix, dermatologist, Jerusalem] who no doubt would send his apologies for absence in reply ...

23 January 1968
Time in my case is not very important though on my small jobs I am punctual.

My granddaughter ($2\frac{1}{2}$) is ordinarily in and out of the place [Royal Academy] a good deal and throws her weight about there, shouting welcome at various old friends from ex-presidents, RAs, girl secretaries, doormen and so on.

30 January 1968
My daughter Jane received some literary instruction long years ago from David Cecil, C.S. Lewis and Coghill and she thinks she knows what children like from five to seven.

6 January 1969
... I got the Vaughan Williams Sea Symphony for myself a few days ago knowing nothing about it but having heard it once in the Queen's Hall rather a long while ago.

4 March 1969
I am under the impression that from the beginning of the Hitler movement in Germany progress of any kind began to slow down, but that it picked up 20 or so years ago ... could you let me know what the highlights have been, and how high.

17 May 1969
... Al Kligman [dermatologist, Philadelphia] told the Matron [at

Utrecht, Holland] that he was looking for a wife and he would like to know her better.

23 June 1969 (After a visit of Dowling Club to South Africa)
... I now know all your children quite well I feel. I don't believe any could be naughty even under strong provocation.

... I found two nieces in Cape Town, and we all went to the Cathedral to find the choir. As good as the pre-1926 days after which it rather snuffed out. The present man is called Barry [Smith], in his 20s, and obviously first class as an organist and choirmaster.

1969 (Proposed visit to London)
It is good news to hear ... that you are thinking of coming to this rough shack to lead the simple life ... I have a Beckstein piano ... 'by appointment' whatever that means. With various German Emperors and Empresses, one called Frederick, and of course Queen Victoria, so belongs to an age you are interested in.

23 January 1970
... You are too good to me. The pictures of Elizabeth are splendid. She is the most beautiful little girl as well as good, and I love being an honorary relative.

... What a marvellous city Cape Town was and remains in places. I am sorry you are not there because I might so to speak go home occasionally.

... We are all sick of Wilson [Prime Minister, Harold] and his kind, the demonstrators, the restless students etc, etc. and getting rid of Wilson & Co is a great relief.

10 July 1970
I rather like the thought of going to Denmark [for the George Club visit] by sea because I like that sort of travelling.

7 July 1971
It was the Beethoven Mass that you saw in my cupboard and it belonged to Vickers [Renwick, dermatologist]. I could not get on with it or with the Bach B minor which I heard first in the Queen's Hall some years ago. But I do like the St Matthew Passion perhaps because it suits the story so beautifully. I got your Fauré nocturnes ... Having played

them over several times . . . I am trying to get the hang but don't think it is really easy music.

The Lebanon was a very good visit to an affair called 'Middle East Congress of Medicine'. Amal Kurban [head of dermatology at the American University of Beirut] is very high class . . .

17 February 1972

I believe I could remember the Chandos voice singing Songs of Araby etc. I don't think Ada Crossley ever came near us and I never saw her.

24 June 1973

. . . I work on only one day a week and spend a lot of time reading which I much enjoy. From the more difficult stuff like Karl Popper to biographies, letters, classics, and so on. The latest Woodham-Smith — Queen Victoria — is most gripping.

. . . I heard from George Wells that your book is out and well reviewed in 'Science'. I am to have the loan of it from him in due course. All the same I would like to have one for myself.

. . . I have given up attending meetings being too deaf and dumb, while for the social side I rely largely on Edward [Wilson Jones], Ken Sanderson, Chas Calnan, whose wife Jo asks me to dinner now and again which is very nice.

10 December 1973

H. [Humphrey] R. Raikes [principal of Witwatersrand University] . . . I shared a study with him at school, and I even spent a weekend at his home in a parsonage in a Kent village . . . I found it hard-going. I often wondered how he had fared, until I found him in the Hofmeyr biography . . . He always looked as if a hard push would break him. I shared a cabin with Hofmeyr* on one of the South Africa–Oxford

---

*The Hon. Jan Hendrik Hofmeyr (1894–1948) CMG, DCL (Oxon.), was a very distinguished South African politician, administrator and writer. He spent the years 1914 to 1918 as a Rhodes Scholar at Balliol College, Oxford. His biography by Alan Paton was published (Oxford University Press) in 1964. Paton wrote 'on 20 September 1913, on the Royal Mail Steamer *Saxon*, he and his mother set sail for England, Oxford and Balliol College. He was now wearing long trousers!'

Hofmeyr's mother was dominating and Dowling must have felt in sympathy with him in his mother-possession.

JUDGE BLACKWELL: Why didn't you let the boy marry?

journeys: Mum being on deck of course and much in evidence. I could think she must have been a disaster or at any rate a handicap in many important ways.

There are some good younger people coming up and I would like to be kept in touch as this has always interested me.

17 September 1973

It was a pleasure to have Joy [Schulz] come in every evening and relate the day's events...I told her on her arrival that I did not want her around in the kitchen, her answer to that being to go straight to the kitchen and clean it all up, and to provide a very expensive kettle with a whistle.

Simon...comes in fairly often to play his piano which he does better than I expected him to do. Ronda Sanderson lent him a book of exercises, Dohnanyi, very good he says but I never heard him doing them.

4 January 1974

'Prisca' [Mrs E. Barrow-Dowling], daughter of a C. of E. Vicar, also a 'Nightingale' [nurse] of the time when St Thomas's Hospital relied heavily on the C. of E. and put the fear of God into its daughters.

I don't know if the Raikes family was pious or not, but I think they were extreme examples of a traditional system now out of date by which the parson and family dominated village life. Using the platform at meetings for repose [Raikes often fell visibly asleep] seems to show a sense of values...

13 April 1974

I most fully agree of course that the English church choir singing is quite special and beautiful in a unique way and the music is just as special.

...Personally I can think of nothing more dreadful than working in Johannesburg.

MRS HOFMEYR: I never tried to stop him marrying. If the right girl had come along, I'd never have stood in his way.

JUDGE BLACKWELL: You knew the right girl would never come along, so long as you were alive.

ANOTHER QUOTE: You are not correct in saying I live with my son. My son lives with me.

May 1974

In Holland ... the programme was mostly over my head. They have professional biochemists ... who can talk their stuff for hours on end without stopping. Kogoj [dermatologist] loved his return to South Africa and is full of affection for his ex-colleagues bar one.

February 1975

My son Tom and elder daughter are really very good — designing and making frames; they like the artisan side of art. She attributes my general unbelief to too much familiarity with choirs and organ lofts.

My brother was a superb choir singer with a deep baritone. Sophisticated female ears lapped up his phrasing, and so did he.

29 March 1975

I don't think I ever knew a note of Granville Bantock's music. You do indeed inhabit that world and may well be as expert as anyone living on English music of that period. I shan't forget something going wrong with a string part at the Festival Hall which you and the Times critic noticed and no doubt the conductor.

My heart seems all right but I take a daily dose of Propranolol and Frusemide and I make no effort of any kind.

29 October 1975

I don't see anyone in these days and I'm poorly informed about what is happening. I have been told that Etain [Cronin] is writing a great book and I am sure she would do this well.

Here the incoming correspondence ceased. On 3 June 1976 George Findlay received two cables: 'Uncle Geoffrey departed peacefully last night. Ian', and 'Dear Uncle Geoffrey died Monday. Funeral Friday 4th. Love Calnans'.

FURTHER LETTERS

Xmas card

David Presbury and wife are in a state of pleasurable excitement about joining a South African dermatologist. They could be right.

To Fred Scott

Thank you for the splendid Basuto shoes. I much enjoy having them.

5 December 1971 (Appearance of the 80th birthday tribute — the Dowling Festschrift: Br. J. Dermatol. *Supplement no. 7 (1971))*

I don't know how to thank you for the South African Festschrift. It is a total surprise and an overwhelming honour to which I am not entitled. Anyway, I have got it and am filled with the grossest self-satisfaction. I am very happy to see that there appears to be no overwhelming difficulty, the dermatological language being what I am used to and the things written about not outside my comprehension.

David Whiting came to a party...Ronald Marks was the barman and very good at it.

[Later]...The more I go through the superb extra edition of the BJD [*British Journal of Dermatology*] the more I am certain that it is superior to all previous issues. I am reading as quickly as my faculties permit which is not fast.

[Later]...Regarding that marvellous book I continue to feel dazed with admiration and to be contentedly inflated. Ryan thinks it an extraordinary achievement. I much like the picture of Teawater and me and am very very proud...the BJD South Africa book is superb. I ooze pleasure and self-satisfaction.

22 August 1973 (on receiving Dr Robert Broom FRS, Paleontologist and Physician *by G.H. Findlay)*

Thank you for your book...I wanted to read it when I could without stopping. Knowing nothing about paleontology and allied sciences I was sure I would have some difficulty over this. Not at all. I have read it in two days word for word and I have enjoyed every minute. Every word about this super chap is gripping. He seems to have been either very poor or close to poverty all the time and not to have been too distressed about this...It is really a big achievement and the publishers have done extraordinarily well; it could not be done here for the price.

20 August 1961 — To F.P. Scott, dermatologist, Bloemfontein, who had sent him D.C. Boonzaaier's book of caricatures of old Cape Town residents

I am thrilled with the book...the pictures are of my elders and many must be quite unknown to any but elder South Africans today...Quite apart from my father, whose picture is excellent, there are quite a number of characters whom we knew...the pictures are good and pretty sympathetic as Merriman said, and they tell you something about each of the characters. Denholm Walker look convivial and that was indeed his handicap. He once had the misfortune to say to one of his daughters from the head of his supper table: 'Gladys say when', when 'Gladys say grace' was intended.

18 August 1975 — To Joy Schulz, dermatologist
I have adopted your lunch routine, roasting a good big chicken weekly or so, and keeping some good cheese and a supply of lager. I have it in the early afternoon and enjoy it, and look forward to it . . . Time for my chicken and beer.

1973 — To Joy Schulz
I am at the moment quite absorbed in *Hofmeyr* by Alan Paton. I have reached the point at which he returns on the *Windsor Castle* in 1914 for his second year at Oxford. I shared the cabin with him on that voyage, but that interesting fact is not mentioned in this biography. His mum was with him as always.

1974 — To Joy Schulz
Presbury is getting on well . . . and getting a lot of practice which he will, as he is gifted in that way. I feel sure he will settle and of course you can be sure that he is missing nothing here.

5 September 1974 — To Joy Schulz
I no longer go to St John's so I am quite out of touch with the ex-colleagues. Malcolm Greaves is the new professor and he is certainly the best we have for the job and ought to do it very well indeed.

1974 — To Joy Schulz
You come to the house whenever you like . . . and look after yourself for a few days. An ample supply of victuals would be left as well as gin and tonic etc. At any rate you would not have to spend time and nervous energy looking for a roof . . . there is a cat which seeks food twice a day. This will be left in the fridge except for some pellets called 'Cupboard Love' which she will eat if very hungry.

1975 — To Joy Schulz
I suffer quite as much . . . from the letter writing syndrome, and as the days creep on my suffering increases steeply. My son Simon doesn't

suffer. He just doesn't write letters ... My time will be up in six more sessions, one weekly. I'm glad to pack up.

I am very sorry about Alan Menter's defection, and the more so in that no one would induce me to live and work in the States where, however, I have never been.

1970 — To George Findlay
It does seem to me that you are rushing along the road to ruin at great speed, but all the same I don't think advice from me would do any good [a financial donation had been made].

1970 — To George Findlay: comments on Chris Barnard's autobiography
I am reading it avidly and with great interest and enjoyment, perhaps with all the more pleasure for knowing the terrain which makes it so easy to go along with the writer all the way. He seems quite a simple straight character, like so many South Africans, and to speak his mind and heart in the simplest language and very vividly all the time.

1969 — To George Findlay
Why must we be so aggressively self-righteous, deservedly the most unpopular people in the world — so said some important chap in the *Times*, forgotten who.

1970 — To George Findlay
I played truant in Cape Town from a meeting ... for the sake of another look at Simonstown, which literally remains the same as always, with VR on the pillar boxes, and the colonial naval residence, as when the colony was well governed.

Chapter 18
The Finale

DOWLING'S remarks could be crisp and dry, but always meaningful. George Findlay wrote:

'We will bring your god-daughter to visit you in 1977,' my wife said to him in 1975.

'I hope I'll be around.'

'You must be.'

'Well, I'll try.'

Some months later Ian Whimster let George Findlay know that Uncle Geoffrey was dead. On 14 June 1976 he received an eight-page letter from Whimster telling him more.

Letter to George Findlay from Ian Whimster

...The very least I could do was to keep you informed by cable. I was able to phone Leo and Mabs Jansen in Utrecht... Your home and theirs were his two dearest overseas homes-from-home. And as you know he was Hon. MD of Utrecht as well as of Pretoria — and equally delighted by both.

Now let us fill you in on the details. Uncle Geoffrey had not been well for around the last six months. But he kept pretty quiet about it, except to a very small group of 'closests'. He was having good days and not-so-good days. And there is now no doubt he had made his own correct diagnosis — but charac-teristically and wisely decided to let nature take its course, and not be 'messed about with' at his age. By very happy coin-cidence, the occasion of this year's Dowling Oration and Dinner, held in Oxford, was during a 'good' phase. He was there, his real self, enjoying every moment of it as much as always. In fact during the course of the Oration he gave forth one of his classical heard-all-over-the-room 'sotto-voces' that none of us present will ever forget. The Oration ceased for about a minute until the applause had died down. And at the Dinner afterwards, Renwick Vickers, in proposing his toast (and knowing that it was to be his last dinner) gave us the perfect 'premature eulogy'. That was in April.

Since then I had dinner with him once more — again on a 'good' day.

If anything were right in this world surely this universally beloved old man should have been given the blessing of being able to just go to sleep in his own bed one night — and simply stay asleep. But it was not to be so. (And who are we to judge anyway.) As things turned out GBD was to endure a few days (mercifully few) of discomfort, pain and — 'humiliation'. Yet even this, deplorable as it seemed, gave him a few more opportunities to express himself.

One night he became acutely ill and was taken to Charing Cross Hospital (God only knows why — except that it happened to be nearer than St Thomas's). There they made the correct diagnosis of obstruction and immediately got a drip set up. It was only an hour or so before Hugh Wallace heard of this and instantly ordered his transfer to St Thomas's. This transfer was agreed to, of course, and an ambulance was summoned. (La was with him at the time and I had this account from her.) *They* said he must go to St Thomas's in the ambulance drip-and-all. *He* said he wouldn't go to *his* hospital with one of *their* drips at *any* price — and ordered the nursing staff to remove the drip forthwith. There followed a period of argument, during which La tried in vain to convince the Charing Cross staff that if her father said he wasn't going to St Thomas's with a Charing Cross drip – he *wasn't*. But they weren't convinced. So he turned finally to La and said that they would have to do it themselves, which they did. He undid the bandage and pulled out the needle. Blood everywhere. La mopped it up.

He arrived in St Thomas's shortly after and of course behaved like a lamb from then on.

I saw him the next day. He was physically in a terrible state, blown up, hiccupping and dehydrated as hell. But cerebrally his old self. As I entered the room (the very best one in the new building) I started gingerly making tentative enquiries about how he was feeling. He waved all this aside — it was just a 'bloody-nuisance-but-they-were-going-to-put-it-right-in-the-morning' — in a matter of seconds. And before I could get another word in he was raving about the marvellous view from his window — 9th floor, looking directly on to the river and Parliament Buildings opposite, with nothing in between.

I agreed and set out to go over to the window to have a good look. But he pulled me back and started another rave about my lymphangioma article in the BJD which he had read the week before. And it was clear that he had grasped every word of it. And the next 10 minutes I was subjected to an intensive *viva* on the whole subject — and on how the follow-up was going etc, etc, etc. That from a mortally ill man who knew he was mortally ill. That interview was terminated by the arrival of daughter Jane.

The next morning Lynn Lockhart Mummery opened him up. He found a massive tumour in the descending colon — with a peritoneum liberally peppered with secondaries and a liver that was one-third liver and two-thirds metastatic tumour. (It grieved me particularly that a liver which had excelled all others I know at metabolising alcohol without damage to itself, to such an incredible extent for so long, had to succumb finally to such an unworthy end.)

Anyhow, Lynn made a colostomy, and did nothing else. George Wells and Paul Naylor and I talked to Lynn at lunchtime and it was agreed unanimously that no more should be done. Just analgesia and sedation — and all our fingers crossed for a pulmonary embolus or cardiac failure (he had after all been kept going on cardiac drugs for the last couple of years).

I went to see him the day after the laparotomy. He was terribly ill and very (thank goodness and St Thomas's) heavily sedated. But in spite of all that, the 'Old Man' — 'The Headmaster' — 'Uncle Geoffrey' was still there. As I sat by his bed and held his hand, he awoke for a minute — then dropped asleep for the next minute. He told me that he was much more comfortable after the first operation and could hardly wait for the second. (He wasn't kidding anybody but he had to keep up appearances.)

When I phoned the ward the next day he was very chesty and almost comatose. I went up there but by then they had summoned all the family. He was unconscious, and they weren't pushing the antibiotics too hard.

An hour later he had gone — as he wanted to go.

The funeral was advertised in the press as 'Private'. They didn't want the whole of St Thomas's staff and British Dermatology there. Nor did they want just half-a-dozen relatives. So they phoned a small group of selected individuals and invited them. I was honoured to be amongst that chosen few.

The funeral service (cremation) was exactly as he would have wished. Nothing religious about it in the accepted sense. But everything human, practical, sincere and philosophical. The service itself consisted 90% of a very competent organist playing Bach. And 10% the St Thomas's Chaplain briefed by Hugh Wallace saying exactly the right things.

The whole affair had the atmosphere of a Thanksgiving Ceremony, and nothing funereal.

Afterwards some of us went back to La's house and had a joyful afternoon tea. Our beloved Great Man — as 'Daddy' or as 'Uncle Geoffrey', as GBD or as 'The Headmaster' — had at last found his way to peace. There simply wasn't anything to be sad about. He may be physically absent from now on — but so after all are Michelangelo, Galileo, Pasteur and a good few others. But they haven't managed to die yet.

By his own wish there was no memorial service. 'Memorial services are for the wives,' he said. And sadly he hadn't one.

Numerous obituaries and tributes poured in from all over the country, as well as from Holland, Poland, Italy, Belgium, South Africa, the United States, Yugoslavia, Israel, Australia and New Zealand.

One of the most touching was from Alice Fawcett, whose father had been so kind to Geoffrey Dowling when he first came to London from Cape Town.

2 June 1976

My Dear Tom, Jane, La and Simon,

Tom has just phoned me and I feel so very sad, not for him as I know that the time had come for him to go, but for you all and for me. He has been there all my life, as he has been for you all, and I loved him dearly.

He was so wonderful to me when I was a child and when I was growing up, and when he married your mother. I was always part of your home. My first day of the holidays was always spent at Battersea. He loved you all and you loved him, and you were all so good to him when he got old.

No one else (except my Dad) had that beautiful smile when he first saw you — I can't believe that I'll never see him again on this earth, and yet I can . . . I knew when I saw him the other day that it might be the last time. What a good thing that I came up and that we had a happy Family Party together.

I am so thankful that he did not have to suffer long and he died peacefully. He had had such a satisfactory and satisfying life in so many ways, being so interested in his work and being able to work till comparatively recently. He got a tremendous pleasure from his family and from music and from going to art exhibitions. You will all miss him terribly and if I can't be with you on Friday, my thoughts will be very much with you.

He and your mother were always so sweet to my parents, and when the latter died, they were there to support me. How many happy holidays I spent with you and no one can take those memories away, even if I am crying now.

My love to you all

Alice

The news of Dowling's death was given to members of the Dowling Club by Dr Terence Ryan in a letter dated 2 June 1976. It well illustrates the feelings and special relationship with the Club and its founder.

2 June 1976

Dear Member,

G.B. Dowling died peacefully at St Thomas's Hospital on Tuesday, 1 June. He had been in poor general health for several months but did not need in-patient care until one week before his death. Hugh Wallace has kept me in touch with recent events and it is clear that GBD had firm views about what we should do after his death. On many occasions he talked to Hugh and sometimes to myself about the Club, the Oration and the funds that provide travel expenses for the young. He regarded these as important and funerals and memorial services as unimportant.

The funeral will be a family event and no memorial service is planned.

G.B. Dowling enjoyed the activities of the Club. During the last year visits to Wells and Oxford pleased him, and the large attendance at the George during the Winter assured him of the Club's vitality. It has been fun for me to hear he was happy with our choice of President and Secretary for the coming year as well as with the Orators and various other schemes planned in his name. He believed that all these brought enjoyment and stimulation linked to Dermatology.

Liveliness and creativity activated by his Club is the kind of memorial he would have liked. Next week we are indulging in just the kind of programme that pleased him most. Only two weeks ago he decided not to go with us to France just in case one of us felt obliged to give him too much attention. I am sure that we should look forward to the future of his Club and be grateful for the life rather than be saddened by the passing of Geoffrey Dowling.

Yours sincerely
Terence J. Ryan
Hon. President, Dowling Club

Chapter 19
Immortality

MAN HAS believed in immortality since the beginning of his existence and development over thousands of years. The concept of immortality as life after death is more widely held as a belief the more primitive the society.

But for anthropologists there are two concepts of immortality. One is the religious belief based on a faith that there is an after-life, a belief which Ashley Montagu* says is the majority view in what he calls non-literate societies. The other is a belief in 'the vicarious life', which Montagu terms the belief in immortality in literate societies.

The concept of vicarious existence is not new. It is at least as old as Buddhism. It is well expressed by Samuel Butler† in *Erewhon Revisited*. Speaking through his characters, Butler gives us a view of immortality to which every man may subscribe, and one may opine that it is a viewpoint which all mankind will one day universally embrace. A great part of mankind has already gone a long way toward doing so. For 25 centuries the Chinese have believed in this form of immortality of achievement or worth and in the immortality of the spoken or written word, or, as Hu Shih has put it, the immortality of the three Ws, worth, work and words.

But, as Hu Shih has pointed out, the conception of immortality embraced by the three Ws is too aristocratic, too exclusive. How many people can achieve or feel that they can achieve immortality in this way? Relatively few. Furthermore, this doctrine fails to furnish a negative check on human conduct. If it is to work, we need a conception of immortality to which all men can feel heir. What we need is not an aristocratic but a democratic conception of immortality, a belief in the truth that everyone is immortal in the sense that whatever men do lives on somehow, somewhere, somewhen. This is the religion of social immortality, the social physics of vicarious existence. By the measure of the conception of social immortality, every man is responsible for

* Ashley Montagu, *Immortality*, Grove Press, New York, 1955.
† Samuel Butler, *Erewhon Revisited*, 1901.

everything to everyone else, for, in the golden and immortal words of John Donne (1572–1631):

> No man is an Island, entire of itself; every man is a piece of the Continent, a part of the main; if a Clod be washed away by the Sea, Europe is the less, as well as if a Promontory were; as well as if a Manor of thy friends or of thine own were; any man's death diminishes me, because I am involved in Mankind; And therefore never send to know for whom the bell tolls; it tolls for thee.

This is the immortality which Geoffrey Dowling achieved, and the vicarious life which he bequeathed to us and succeeding generations of dermatologists in Britain.

How did this boy who came to London from Cape Town at the age of 12 develop into the greatest dermatologist that Britain has produced in the twentieth century?

Genetics must have played some part. His parents were both professional musicians of distinction. Yet all direct parental and family influence virtually ceased at the age of 12. He originally wanted to become a naval officer. When frustrated in that direction he was able to devote himself to medicine and then to dermatology, through the help and inspiration of his guardian, Dr John Fawcett.

His childhood years in England were full of unhappiness and loneliness. He was no stranger to adversity. But adverse circumstances may have completely different effects on different people. For some it produces hardness and an uncompromising personality. In others it induces deep feelings of compassion and an attitude of caring. It had the latter effect on Geoffrey Dowling.

One can only guess at the details of his childhood. In his years of adolescence at 66 Wimpole Street, the Fawcetts had no children of their own, and hence no experience of parenthood. John Fawcett was a man with a very strong work ethic, and this must have been instilled into the young Geoffrey. The life of a London physician in those days required a lot of reading and study in the evenings. And so Geoffrey would have known many hours of childhood loneliness in his own room, reading and thinking. He became a keen reader, and remained so all his life.

During this time he acquired and developed his character and personal qualities. The principal ones were humility, integrity and honesty. These were what attracted the dermatology registrars to him in later life. They always knew that, if they asked him a question on medical, personal or other matters, they would receive 'nothing but the truth'.

And there was his special quality of kindness. He had an inability to hurt. In the Fawcett household he would have learnt obedience and never to complain. He learnt to eat and enjoy everything put before him and in later life would always be a most appreciative guest.

He acquired an excellent memory and astute powers of observation. He was always sensitive to the needs of others and their feelings. His strikingly bright eyes would see everything; and they could express silent words of sympathy and solicitude.

He was incapable of humiliating anyone, even though he could so clearly see personal faults and weaknesses in others. He seemed immune to feelings of envy, jealousy or selfishness. He was an excellent judge of character.

He abhorred privilege, speculative ideas and pretentiousness, whether in medicine, politics or anything else. He was a realist, a pragmatist.

His experience of two years in the army, including active service in France during the First World War, had a very strong impact on his character. He returned with a determination and resolve to succeed and excel, and with a maturity which gave him the confidence to know that he could do it.

At Guy's Hospital as a student and then a junior doctor, he made some particular friends, such as John Conybeare and Robert Macintosh, to whom he remained close all his life. When he moved from Guy's to St Thomas's Hospital, he was at first rebuffed and must have felt very depressed. But his dedication to integrity and excellence gradually overcame all opposition, so that in time he became one of the most popular and respected members of the staff there. His distinction was recognized by all his colleagues.

His facility for friendship was most appreciated by the junior doctors, in medicine and dermatology. At Guy's Hospital he was seen to be an excellent teacher. After 20 years of sheer hard work as his own teacher, he made himself the best dermatologist of his generation. At the end of the Second World War at St Thomas's Hospital, he alone saw the opportunity to change British dermatology and eradicate all the shortcomings of previous generations. His vehicle was a journal club, known as the George Club and later the Dowling Club. Admission was open only to junior dermatologists, but open to any one of them.

The result was the extraordinary camaraderie which we all enjoy in British dermatology today. He transmitted his own qualities of tolerance and friendliness not only to the British registrars, but to any temporary visiting dermatologists from overseas, and especially to those from Commonwealth countries. He recognized the particular qualities of doctors from Australia, New Zealand and South Africa.

In his time he received all the honours possible in his specialty, such as the Marchionini Gold Medal from the German Dermatological Society, and two honorary doctorates, from the Universities of Utrecht and Pretoria.

Perhaps the greatest evidence of his immortality has been the progress of the Dowling Club since his death in 1976. It is now bigger and stronger and more active than at any previous time. It includes virtually all the younger dermatologists in Britain and is a truly national organization. It will go on for ever.

How did he do it? He had all the personal requirements for success in medicine, the first of which is a prime motivation for success, to want it. There is no doubt that he came out of the First World War with a strong will to excel, passing all his qualifying and higher examinations effortlessly. From apparent obscurity he soon became noticed and recognized by his contemporaries as well above the average. Secondly, apart from a few incidents, he had the gift of good health and especially stamina. Most importantly, he was able to do with less than eight hours sleep at night. Few people with chronic illnesses such as asthma or duodenal ulcer can last the course to obtain success, although there are exceptions.

Thirdly, he had considerable personal discipline. He was devoid of excessive appetite of any kind, whether it be food or drink or women or money. He could enjoy them all but was never seduced by them.

And, fourthly, he was blessed with an even temperament. He could be tolerant, but never of incompetence or arrogance. He could be irritated and angry, but never lost his temper. He took great care to avoid confrontation, and would never enter any conflict unless he was certain to win. If he received any rebuff, he was able to let it pass over him, as also, when blown off course by some adverse event, he was able quickly to return to his original plotted path of progress towards his objective.

Almost no man can remain immune from the corrupting influence of personal power, when it is continued for long enough. The special quality which protected him from such influence was a total absence of conceit. For he was certainly not unaware of his popularity, amounting to adulation, among the registrars and young dermatologists who had contact with him. His power, influence and reputation were enormous, and unequalled by any other dermatologist. Yet no trace of conceit was ever detectable. Such striking absence of conceit in a leader can be expected to attract envy, and this was true in Dowling's case, but he never paid attention to it. He knew that his best attitude was to ignore it, and did not even acknowledge its existence.

To have talent and the qualities required for success is, of course, not enough. The results depend on how they are used. Many people with talent fail to obtain success, in medicine and in many other human activities. In knowing how to use it Geoffrey Dowling had something in common with Sir John Harvey-Jones, the former chairman of Imperial Chemical Industries. Sir John was a Royal Naval Officer in 1947 serving under the British Commanding Officer in charge of dismantling the German dockyard at Wilhelmshaven. At the end of his appointment, the Commanding Officer wrote, 'Lieutenant Harvey-Jones is an able officer, who knows how to make things happen, albeit tactfully.'

These words are an excellent summation of Geoffrey Dowling's special qualities. He had the most extraordinary facility to 'make things happen'. Like Harvey-Jones, he preferred to work with people rather than over them, and entrusted all his faith and hopes in young people, whose abilities were so frequently underestimated and under-used. He expected every senior registrar to be better than his consultant, since some piece of knowledge which had taken a senior person five or ten years to acquire could be given to or assimilated by a junior in half an hour.

Two contradictory statements are frequently made about Dowling:

'As a teacher he was a non-starter.'

'He was the greatest teacher of his generation.'

The explanation is to be found in the method and what he taught. He never aimed to teach what could be readily learnt from books and journals. Rather, he was a teacher of ideas. He was a sower of seeds, and he sowed the seeds of ideas about dermatology in the minds of young dermatologists, in whom the soil was more likely to be fertile. There is no doubt that the young registrars went on thinking and talking about his remarks long after he had gone. Many scientific papers were subsequently published by them, but Dowling's name rarely, if ever, appeared under the authorship. He knew he had given them the original idea, and he was not resentful.

Geoffrey Dowling's place is assured in British dermatology as a kind of philosopher or political thinker, with the charismatic quality of a guru. Most dermatologists at the present time in Britain are unaware of how their approach to their subject has been changed from that of preceding generations by this one man, who was characterized by absolute honesty and integrity, a complete absence of conceit, and an ability to plant ideas in fertile minds.

He has achieved immortality and his name will live for ever.

Index